MAGNETIC RESONANCE IMAGING

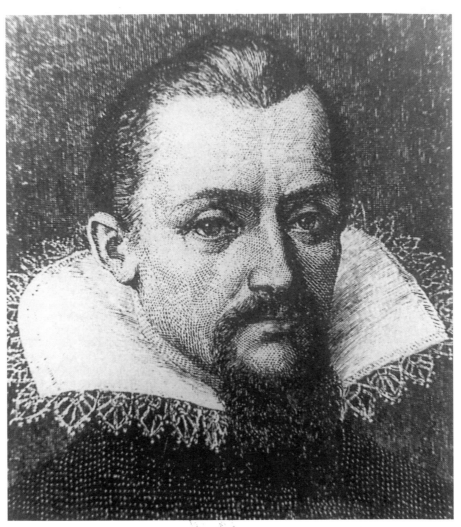

Johann Keppler (1571–1630)
Imperial Mathematician

MAGNETIC RESONANCE IMAGING

Mathematical Foundations and Applications

WALTER JOHANNES SCHEMPP
Lehrstuhl für Mathematik I
University of Siegen
Siegen, Germany

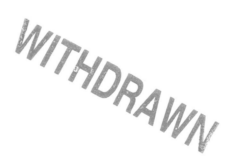

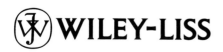**WILEY-LISS**

A John Wiley & Sons, Inc., Publication
New York · Chichester · Weinheim · Brisbane · Singapore · Toronto

Library of Congress Cataloging-in-Publication Data:

Schempp, W. (Walter), 1938–
    Magnetic resonance imaging : mathematical foundations and applications / Walter Johannes Schempp.
        p.   cm.
    "A Wiley-Liss publication."
    Includes index.
    ISBN 0-471-16736-3 (cloth : alk. paper)
    1. Magnetic resonance imaging.   2. Magnetic resonance imaging—Mathematics.   I. Title.
RC78.7.N83S37   1998
616.8'047548—dc21   97-48760
                                                        CIP

Printed in the United States of America

10 9 8 7 6 5 4 3 2 1

As but a small indication of my appreciation, this volume is affectionately dedicated to my academic teacher and mentor

Professor Dr. Karl Zeller
Tübingen

on the occasion of granting to him the degree of Doctor Honoris Causa by the University of Siegen on February 2, 1995. He deserves far more.

CONTENTS

FOREWORD

Science has to do with the description and the modeling of nature as observed. Observations, however, are inherently local: They are of the here and now—to that extent they are unique and therefore nonrecurring. On the other hand, we have the ability to imagine and to represent what we observe, to face the future as it happens in the light of the knowledge born of the past. Clearly, our imagination has greater scope than what the immediate context of observation provides: It is indeed a feature of our thoughts that they are inherently global, that is, independent of what there is or happens locally. So, the art of the scientist is to bring global notions to bear on local events. This means, *inter alia*, that concepts are to be severely constrained by observational criteria if our concern is to represent nature as it is rather than simply as we like to imagine it. To this end, one looks for *patterns* among singular observations—whence the notion of a *law of nature*. The term "law" is used to convey the fact of a perceived *invariance* across local contexts of observation, as an expression of the sense we make of what is observed.

To bring the conceptual to bear on the observable, given the difference in scope between them, requires that they be carefully interfaced in the language of representation. The chief contribution of the scientific revolution of the sixteenth and seventeenth centuries has been the creation of languages dedicated to a single use, that of representing what there is in an unambiguous way. In such languages, the interface between concepts and observations is a mathematical syntax. Patterns of events are then represented by morphisms deployed in some appropriate *semantic space*, for example, a phase space. The semantic variables, for example, the phase variables, are next projected onto a corresponding *observation space* wherein the observable events are to be found. In this process, to any possible value of each semantic variable s a *measure* set $m(s)$ in observation space is made to correspond. Thus, to each computed value s_c of s there should correspond some observed values

$s_0 \in m(s_c)$ satisfying a variety of constraints governed by the strategy of observation, which includes, among other things, the theory of the means of observation, itself independent of the theory governing the patterning of the events observed.

Developments in particle physics in the last three decades have shown that there is an important difference between contexts of observation based on the energy required to observe what there is. In particular, they have shown that the energy differences were of such a magnitude as to form distinct and reasonably well delineated *strata*, or levels. Further, it was found that adjacent strata in hierarchical systems were largely decoupled by contrast with the way systems belonging to the same energetic stratum interacted—whence the view that there are, broadly speaking, two very different kinds of interactions, depending on whether they take place within a single energetic stratum or not. In either case, observed patterns emerge, from which the notion of two different types of laws in nature was got. Let us briefly examine how these laws are to be represented.

The first type of laws correlates events resulting from interactions confined to a specific energetic stratum, the *intralevel interactions*. They are expressed directly in terms of the observable events. For example, Keppler's laws of planetary motion and Galileo's law of free fall are expressed in terms of time and space measurements. It is this spatiotemporal feature which justifies the claim that this is a law of nature and not simply a *law of science*. The original global character of the pattern is *universalized* in the representation of the law and made applicable to all relevant observational contexts, its projectibility onto any particular context affecting only the initial conditions and not the invariant pattern. The manner in which the semantic variables are related by the morphism unveils the symmetry properties of the particular law.

It is a characteristic of the interactions taking place within each energetic stratum that they all satisfy the same set of symmetry properties. Such symmetries are of a more general form than the laws, leading the laws to be represented by the symmetry groups that characterize them. These symmetries, which are specific to a given energetic stratum, are referred to as *dynamical symmetries*, by contradistinction with the *geometrical symmetries* which are not specific to any one set of interactions (such as the conservation laws for energy, angular momenta, etc). Further, geometrical symmetries are expressible in terms of observable events, while dynamical symmetries are not; the relation they bear to the laws is similar to the relation that the laws bear to the events. So much for intralevel interactions, the laws that govern them and the symmetries they exhibit.

The second type of law correlates *different kinds of events*, resulting from interactions between systems belonging to different energetic strata. These *interlevel interactions* cannot be expressed in terms of events, due to the observed energetic gap and consequent loose coupling between adjacent energetic strata.[1] The matter may be put thus: Dynamical systems have an *internal dynamical régime* and a set of *external characteristics*, such as electrical charge and nuclear spin, that enable

[1] S. S. Schweber, "Physics, Community and the Crisis in Physical Theory," *Phys. Today*, November 1993, 34–40; T. Y. Cao and S. S. Schweber, "The Conceptual Foundations and the Philosophical Aspects of Renormalization," *Synthèse* 97/1 (1993), 33–108.

them to interact with other systems having similar properties. These external characteristics provide a system with, among other things, its identity relative to other
systems in the same energetic stratum. They are *causally* related to the interactions
which are responsible for the internal régime of the system, and so are *endogeneous*.
For example, the properties of the atom of hydrogen, e.g., its chemical identity, are
due to the intralevel interactions taking place between its constituents, the proton
and the electron. In a similar vein, mental activities are commonly thought to be
causally related to neurological events sited in the human brain, and so on in all
natural hierarchical systems.

The chief factor militating against the expression of these laws directly in terms
of events is the presence of the energetic gap between the strata that the causal interactions bridge, leading to the absence of observable type–type connections between
individual events internal to the system and those external to it. Ordinarily, the representation of a causal interaction should link cause and effect by a morphism showing
how the former relates to the other. Since, in the case of interlevel interactions, the
causal events belong to a different energetic stratum from the one in which the effects are observable, a causal morphism should have two semantic domains instead
of one, with the consequence that its universe of discourse could not be considered
semantically homogeneous. Therefore, interlevel morphisms cannot be represented
in the same manner as the morphism representing causal relations within a single
energetic stratum.[2] A reductionist strategy, whereby the endogeneous characteristics
of the emergent stratum are redescribed as properties of the underlying substrate,
would leave the observed energy gap between the related strata unaccountable.

Nonetheless, many researchers proceed on the assumption that a computational
strategy will eventually succeed in bridging the energetic gap between two related but
disjointed strata and thereby yield the causal morphism linking them. The attitude is
based on the belief that all natural processes are computational and on the hope that the
point will eventually be reached when the capability of the technology and its desired
performance will be evenly matched. This hope is likely to prove unreasonable.

First, the claim that all natural processes are computational in character is an
empirical one and so stands in need of observational support, of which none has yet
been given. Computer simulation is not in general equivalent to the observational
validation of claims about nature, nor does it usually suffice as theoretical validation.
Its justification lies elsewhere, in its usefulness for certain tasks (e.g., robotics or
expert systems). Second, the fact that computational strategies are deployed by means
of algorithms, which are widely taken to be equivalent to effectively computable
recursive functions, stands in the way. For these functions have a single semantic
domain, so that whenever they are applied to real systems, that is, to systems of
observable events, the semantic variables are to be interpreted uniformly, preserving
a homogeneous universe of discourse. In such applications, *semantic homogeneity*
means that both inputs and outputs are *projectible* onto the *same observation space*.[3]
However, this is one of the conditions that the partial decoupling between different

---

[2] E. P. Wigner, "The Problem of Measurement," *Am. J. Phys.* 31 (1963), 6–15.
[3] On a related matter, see a recent review by Freeman J. Dyson in *Nature* 380 (1996), 296.

energetic strata rules out. It is also the reason why computational strategies are successfully exploited only in the simulation of interactions within a single energetic level of observation and why there is not a single instance of their having been used successfully to simulate any of the interactions between events occurring in energetically different strata.

However, another approach is possible, based on the eminently reasonable proposition that the link between different energetic strata represented by symmetry groups is best sought in some appropriate Lie group transform. And since it is not possible to correlate events directly across energy gaps, the observer always being on one side of the gap, one may try to correlate the geometrical patterns they form in each energetic stratum as a result of the interactions they are subjected to and of the laws they obey, rather than in terms of the interactions themselves. The difficulty, however, like the devil, lies in the details.

It is the singular merit of Professor Walter J. Schempp to have conceived and spelled out the details of this *new* strategy for linking patterns of observables constructible within different energetic strata. In this work, which is focused on a particular case of great interest and scientific sophistication, he has detailed in a masterful way the underlying mathematical structure of the causal connection between micro- and macrolevels in nuclear magnetic resonance imaging (NMRI). But there is more to this book than an admirable and complete treatment of the NMRI hierarchical system by the method of unitary representations of transversally *stratified* Lie groups induced from one-dimensional representations of closed normal subgroups and the associated reconstructive *symbolic calculus* in the Weyl theory of pseudodifferential operators. The greatest value and the most promising feature of this truly remarkable book lies elsewhere, in the *extremely ingenious* new strategy which the author employs to relate the *patterns of observables* found in the different energetic levels rather than the individual events. The value of the strategy is due primarily to the fact that it is not specific to the particulars of any one pair of dynamical strata and is therefore fully exportable.

The promise is nowhere greater than in the study of evolutionary systems, which is notoriously deficient in scientific rigor. Any two adjacent strata in an energetically complex hierarchy are bound to have characteristic features distinguishing them from any other interacting pairs, a phenomenon ubiquitous in emergent systems. This means that it is unreasonable to hope for the development of a single language satisfying normal scientific constraints, capable of spanning the whole evolutionary spectrum, from the simplest systems studied in particle physics to the most complex organisms and their ecological milieux. What Professor Walter J. Schempp offers us here is something far more practical: a *general mathematical strategy* for the representation of causal interactions across energetic gaps applicable to all such cases.

This mathematical strategy is deployed in two stages, the first of which consists in the generation of an objective (i.e., not observer indexed), geometrical (i.e., continuous) representation of the relevant pattern of observables in the causal layer. In the case of NMRI, this means getting a *synchronous spatiotemporal pattern* of the behavior of protons' spin angular momenta under magnetic stimulation. In this, the author follows the *geometrical quantization* strategy first developed by one of his distant forebears, Johann Keppler (1571–1630), in the process of determining the global shape of planetary orbits by the area law without the benefit of a theory of gravitation which had yet to be formulated. Instead of the Newtonian causal interaction, the Kepplerian dynamics of physical astronomy centered on the sun is in terms of *magnetic* attractive forces which control *spatial* frequencies in the orbital plane rather than accelerations. The magnetic hypothesis of planetary motion includes the assumption that the magnetic axis of the planet maintains a constant direction at right angles to the orbital plane through the sun, to provide geometrical symmetry about the apsidal line through the ability of the magnet to control *direction* in the three-dimensional projective space.

The second stage consists of the transformation of the geometrical pattern from the stratified *causal group* into the corresponding geometrical pattern in the *emergent* layer, where it can be analyzed further as needs arise. The result is a mathematically rigorous representation of an interlevel causal interaction, the only one yet devised and fully deployed in the literature. It is clearly articulated, a quality essential to its applicability to, and general usefulness for, other areas of research, a consideration not without merit given that its scope is far greater than the focus on synthetic aperture radar (SAR) high resolution imagery and NMRI would indicate.

We are indeed in Professor Walter J. Schempp's debt for having produced this methodologically seminal text which marks a turning point in the effort to understand a most important type of natural law, the one specific to the processes of energetic complexification inherent in systems hierarchies. For the nature of causal relations across energetic boundaries is undoubtedly the single most pressing issue facing theoretical science today. It is to be hoped that the publication of this book, in which *Schempp's strategy* is deployed with such penetrating insights, will help to make it the instrument of choice for research on emergence: The time is none too soon.

GEORGE L. FARRE
Georgetown University

PREFACE

Mensch, streckh deine Vernunfft hieher / diese dinge zu begreiffen.
—Johann Keppler (1571–1630)

What these people do is really very clever. They put little spies into the molecules and send radio signals to them, and they have to radio back what they are seeing.
—Niels Bohr (1885–1962)

There is nothing that nuclear spins will not do for you, as long as you treat them as human beings.
—Erwin Louis Hahn (1949)

In order to understand the principles of MR imaging, one must successfully navigate through an elaborate structure whose essence is very much like a mathematical subject.
—Alfred L. Horowitz (1995)

The essence of technology is nothing technological.
—Martin Heidegger (1889–1976)

The sense we make of the world is governed by our conceptual means. More specifically, sense is made of nature by projecting a conceptual structure onto observed events.
—George L. Farre (1997)

The general philosophy shared by the majority of scientists is that the frontiers between the various disciplines of science are only conventional. The borders change according to the state of the common human knowledge base, the understanding of nature, and the digital computer performance *in silicio* currently available. Mathematics is playing an ever more important role in an understanding of the physical and biological sciences "from the inside." It provokes a blurring of boundaries between various scientific disciplines and a resurgence of interest in the modern as well as the advanced classical methods of applied mathematics.

Particularly fuzzy are the interfaces between physical and biomedical sciences. The tendency in quantum information technology and quantum computing research to achieve a physical implementation of deoxyribonucleic acid (DNA) computers is a strong indication that these boundaries can be penetrated by an application of mathematical methods to the quantum dynamics of biomedical phenomena. The experimentally well-established fact that transient phase locking of high frequency oscillations in biological neural networks is a result of the dynamical changes in the cross-correlation between the coherent firing of two neurons following a salient sensory or behavioral event is another indication that mathematics remains the *only* lingua franca presently available that allows to relate biomedical phenomena to quantum dynamics via the computerized techniques of advanced Fourier analysis and synthesis.

It should be emphasized, however, that the application of the mathematical language of noncommutative Fourier analysis to the dynamics of biomedical phenomena by the trace filter encoding of quantum holography does not imply a reductionist strategy. A strategy of reducing biomedical phenomena, encoded by genetic information, to physics has been most prominently outlined by Erwin Schrödinger (1887–1961) in lectures entitled *What Is Life?* delivered under the auspices of the Dublin Institute for Advanced Studies at Trinity College, Dublin, in February 1943.

Theoretical physicist Schrödinger did not at that time realize that the nuclear spin dynamics could be tuned in to the trace filter encoding of the quantum information of spectroscopic samples *in vitro* and of the living cells of soft tissues *in vivo*. At that time he was neither aware of a nuclear magnetic resonance (NMR) method of spatially discriminating the region from which the free induction decay is obtained nor did he realize that the resolution of resonance lines would be the key to the spectral localization procedure of NMR coherent tomography. That unexpected revelation would come from a visionary physician by the name of Raymond V. Damadian, but it would not arrive for another 34 years, more than 80 years after Wilhelm C. Röntgen's landmark discovery of X-ray imaging. Damadian's radiodiagnostic breakthrough in 1977, however, would not be possible without the theoretical foundations of quantum physics independently developed by Schrödinger and Werner K. Heisenberg (1901–1976). Specifically Erwin Schrödinger's concept of coherent state turned out to be of wide-ranging importance for the interface of classical and quantum physics. His way of reasoning on the physical aspect of the living cell exerted a strong influence on the modern philosophy of reductionism and touched off a flurry of activity in the unification of the sciences.

Today, the limitations of the reductionist strategy in science has become apparent. The value of implicit "tacit" personal knowledge that resists to be expressed in terms of mathematical physics is nowhere greater than in clinical medicine. Its special contribution to such studies is the construction of the *semantic filter bank*, which is an essential ingredient of the observations, evaluations, and interpretations in all areas of science, including biology and medicine. This filter bank is of an individual character and a product of time history. It is determined by recorded experience and cannot be hardwired in any information processing system. Thus the reasoning and action of the experienced diagnosticians are not about to be replaced by an expert system emulated *in silicio*.

Although radiology and its subspecialities have the strongest technological influence and the highest computer intensity among the disciplines of medicine, clinical radiodiagnostics forms a classical paradigm for demonstrating the convergence of the implicit tacit personal knowledge, tending from the historical roots of recorded experience to the final mathematical theory. The coexistence of a quantum mechanically based mathematical theory of clinical magnetic resonance imaging (MRI) and the semantic filter of the diagnosticians' expertise for radiodiagnostic evaluations and interpretations form a fascinating aspect of this discipline. The present book, which has its origin in the practical work done at various centers of radiodiagnostics, tries to trace this coexistence. In essence, it is written as a challenge to the reader, to complete his or her theoretical knowledge by acquiring practical experience and to make acquaintance of more advanced MRI diagnostic techniques.

Over the last decades, considerable interest has developed in the application of quantum physics to *macroscopic* systems where a small number of collective degrees of freedom show quantum behavior. Specifically, the computation information processing capability of quantum dynamical systems, which has been of theoretical interest, has now become of great practical importance because of the promise of nuclear spin ensembles for representing quantum computation information about spin density flow and molecular sites on spatially discriminated chemical composition.

In the quest to build a quantum computer, ensembles of nuclear spins are particularly attractive to quantum engineers because of their extremely good isolation in bulk samples from electronic and oscillational perturbations that can lead to environmentally induced phase decoherence of the trace filter response. The routine use of electronically programmed electromagnetic hard pulse trains for probing and tuning *spin isochromats* (literally, "spin wavelet packets of the same color") in bulk samples points to the promise of nuclear spin ensembles for representing quantum computation information by NMR spectroscopy.

A prominent and fascinating aspect of the technology of ensemble quantum computing is its wide range of applications, which include biochemistry and biomedicine. As one of the earliest achievements in the evolving discipline of quantum engineering, modern NMR spectroscopy extended far beyond the early fields of nuclear physics and chemistry. Now it is extensively used as a computer-intensive, *noninvasive* method of obtaining high resolution clinical images and studying tissue metabolism *in vivo*. Clinical MRI is able to provide the fundamental principles of diagnostic imaging, high soft tissue contrast, noninvasive reproducibility of image quality, good conspicuity of pathology, and comprehensive imaging information. The unfortunate distinction between NMR spectroscopy and MRI diagnosis, resulting in part from the patchwork implementation of NMR spectroscopy on clinical MRI scanners, will become less apparent with the increasing availability of integrated NMR/MRI scanner systems. Beyond this practical application, the clinical NMR/MRI scanner provides an invaluable model of stochastic analysis. Actually it forms a Ornstein–Uhlenbeck laboratory for the research on geometrical pattern emergence (Figure 1).

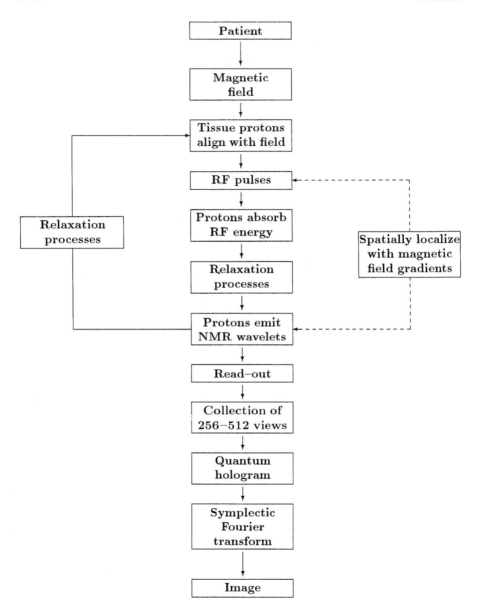

Figure 1. Simplified flowchart displaying the main principles on which a clinical MRI scanner is based. The reconstructive process from multichannel phase histories is through probing the magnetic moments of nuclei employing strong magnetic flux densities and radiofrequency (RF) radiation. The whole process of clinical MRI is based on perturbing the equilibrium magnetization of the object with a train of RF pulses and observing the resulting time-evolving response wavelets produced in a coil. In the read-out procedure, the symplectic Fourier transform algorithm reflects the basic structural feature of the MRI modality. This symplectic affine structure is attached to the coadjoint orbit leaves associated by the Kirillov correspondence to the unitary dual $\hat{G}$ of the Heisenberg nilpotent Lie group G. The HASTE (half-Fourier acquisition single-shot turbo spin-echo) technique takes advantage of the symmetry properties of the symplectic Fourier transform.

In NMR spectroscopy, the Larmor precession spectra of the spin isochromats under the influence of the longitudinal spin–relaxation process, are at the core of the NMR trace filter response. The active arrays of nuclear spins representing quantum bits ("qubits") can be tuned and controlled in a multitude of different ways in space and time in order to extract, by a plethora of quantum computational methods, information about molecular structure and molecular motion. However, any conclusions that are reached *in vitro* must eventually be confirmed by observations made *in vivo*.

The NMR trace filter response wavelets are very rich in measurable characteristics, including initial phase, local precession frequency, and rate of amplitude recovery and decay, that reflect the nature of molecule ensembles in bulk samples, the structure of their environments, and the way in which the molecules interact with them. Due to the abundance of quantum computation information contained in the NMR trace filter response wavelets, redundantly recorded and rearranged in quantum holograms, the MRI modality has a tremendous flexibility. Nevertheless, the amount of quantum information that can be extracted from even highly precise measurements of the phase coherent wavelets is limited, because the act of observation irreversibly alters the quantum system forced into the observed states. The art of high resolution NMR spectroscopy fascinates with its spin choreographic strategies destined to overcome at least some of these inherent limitations.

What has made NMR spectroscopy and clinical MRI such prominent and exciting techniques? One fundamental reason is that quantum computing by NMR spectroscopy and clinical MRI are underpinned by *deceptively* simple ideas. In quantum computing by NMR spectroscopy, single molecules form independent quantum exclusive-OR gates. Due to the distinct resonance frequencies in a two-spin system, the quantum XOR gate allows to flip one of the spins by a single selective radiofrequency (RF) pulse without tipping the other spin. Each of the spins in every molecule identically across the macroscopic liquid sample at room temperature is externally tuned in and controlled via electronically programmed RF pulse trains, as in a synchronized, single-instruction parallel computer, to perform modulo-2 addition of two qubits. It is this capability of being fully programmed by electronic means which actually makes the difference between NMR and DNA computers.

Until now, due to the limitations of current technology, only very small problems have been solved in quantum computing by the pure states of *single* spin systems. In the course of NMR spectroscopy and an image formation process, however, the *ensembles* of nuclear spins within the sample are excited by programmed hard pulse trains with a central frequency at the RF range. Spatially varying magnetic flux densities are trace-filter-encoding the positions of spin isochromats by the Larmor spectra of precession frequencies. The spectral localization of the trace-filter-encoded nuclear spin density is performed by the superposition of affine linear magnetic field gradients which are Mellin transformed with respect to the laboratory coordinate frame of reference. After elimination of the dispersive components of the Larmor precession spectra by the purging processes, the planar *traces* of the excited Heisenberg helices are rearranged in a form of *circular* grating arrays. The ensuing quantum holograms organize the recordings of the Mellin transformed time histories via the superpositions of *coexisting* linear gradients during the acquisition of NMR trace filter response wavelets. The final image is then reconstructed via a quantum holographic sweep from the trace-filter-encoded differential phase and local frequency coordinates of the circular grating array in the laboratory frame of reference.

The holographic procedure performed by the clinical MRI scanner systems implies the existence of phase-locked, synchronized neural networks. These synchronized networks represent the internal interference effects masked in the bulk sample. Their calculations are based on quantum parallelism at the spin isochromat level. In most clinical applications of MRI, the NMR trace filter response wavelets originate from the spin isochromats of the hydrogen nucleus, which is a single proton. Under typical NMR imaging conditions of an external static magnetic field to partially overcome thermal randomization, the fraction of contributing proton ensembles is small at room temperature, while the rest of the spin isochromats take on random orientations within the macroscopic sample. Boltzmann statistics show that, for protons at room temperature, the difference in equilibrium alignment versus antialignment is not obvious, being only of the order of one part in a million and, considering such a statistic, it is an amazing application of coherent quantum *stochastic* resonance that the spin isochromat calculations are detectable in bulk samples.

The spin–relaxation weighted scans are amplified to the macroscopic system level via coherent quantum stochastic resonance as a form of classical parallelism. Soft tissue NMR images of astonishing contrast resolution are obtained from the trace-filter-encoded quantum information. With specialized ultrafast approaches and upgraded bipolar gradient and faster receiver hardware, the MRI scans can be acquired in as little as 20 ms and entire multislice studies in 20 to 60 s. The stringent technical requirements for ultrafast imaging modalities have limited their development until recently. Their evaluation, however, can be of extremely high *diagnostic value* provided the radiodiagnostician disposes of the appropriate semantic filter for an accurate interpretation in the case reading room. In this way, important insights into the metabolism of normal and diseased cells are made possible at the macroscopic system level by the use of chemical shift imaging techniques and various other liquid state NMR methods.

From the cognitive point of view, one can speak of the visualization computation of quantum information, more precisely, of a wave of geometrization which for the first time is extending far beyond the boundaries of medical radiodiagnostics to cover the emergence of the *foliated* energetic structure of observation. In clinical MRI, the tomographic slices are the *substrates* for the NMR trace filter encoding procedure of quantum holography. Now that clinico-morphological structures can be visualized within the anatomy with high resolution MRI, scout scans should be used to orient the tomographic slices according to the actual cross-sectional structures. Anatomy can best be understood and abnormalities best recognized in an axis that makes sense of how the organs are organized. As in all clinical imaging modalities, however, understanding the normal development of morphological anatomy is a fundamental step to recognizing the abnormal clinico-morphological structures through imaging.

Given the expense of clinical MRI equipment and the reluctance of clinical radiologists to complete the training necessary to become an experienced NMR spectroscopist, one might properly ask what virtue a radiodiagnostic imaging method possesses of a sophistication comparable to spaceborne synthetic aperture radar (SAR) high resolution imagery. Such virtue lies in the fact that the MRI modality has proven to be an extremely sensitive and increasingly specific modality for *in vivo* diagnostic whole-body scanning. Although it is still in its infancy, the intrinsic flexibility brought clinical MRI far ahead of X-ray imaging or ultrasonic imagery within the medical diagnostic image industry. It is expected that the availability of superconducting magnets cooled with only liquid nitrogen will make MRI scanner systems affordable to even small centers of radiodiagnostics.

A unique property of MRI, compared with other clinical imaging modalities, is that a multitude of independent NMR parameters over a wide range can be utilized to acquire an unsurpassed range of image contrast. The intrinsic parameters include, *inter alia*, spin density, longitudinal and transverse spin–relaxation rates, chemical shift, diffusion, and magnetization transfer. In this way a whole new science has been created which revolutionized radiodiagnostic medicine and biomedical research. The potential of this new science is just beginning to be realized. The noninvasive nature of NMR imaging, an overriding concern in diagnostic medicine, contributes to the great value of the MRI modality in the antemortem diagnosis, with improvements and discoveries coming "on-line" at a rapid pace. Its future seems so fruitful that speculative imaginations need not so much to be unleashed as restrained.

The longer one is used to running a clinical MRI scanner, the more its structure resolves into mathematical concepts. In fact, this is an experience shared by everybody interested in a deeper understanding of the nonlocal quantum phenomena. Therefore, the author has long felt the need for a text which addresses the structure–function problem of computerized pulsed Fourier MRI in terms of transversally stratified Lie group actions because the wide-band spectra occurring in computer-intensive noninvasive medical radiodiagnostics form a challenging trace filter problem for noncommutative Fourier analysis and the associated *orbital calculi*. As a consequence, the concept of *trace* in its various functional analytic and geometrical contexts penetrates the present text. The trace forms the pivotal concept of the projective geometrical analysis approach to clinical MRI.

The orbital calculus of the simply connected, three-dimensional, two-step nilpotent Heisenberg Lie group G represents a powerful functional calculus for the canonical commutation relations of quantum physics. Because even the texts dealing with the MRI instrumentation function from a system-theoretic perspective are plagued with the problem of obscuring the gauge structure of the Larmor precession spectrum and the free induction decay, the language of the orbital calculus of G seems to be the only universal language available allowing for a satisfactory presentation of the structure–function problem of clinical MRI.

The transversally stratified Heisenberg Lie group G forms the sub-Riemannian analogue of the flat Euclidean vector space. Actually G serves as a *paradigm* for the theory of sub-Riemannian manifolds. The author is tempted to say that an understanding of harmonic analysis on G is indispensable to appreciate the applications of wavelet methods and the quantized calculus on the quotient projection

$$G \longrightarrow G/\text{center}$$

to the fields of NMR spectroscopy and clinical MRI. The passage to the differential phase and local frequency encoding transverse plane G/center, the quadrature demodulation of filter response wavelets, as well as the reconstructive read-out procedure of quantum holograms by means of the trace filter sweep of quantum holography are the key steps to an understanding of pulsed Fourier NMR spectroscopy and clinical MRI.

It is of equal importance to adopt the converse point of view. The Heisenberg group G forms a central extension of a real two-dimensional symplectic affine vector space, the translations of which derive from the transitive Hamiltonian action of G. In terms of projective geometry, the transitive Hamiltonian action of G derives from transvections.

Although the one-dimensional center of G has been factored out by the trivial fibration G/center, the *center* of G plays, via the driving oscillator and the central spectral transform of the left-invariant sub-Laplacian differential operator $\mathcal{L}_G$, a central role in the mathematical model of pulsed Fourier NMR spectroscopy and clinical MRI. Indeed, the natural symplectic affine structure of the flat radial cross section G/center derives via the natural planar connection from the group of isometries of the sub-Riemannian geometry of G. It allows to translate the Larmor frequency equation for the precession dispersion of spin isochromats into the language of *subelliptic* geometrical analysis. The principal *symbol* on the cotangent bundle $T^\star(G)$ of the Hörmander sum of squares $\mathcal{L}_G$ provides the Heisenberg helices as the nonresonant geodesics of G under the natural left invariant sub-Riemannian metric of G. Indeed, this metric, which is left-invariant under the transitive Hamiltonian action of G, is obtained as a subelliptic bundled form on the tangent bundle $T(G)$ from the principal symbol of the left-invariant sub-Laplacian differential operator $\mathcal{L}_G$ on $T^\star(G)$ by the involutive Legendre transformation

$$T(G) \longrightarrow T^\star(G).$$

The isometries of the sub-Riemannian manifold G allow to tune in the grating arrays of the traces of Heisenberg helices in order to perform the tracial encoding of image contrast within the quantum hologram inside the transverse plane G/center.

In terms of Lie group theory, the elliptic non-Euclidean line geometry of the canonically foliated three-dimensional superencoded projective space

$$\mathbf{P}\big(\mathbb{R} \times \mathrm{Lie}(G)^\star\big) \qquad \mathbb{R} = \text{stratigraphic time line}$$

governs the trace encoding procedure and quadrature demodulation of filter response wavelets, the spin echo refocusing in the rotating coordinate frame of reference and the gradient echo rewinding in the laboratory coordinate frame of reference, and the reconstructive read-out process of the Fourier NMR spectroscopy and clinical MRI modality. The spin echo refocusing and the gradient echo rewinding procedures are based on genuine quantum self-interference effects. Due to the projective immersion, the primary axis is no longer time scale but the direction of the coexisting differential phase encoding linear magnetic field gradients with respect to the laboratory coordinate frame of reference. The Mellin transformed gradients control the spin–relaxation weighted Heisenberg helices via the direction of a projectively immersed bundle of parallel lines in the laboratory coordinate frame of reference. In this way, the functor **P** closely *binds* the stratigraphic time line $\mathbb{R}$ via resonance to the line geometry of the stack of planar leaves $\mathcal{O}_\nu$ ($\nu \neq 0$) defined by the canonical foliation of the super-encoded projective space $\mathbf{P}(\mathbb{R} \times \mathrm{Lie}(G)^\star)$. Therefore **P** provides the space–time manifold in the sense of the space–time analysis of Immanuel Kant's *Critique of Pure Reason*. The compact and connected real projective plane $\mathbf{P}(\mathbb{R} \times \mathcal{O}_\nu) \hookrightarrow \mathbf{P}(\mathbb{R} \times \mathrm{Lie}(G)^\star)$ allows for an *antipodal-spherical* visualization of the spin dynamics.

In NMR spectroscopy and clinical MRI, time is not merely a parameter line of clock transitions which serves the *logical* control of defining a systemwide sequence reference for the successive instants at which the state changes in the MRI scanner system may occur. An example for state changes is the spin–relaxation weight control of spin isochromats the timing of which provides the contrast control of MRI. The punchline is that, due to the functor **P**, the systemwide time reference becomes an integral *geometrical* part of the *synchronous* MRI scanner system itself. The functor **P** simultaneously serves the physical purpose of accounting for element and wiring delays (Keppler denotes the concept of delay by the technical term *mora* = $\mu \acute{o} \rho \alpha$) as well as their geometrical symmetries in the paths from the output to the input of clocked elements. The temporal switching as well as the rewinding of Mellin transformed linear magnetic field gradients represents such a physical embodiment of the timing process by which the stratigraphic time line $\mathbb{R}$ no longer forms the primary axis of the free induction decay response but forms the Mellin transform along the directions of the linear magnetic field gradients. In this sense, timing is everything in the NMR trace filter encoding.

The ability of the stratigraphic time line $\mathbb{R}$ to serve two masters, logical control and physics, has a certain elegance and conforms to an established tradition of parsimony in the use of active elements in the design of synchronous systems. In MRI scanners the active elements are the spin packets, or synonymously, the spin isochromats. The quantum holographic read-out of their spin–relaxation weighted density from the planar leaves under their rotational curvature is performed via the confocal observation plane at infinity,

$$\mathbf{P}(\mathbb{R} \times \mathcal{O}_\infty)$$

consisting of Damadian's resonance "sweet spot" arrays. The symplectic Fourier transform as a bank of filters is particularly well adapted to the parallel reconstructive amplification process from the plane of emergence. The emergence of geometrical patterns arises by coherent quantum stochastic resonance associated to the chaos decomposition via the central representation disintegration.

The geometrical symmetry properties of the symplectic spinors associated to the coadjoint orbit picture leads to the implementation of the Kepplerian stratification strategy of phase-sensitive quadrature detection and the tracial reconstructive calculus of Weyl *symbols* of pseudodifferential operators. Its application to NMR spectroscopy offers a fascinating intellectual study of sub-Riemannian geometrical symmetries in the spirit of Keppler. The deep context of the Kepplerian dynamics of physical astronomy on one side and the Clifford parallelism of the three-dimensional elliptic non-Euclidean space $\mathbf{P}\big(\mathbb{R} \times \mathrm{Lie}(G)^{\star}\big)$ on the other justify the projective viewpoint adopted in this ray-tracing approach.

Due to the powerful applications of subelliptic geometrical analysis on the transversal Heisenberg group stratification G/center to computerized pulsed Fourier NMR spectroscopy and clinical MRI, the mathematician Lewis A. Coburn renamed the Heisenberg group G and coined the term "NMR group" at the Conference on Pseudodifferential Operators and Microlocal Analysis, held in the Mathematical Research Institute Oberwolfach in the spring of 1997. This group provides the mathematical basis of the emerging field of quantumography, which extends both holography and computing to the quantum emulation of cognitive systems.

Methodologically, the multidisciplinary approach to a geometrical understanding of the quantum phenomena of biomedical research requires an emphasis on the explanatory and informal aspects. It incontrovertibly requires the avoidance of a linear organization of the material in the traditional theorem–proof style of mathematical texts and suggests a *cyclic* repetitive approach. Hopefully, the pedagogical advantages of the cyclic style of presentation will outweight its mathematical inefficiencies.

Unfortunately such an approach does not imply that the tools of elementary mathematics are sufficient for a deeper understanding of NMR spectroscopy and clinical MRI. The standard bra–ket formalism of quantum mechanics is not well adapted to a treatment of the MRI modality because it does not reflect in the inherent subelliptic geometry of energetic strata or the geometrical symmetries exploited in quantum computing by NMR spectroscopy and clinical MRI. Due to the richness and depth of the mathematical foundations of MRI, the well-known warning that each formula will cut down the medical readership must be unheeded: There is no alternative to the mathematical formulas of wavelet analysis in the study of the sub-Riemannian geometrical symmetries inherent to harmonic analysis on the Heisenberg Lie group G and the transition from the cotangent bundle $\mathrm{T}^{\star}(G)$ to the unitary dual $\hat{G}$ in order to successfully exploit these symmetries.

The book deals with the elaborate structure of Fourier MRI from the Lie group representational point of view. Neither is it a text freeing the reader of mathematical formulas of the introductory type that most radiological monographs on MRI prefer to include for the benefit of the medical readership nor does it provide a type of compilation promising that the reader can find almost everything he or she always wanted to know about NMR physics but were afraid to ask. According to the structural strategy of exposition, important concepts are introduced and presented again in increasingly sophisticated form, as the need for a formal treatment of the Lie group representational structure governing pulsed Fourier MRI develops and the frame of reference becomes firmer and broader.

In teaching courses on Lie groups, Lie algebras, and Fourier analysis to first-year graduate students at the Universities of Bonn, Mannheim, and Siegen, the author's main guideline was twofold: to provide the students with a clear and logical presentation of the basic concepts and principles and to present the fundamentals without remaining exclusively in the territory of pure mathematics. In order to meet these objectives and to keep the discussions concrete, he attempted to include a variety of illustrative applications. Among these are functional analysis, including distributional kernel theory, approximation theory, orthogonal polynomials, and numerical analysis on one side and classical and quantum dynamical systems, projective, symplectic, and differential geometry of foliations, as well as image processing and photonics on another side. In this multidisciplinary approach, the students have been motivated through applications that demonstrate the unifying role of mathematics in various other disciplines, including quantum physics, quantum computation, electrical and quantum engineering, system theory, cybernetics, computerized vision and visualization, robotics, as well as computer-assisted radiodiagnostic medicine and surgery, without doing all of them the justice they deserve.

Given the scientific sophistication of the multifacet topic, the present book has a long history. The mathematical conception of quantum holography in the context of three-dimensional projective geometry and its application to Fourier optical processing of SAR images were actually designed before clinical MRI was introduced into the Radiology Departments of Clinical Centers as one of the most exciting and valuable applications of quantum holography. Based on SAR high resolution imagery, the symplectic spinorial mathematics of quantum holography was developed independently of the application to photonic holography and clinical MRI and unwittingly of Nicolaas Bloembergen's spectroscopic contributions at optical frequencies to the evolution of the MRI modality. Because the author was unaware during that phase of his studies of the photonic work done by the Nobel laureate Dennis Gabor unaided by the laser in 1948–1951, he reinvented photonic holography as an application of the discrete series *trace* formula of quantum holography. This formula is a direct extension of the trace formula for irreducible representations of compact topological groups to irreducible unitary linear representations, square integrable modulo center, of locally compact groups.

The mathematical treatment of photonic holography was not restricted to the standard coherent state analysis of square integrable, holomorphic and anti-holomorphic functions of the Paley–Wiener type on the complexified cross section G/center. The *coadjoint orbit* visualization of the Stone–von Neumann–Segal theorem suggested a layered structure for the holographic memories to be used in laser-controlled photonic computers. In coherent photonics, stacks of photorefractive substrates are appropriate for the construction of the high density memory layers, but the mathematical approach to stratified holographic data storage needs to be completed by a treatment of the phenomenon of phase coherent wavelet *collapse*.

Concerning the organization of this book, the teaching experience has been that when a large volume of complex information originating from different disciplines must be assimilated and organized in context, some intentional repetition of the central conceptions can greatly help. This holds even more when the communication between the different disciplines involved still has to be established, and clinical questions of radiodiagnostic accuracy are added with each new advance in the continuing time evolution of clinical MRI technology. Therefore introductory material to acculturate the reader to clinical MRI concepts is included. Different paths of approaching the structure–function problem of computerized pulsed Fourier MRI have been chosen in order to stress the analogy to SAR high resolution imagery and to reinforce the theoretical aspects.

But why restrict the discussion to NMR spectroscopy and clinical MRI? The reason is the paucity of mathematically based reference material in this area. Of course, a book aimed at developing the mathematical foundations and applications of the highly sophisticated MRI modality cannot begin from scratch. For an in-depth understanding of the material, the book assumes basic knowledge of the fundamentals of general Fourier analysis on noncommutative, simply connected Lie groups at the L^2 and distributional levels. In view of the fact that in the field of NMR spectroscopy the time-honored continuous wave techniques have been replaced by synchronized pulse train methods to elucidate molecular structure and chemical dynamics, the extension from the L^2 level to the symplectic spinorial level is imperative for understanding the spectral localization procedure of computerized pulsed Fourier MRI and the trace filter encoding performed by wide-band RF spectra. Indeed, distributional kernel theory is indispensable to appreciate the trace filter sweep of quantum holography. The scanning in the canonically foliated, three-dimensional projective space $\mathbf{P}(\mathbb{R} \times \text{Lie}(G)^\star)$ is performed by the leaf select Pfaffian P_G. The $\mathbb{R}$-linear form P_G on the one-dimensional center of the Heisenberg Lie algebra $\text{Lie}(G)$ allows for tomographic slice selection in the longitudinal direction. Only those spin isochromats which are localized within the slice-select scan plane are on speaking terms.

The Lie functor $\text{Lie}(\cdot)$ is in loose coincidence to the fact that the first commercial MRI scanner was installed in the radiology offices of Doctor Lie and Associates in Cleveland, Ohio. For the past six years, it has been both the author's passion and burden to establish that the most demanding noninvasive radiodiagnostic imaging modality presently available not only is in the spirit of mathematics but actually represents a new direction in subelliptic geometrical analysis and stochastic analysis which surprisingly admits strong roots in the Kepplerian dynamics of physical astronomy. The manuscript has been written in encompassing compassion on the patients presented to the author on the scanner couch when he practiced as a radiology fellow at various departments of MRI in Europe and the United States. Their disorders, most often severe diseases, developmental abnormalities, congenital malformations, or traumas, have been a permanent stimulus throughout the long period of learning, protocolling, correcting, and again learning at the bedside.

The advent of multifacet imaging modalities such as clinical MRI and SAR high resolution imagery is a lesson to those quick-reward pragmatists who feel that basic research should be severely restricted and applied research should reign supreme as the sure and only way of making science useful. According to the philosophy that both lines of research should have their appropriate places in science, the message of the book is that geometrical symmetries inherent to the coadjoint orbit visualization are at the base of quantum computing by Fourier NMR spectroscopy and clinical MRI. Suppressing fundamental research on quantum information technology and quantum computing by the acknowledged limitations of current technology or the impatience of short-sighted pragmatists would impose great damage on the future development of science.

If ever there was a strong argument for the long-term benefit of interdisciplinary research, it is the advent of computerized pulsed Fourier MRI. Try to accept the extended knowledge base for now as part of the spin–relaxation weighted sub-Riemannian geometry to design and apply more advanced clinical MRI techniques for the benefit of humankind.

There are clear attractions in using noninvasive imaging methods for the study of living systems. No other recent imaging modality has had as significant an impact on how to noninvasively image cross sections of the human body as has MRI. Although Damadian's original goal of fast and easy cancer screening has not been fully realized using spin–relaxation weighted scans of water and lipids, it can only be assumed that the progress in clinical MRI will continue and that there are many more improvements and discoveries of new clinical applications around the corner. The rewards for such improvements and expansion of knowledge of clinical MRI make the commitment a joy.

WALTER JOHANNES SCHEMPP
Universitaet Siegen

ACKNOWLEDGMENTS

You do not know anything until you have practiced.
—Richard P. Feynman (1918–1988)

Das menschliche Erkennen ist ausgehend von der Tatsache zu betrachten, daß wir mehr wissen, als wir zu sagen wissen.... Der Akt, mit dem eine mathematische Theorie mit ihrem Gegenstand in Beziehung gesetzt wird, ist eine implizit vorgenommene Integration. Eine Theorie kennt man erst dann wirklich, wenn man sie verinnerlicht und ausgiebig zur Deutung von Erfahrungen verwandt hat. Daher gilt: Eine mathematische Theorie kann nur so errichtet werden, daß sie sich dabei auf ein früheres implizites Wissen stützt, und sie kann nur in einem Akt impliziten Wissens als Theorie fungieren, nämlich so, daß wir uns von ihr aus der früher erworbenen Erfahrung, auf die sie bezogen ist, zuwenden.
—Michael Polanyi (1985)

One of the attractions of clinical MRI is the interdisciplinary nature of its techniques and intrumentation. Taking into account the astonishing broad range of disciplines which clinical MRI covers, the author owes much to the entrance of quantum mechanical ideas into computer science and the art of electronics, the introduction of signal-theoretic and image processing methodologies into mathematics, the fascination exerted by Doppler radar remote sensing technologies such as SAR high resolution imagery, and the exciting ideas developed by the on-going dialogue between cognitive neuroscience and mathematics. This approach to the missing science of consciousness is supported by neurofunctional MRI experiments which are able to provide shadows of the mind.

The author gratefully acknowledges the experienced practical advice provided to him by the scanning MRI technologists and operators of the Felix Riedel Center for Continuing Medical Education in Jona, Switzerland, and Philadelphia, Pennsylvania, and the Fondazione di Studi Universitari in Lugano, Switzerland; during practical sessions of clinical imaging at the General Electric Signa 0.5-T superconductive magnet scanner system; and at the Istituto di Radiologica, Università "La Sapienza," Policlinico Umberto I in Rome, Italy. He is grateful for the hospitality extended to him by the Departments of Radiology of Stanford University School of Medicine at Stanford, California; the University of California School of Medicine at San Francisco, California; the Harvard Medical School at Boston, Massachusetts, where parts of this work on neuroimaging, musculoskeletal, and neurofunctional MRI in *theoria cum praxi* has been done; and the Russell H. Morgan Department of Radiology and Radiological Science, The Johns Hopkins Medical Institutions at Baltimore, Maryland, for its teaching of bedside knowledge of MRI diagnostic tests. As a visiting fellow in neuroimaging, musculoskeletal, and functional MRI, the author acknowledges his debt to the MRI staff neurologists for their expert clinical guidance on semantically interpreting clinical MRI scans during sessions in the Case Reading Room at Stanford University Medical Center; the MRI staff technologists of the University of California at San Francisco, Department of Radiology for their practical advice and help; the team of physicists, neuroscientists, and staff MRI diagnosticians of the Nuclear Magnetic Resonance Center of Massachusetts General Hospital and Harvard Medical School for their expert instructions given at the Nuclear Magnetic Resonance Research Laboratories of MGH at Charlestown, Massachusetts; and the staff radiologists in the Case Reading Room of Johns Hopkins Division of MRI for sharing their practical experience during the author's Clinical Preceptorship in MRI. Moreover, the author is grateful to Bruker Medizintechnik GmbH, Rheinstetten, for providing comprehensive information concerning the MRI scanners of the TOMIKON and MEDSPEC series and to Carl Zeiss, Oberkochen, for providing material on the recent development of the computerized (Mehrkoordinaten–Manipulator) MKM neuronavigation microscopy system for framed stereotactic interventions in neurosurgery. The MRI-guided MKM neuronavigation microscopy system actually transposes the spatiotemporal navigational principles of Johann Keppler (1571–1630), Mathematicus Caesareus at Prague, to the field of interventional radiology. The neuronavigation microscopy technique, applied within an open MRI scanner, leads to less trauma and damage to soft tissue. In modern neuroscience, it allows for precise placement of intracranial depth electrodes in epilepsy surgery of focal seizures.

No effort is a solo endeavor. The author's special note of thanks goes to Section Chiefs of Clinical Radiology Doctors Manfred Crone and David A. Bluemke, Ph.D., Doctor Gordon E. Olson, and the late Doctor Karl Ruopp for letting him participate in their medical insights, and to Dres. Ernst Binz, Basil J. Hiley, Koichiro Matsuno, Basil G. Mertzios, Dieter Michel, and Edgar D. Mitchell for letting him participate in their physical insights. He thanks Dres. Peter J. Marcer and Brian Oakley of the British Computer Society for their efforts to include quantum holography as a topic of research into the emerging European Institute of Quantumography. Finally he thanks Father Felix OP for his indulgent introduction into the Aristotelean physics and his help in the imitation of the ancients and his assistants Dr. Ludger Knoche, Dr. Karin von Radziewski, and Dietmar Schneider for their expertise and constantly available assistance with the text system.

In writing this book the author has benefited from the support and encouragement of many people. He wishes to give special recognition and express his special thanks to Professors George L. Farre (Georgetown), Erwin Kreyszig (Carleton), and Karl H. Pribram (Radford). Professor Farre's deep insights into evolutionary systems and his incisive discussions of the energetic structure of observations strongly influenced the group representational approach to quantum computing by NMR spectroscopy and clinical MRI. His generous assistance with a language that is not the author's mother tongue deserves a particular acknowledgment. From its very beginning Professor Kreyszig continously accompanied the publication process with his rich experience, generous support, and invaluable advice. Professor Pribram's expertise stimulated the linkage between quantum holography and cognitive neuroscience. Without their dedicated help and competent advice, the influence of Professors Emmet N. Leith (Ann Arbor) and Bernard Widrow (Stanford) exerted by their stimulating *leitfaden* courses on optical signal processing and neural network engineering, and the visions of Professors Günter Pickert (Gießen) and Karl Zeller (Tübingen), from whom the author had the privilege of learning, this text could not have been compiled.

1

NMR SPECTROSCOPY AND CLINICAL MRI: HISTORICAL AND PHENOMENOLOGICAL ASPECTS

Bloch and Purcell opened the road to new insight into the micro-world of nuclear physics. Each atom is like a subtle and refined instrument, playing its own faint, magnetic melody, inaudible to human ears. By the methods due to Bloch and Purcell, this music has been made perceptible, and the characteristic melody of an atom can be used as an identification signal. This is not only an achievement of high intellectual beauty—it also places an analytic method of the highest value in the hands of scientists.

—Harold Cramer (1952)

Why not use pulsing?

—Nicolaas Bloembergen (1972)

Just as the symphonic score allows the conductor to follow and understand complex actions that the orchestra will perform, the pulse sequence timing diagram allows a better understanding of the actions of MR image formation.... Timing is everything and that is why the representation of the choices of a direction is called a pulse sequence timing diagram.

—Robert B. Lufkin (1998)

Important though the general concepts and propositions may be with which the modern and industrious passion for axiomatizing and generalizing has presented us, in algebra perhaps more than anywhere else, nevertheless, I am convinced that the special problems in all their complexity constitute the stock and core of mathematics, and that to master their difficulties requires on the whole the harder labor.

—Hermann Weyl (1885–1955)

1.1   THE DEVELOPMENT OF COMPUTERIZED PULSED FOURIER NMR SPECTROSCOPY AND CLINICAL MRI: FIRST PART

In electrodynamics, the propagation of electromagnetic fields is described by the Maxwell equations of local field operators operating on flat Euclidean space. It is a well-known result of the quantization of electromagnetic modes in the Heisenberg picture that the Maxwell equations for the free electromagnetic radiation field in the Coulomb gauge can be inferred from the equation of motion for the free photon system. This fact leads to a treatment of laser oscillators.

In the interaction between electromagnetic radiation fields and nuclear sytem, one of the fundamental interactions of nature, resonances play a key role. It was, however, not until Heisenberg and Schrödinger independently set the stage for the development of quantum physics that the finer details of the magnetic properties of materials were elucidated. In 1924 Wolfgang Pauli postulated, on the basis of hyperfine splittings in spectral lines, that an atomic nucleus with unpaired nucleons has a spin and therefore an intrinsic magnetic momentum. In the following year, Samuel A. Goudsmit and George E. Uhlenbeck at the University of Leiden were the first to propose that the electron has its own intrinsic magnetic momentum. This was the theoretical basis of electron paramagnetic resonance (EPR) spectroscopy, which culminated in the ENDOR (electron nuclear double resonance) detection experiment.

Spectroscopy provides direct evidence of *quantization* of energy. Nowhere is this more simply illustrated than in NMR experiments. Textbooks on quantum physics would surely have chosen nuclear spin ensembles as their starting point, rather than atomic spectra, had Fourier NMR spectroscopy been discovered at an earlier date. The resonance lines which are observed in high resolution NMR spectra provide incontrovertible evidence of the transitions between the various energy levels. In contrast to conventional spectroscopy, however, the separation between the energy levels depends upon the applied magnetic flux density. Spatially varying magnetic flux densities which are superimposed on the stationary magnetic flux density in order to resolve the resonance lines are suitable to tracially encode the positions of the spin isochromats. Similarly, the resonance lines of EPR spectroscopy are detected by sweeping the magnetic flux density. The 1991 Nobel Prize in chemistry, awarded to physical chemist Richard Robert Ernst, highlights the importance of computerized pulsed Fourier NMR spectroscopy and its filter bank approach. The explosive development it has enjoyed in the last decade has led to the unfortunate distinction between NMR spectroscopy and clinical MRI.

The dynamical foundation of NMR spectroscopy and clinical MRI was created independently and almost simultaneously in 1945 by two experimental groups. The group at Stanford University worked under the leadership of Felix Bloch (1905–1983). He was a former student and assistant to Heisenberg in Leipzig, a student of Hermann Weyl at the Swiss Federal Institute of Technology (ETH) in Zürich, to Schrödinger at the University of Zürich, and on Heisenberg's recommendation an assistant to Pauli in the early days of quantum physics. The other group worked at Harvard University under the direction of Edward Mills Purcell (1912–1997) and at the Radiation Laboratory of the Massachusetts Institute of Technology, headed by

Isidor Isaac Rabi. Both observations in bulk material were made within a few days of each other so that unknowingly both groups were working against time.

The moment of birth of the temporal magnetic resonance phenomenon was marked by Bloch's fundamental *dynamical* approach of flipping magnetic moments in 1946 ([114], [223]). Referring to the ill-fated experimental attempts of Cornelis J. Gorter, a former student of Paul Ehrenfest and George Uhlenbeck at the University of Leiden, Bloch's approach to nuclear induction reads as follows ([114], pp. 1–2):

> The method of magnetic resonance has been successfully applied to measure the magnetic moment of the neutron and of various nuclei. The principal feature of the method of magnetic resonance is the observation of transitions, caused by resonance of an applied radiofrequency field with the Larmor precession of the moments around a constant magnetic field....

> The first successful experiments to detect magnetic resonance by electromagnetic effects have been carried out recently and independently in the physics laboratories of Harvard and Stanford Universities. The experiment of Purcell and his collaborators is very closely connected to that of Gorter....

> The considerations upon which our work was based have several features in common with the two experiments, previously mentioned, but differ rather essentially in others. In the first place, the radiofrequency field is deliberately chosen large enough so as to cause at resonance a considerable change of orientation of the nuclear moments. In the second place, this change is not observed by its relatively small reaction upon the driving circuit, but by directly observing the induced electromotive force in a coil, due to the precession of the nuclear moments around the constant field and in a direction perpendicular both to this field and the applied r-f field. This appearance of a magnetic induction at right angles to the r-f field is an effect which is of specifically nuclear origin and it is the main characteristic of our experiment. In essence, the observed perpendicular nuclear induction indicates a rotation of the total oscillating field around the constant magnetic field.

> This effect is, of course, most outspoken at resonance (just as the Faraday effect becomes greatest in the neighborhood of a resonant frequency) and, in practice, is noticed by its sudden strong appearance under resonant conditions. It is worth while, however, to point out that the observation of nuclear induction should be possible without any use of the magnetic resonance. Not only a weak r-f field, acting at resonance over very many Larmor periods, can produce an appreciable nuclear change of orientation, but also a strong field pulse, acting over only a few periods. Once the nuclear moments have been turned into an angle with the constant field, they will continue to precess around it and likewise cause a nuclear induction to occur at an instant when the driving pulse has already disappeared. It seems perfectly feasible to receive thus an induced nuclear signal of radiofrequency well above the thermal noise of a narrow band receiver. It is true that, due to the broadening of the Larmor frequency by internuclear fields or other causes, this signal can last only a comparatively short time, but for normal fields it will still contain many Larmor periods, i.e., it will be essentially monochromatic. The main difference between this proposed experiment and the one which we have actually carried out lies in the fact that it would observe by induction the free nuclear precession while we have studied the forced precession impressed upon the nuclei by the applied r-f field. The existence of a resultant macroscopic moment of the nuclei within the sample under

investigation is a common prerequisite for all electromagnetic experiments with nuclear moments. It is in fact a change of orientation of this macroscopic moment which causes the observed effects, and irrespective of the changes of orientation of the individual nuclei which might be induced by a r-f field, their moments would always cancel each other, if they did so initially, and thus escape observation.

Bloch's approach has set the stage for the art of spin choreography ([106], [107]) currently practiced in NMR spectroscopy. By "art" is meant the kind of skillful mastery that comes from an intimate familiarity with the tuning problems of high resolution NMR spectroscopy. The temporal tuning in of spin isochromats forms the prelude to MRI and external qubit manipulation of quantum computing by pointing out the bridge between classical electrodynamics and nuclear physics.

The experimental skill needed to achieve the desired effect in condensed matter is illustrated by the fact that Gorter had attempted to detect NMR scanning signals in a solid at the University of Groningen four years earlier by measuring the influence of nuclear dispersion by thermal changes on the frequency of resonance. Gorter noted ([223], p. 423):

> After a visit to an industrial laboratory, Ehrenfest once exclaimed to me that, although he understood hardly anything of the wonderful techniques being developed in the radio industry, he felt that such techniques might become of great benefit to pure scientific research.

However, the result of Gorter's experimental work done in 1936 and 1942 was negative. The failures to detect NMR are perhaps to be attributed to the fact that Gorter used too pure materials. The relaxation time was so long that the thermal equilibrium was destroyed before the magnetic resonance effect could be detected.

The other successful approach to NMR was stimulated by the challenge of understanding the phenomenon of water absorption of microwaves. Purcell, on leave from Harvard University, was recruited by the MIT Radiation Laboratory to help in the development of radar. Due to this radar background, he emphasized the quantum transitions aspect of NMR. In the landmark paper with his associates Nicolaas Bloembergen and Robert V. Pound, one of the most cited physics papers ever published, Purcell et al. summarized in 1948 the immersion idea of the RF *spectroscopic* approach to NMR as follows ([114], pp. 16–18):

> In nuclear magnetic resonance absorption, energy is transferred from a radiofrequency circuit to a system of nuclear spins immersed in a magnetic field, H_0, as a result of transitions among the energy levels of the spin system.

> The exposure of the system to radiation, with consequent absorption of energy, tends to upset the equilibrium state previously attained, by equalizing the population of the various levels. The new equilibrium state in the presence of the radiofrequency field represents a balance between the processes of absorption of energy by the spins, from the radiation field, and the transfer of energy to the heat reservoir comprising all other internal degrees of freedom of the sustance containing the nuclei in question.

Finally we review briefly the phenomenological theory of magnetic resonance absorption, before describing the experimental method. The phenomenon lends itself to a variety of equivalent interpretations. One can begin with static nuclear paramagnetism and proceed to paramagnetic dispersion; or one can follow Bloch's analysis, contained in his paper on nuclear induction, of the dynamics of a system of spins in an oscillating field, which includes the absorption experiments as a special case. We are interested in absorption, rather than dispersion or induction, in the presence of *weak* oscillating fields, the transitions induced by which can be regarded as nonadiabatic. We therefore prefer to describe the experiment in optical terms.

Due to the different experimental viewpoints adopted, the two experimental groups had difficulties in accepting that they had discovered *dual* effects of the same NMR phenomenon almost simultaneously. The Fourier duality brings the assurance that Bloch's nuclear induction decay mode and Purcell's nuclear magnetic resonance absorption mode actually are equivalent spectral approaches. Both modes, acquired following phase-sensitive quadrature detection, are unaffected by any magnetic field gradient.

The Fourier duality holds rigorously, except at very low temperatures. The *symplectic* structure which is inherent to the mode duality marked the start of computerized pulsed Fourier NMR spectroscopy. It can be expressed by the alternating matrix

$$J = \begin{pmatrix} 0 & -1 \\ 1 & 0 \end{pmatrix}$$

of phase-sensitive quadrature detection, which indicates that the absorption mode and the dispersion mode are $\frac{1}{2}\pi$ out of phase. Their spectra are given by the Lorentzian line profiles in quadrature channels:

- The free induction decay as the NMR filter response wavelet to a $\frac{1}{2}\pi$ pulse excitement of the nuclei of condensed matter is the Fourier transform of the steady state absorption-mode spectrum.
- The nuclear magnetic resonance absorption mode is performed *ex corporis*. In the read-out process, the magnetic resonance absorption-mode information follows from the quantum holographically stored dispersion-mode information.
- Pulsed Fourier MRI uses phase-sensitive quadrature detection of information channels which are represented by affine Lagrangian lines.

Computer technology was not well developed at the time of Bloch's and Purcell's NMR experiments. Its application to pulsed Fourier NMR spectroscopy and SAR high resolution imagery had to wait for the introduction of inexpensive computers in the late-1960s and by the design of the fast Fourier transform (FFT) algorithm for an efficient evaluation of the discrete Fourier transform. It was actually Russell Varian, one of the co-developers of the klystron, which had been incorporated as the master oscillator in practically all microwave radar systems and EPR spectrometers, who first proposed the use of the Fourier transform in order to increase the sensitivity of NMR spectrometers by resonance. Weston A. Anderson, a co-worker of Ernst at Varian Associates, noted ([223], p. 595):

> In 1965 we continued to await the advances in computer technology that would make the process truly practical—after all, what good was a 10-second data collection if you couldn't see the spectra for several days? The plodding scanning method still generated meaningful spectra faster than FT NMR.

> As soon as possible, we ordered a minicomputer. By today's standards, it was slow, and the 4,000 bytes of memory trivially small. However, it enabled us to transform the data and plot it out in a few minutes.

Now, since the day of the $5 analog-to-digital converter (ADC) is here, dedicated FFT processors allow electronic adjustment in quadrature of the phase of reference. Due to Fourier duality, computer implementation of the FFT algorithm allows detection of phase-coherent wavelets whose Fourier transforms represent either the nuclear dispersion or the nuclear magnetic resonance absorption spectrum in condensed matter.

On any given digital computer, a number of factors would influence the choice of the optimal FFT algorithm. These include such topics as relative speed of memory access and floating-point performance, efficiency of computing trigonometric functions whether or not implemented in dedicated hardware, degree of accuracy required, and other factors. Also, special features, such as computing the Fourier transform of a function whose Fourier transform is known to be real valued would affect the choice of a specific FFT algorithm for an optimum of efficiency.

The fundamental principle that the FFT algorithm and its various modifications are based upon is that of decomposing the computation of the discrete Fourier transform of an input data array of finite sequence length N into successively smaller discrete Fourier transforms. Computing the discrete Fourier transform involves $N - 1$ additions and N multiplications of complex numbers plus N integer products. If the computations are performed independently, the total effort to compute the discrete Fourier transform involves N^2 multiplications and $N(N - 1)$ additions of complex numbers, plus some further chores of minor complexity.

The dramatic increase in efficiency is achieved by exploiting the *symmetry* of the complex Nth roots of unity forming powers of the primitive complex Nth root of unity in a look-up table. This symmetry, hence the basic idea of the FFT algorithms, is due to Carl Friedrich Gauß (1777–1855). The savings in multiplications of complex numbers, however, is bought at the price of an increase in the number of additions. This trade-off is typical of this kind of fast algorithms.

In the simplest form when N is an integer power of 2, the FFT algorithms are termed radix 2. The manner in which the successive decomposition principle is implemented leads to a variety of different radix 2 algorithms, however, all modifications with comparable improvements in computational speed. The computational complexity of the algorithms with $\log N$ stages is roughly proportional to the product

$$N \log N$$

rather than the N^2 operations consumed by the discrete Fourier transform appetite, and the input and data arrays are stored by the processor in the same storage location. If memory is expensive and one needs to make the best use of it, this savings can be important.

The in-place computation of the discrete Fourier transform by means of the FFT algorithms made the Fourier transform a truly practical tool of digital signal processing ([260]), and one of the reasons that Fourier analysis is of such wide-ranging importance in digital signal processing is because of the existence of efficient algorithms for the in-place computation of the discrete Fourier transform. Due to the FFT algorithm, for instance, the trend in SAR high resolution imagery is clearly toward digital processing, where it allows to realize the concept of corner turn memory by the trace filter encoding of SAR data ([365]).

The butterfly computations of the decimation-in-phase FFT algorithm as well as its dual variant, the decimation-in-frequency FFT algorithm, admit reversed flow graphs and bit-reversed sorting of the data arrays at the input or on the output, respectively. In the first procedure, the first and last halves of the transform were obtained from the even and odd points in the input array. In the second procedure, the even and odd points are obtained from the transforms of the first and second halves of the input array. These symmetries show up in the flow graphs, and in both procedures a permutation pass is required.

The flow graph of an elementary two-point discrete Fourier transform has a symplectic structure which is given by the corner turn matrix

$$ J = \begin{pmatrix} 0 & -1 \\ 1 & 0 \end{pmatrix} $$

of Pfaffian $Pf(J) = 1$ and purely imaginary spectrum $\{-i, i\}$. The complete flow graphs of the butterfly computation in cascade can basically be implemented along horizontally adjacent lines by the finite Heisenberg group. The purpose of this group is to organize the *reflection* symmetries of the look-up table of roots of unity. This fact is a first cue that *nilpotent* harmonic analysis actually plays an organizational role in Fourier NMR spectroscopy and clinical MRI. It is via this computational detour that Russell Varian indirectly contributed to the Heisenberg group approach to the discrete Fourier NMR spectroscopy. Note also that the alternating matrix J is at the basis of the $\frac{1}{4}$ Number of EXcitations (NEX) technique, which uses only one quadrant of the data acquired from the pulse excitation–acquisition cycles. The penalty for reducing the image acquisition time T_A is a reduction of the signal-to-noise ratio.

The coadjoint orbit visualization of the Heisenberg Lie group G, which is of central importance for the trace filter sweep of quantum holography, is not abundantly helpful in the case of a *finite* Heisenberg group. However, the basic idea of immersing the discrete Fourier transform with its interpretation as a digital filter response into a nilpotent group, the structure of which allows for reduction of the number of time consuming arithmetic operations, is useful for the study of the applications of the real Heisenberg groups. Because the concept of the Heisenberg group is disconcerting even to engineers with a long experience of applying the Fourier transform, the implementation of filter banks by the Heisenberg group should make the Lie group concept more familiar to the electrical engineering community.

The experiment of Bloch's group predicted a transient NMR filter response without giving practical emphasis to the experimental use of RF *pulse* extensions over many periods. The application of pulse trains, however, excites the nuclear spins simultaneously and avoids the waste of time asssociated with the very slow field sweep through resonance and the associated narrow-band filter. Concerning the application of pulse excitations, which actually made MRI possible, the discoverer of the spin echo technique, Erwin L. Hahn, commented on the NMR experiments of Bloch and Purcell ([223], p. 511):

> Purcell and his cohorts were at the forefront of radar pulse technology at the MIT Radiation Laboratory, and yet they did not exploit transient pulse response to NMR. In his pioneering paper, Bloch mentioned that free precession would result after the sudden reorientation of spins by a nonadiabatic field pulse, but did not emphasize that experimentally one could use an RF pulse extending over many periods.

The instant when the driving pulse has already disappeared but the nuclear magnetic induction continues to coexist and to define a rotational curvature of the selected tomographic slice is recorded as an *event* of the NMR protocol on the stratigraphic time line $\mathbb{R}$. As the event line of the systems manager which controls the synchronization of the pulse excitation–acquisition cycles and the synergy of the coexisting linear magnetic field gradients, the stratigraphic time line $\mathbb{R}$ has to be incorporated into the geometrical quantization procedure. The line bundles involved in this projective construction represent the linear gradient *directions* within the embedding superencoded projective space:

- The stratigraphic time line $\mathbb{R}$ allows for synchronization of the temporal repetition periods T_R of the pulse excitation–acquisition cycles.
- The event line $\mathbb{R}$ incorporated into the systems manager controls a recording of the time history via the superpositions of linear magnetic field gradients.
- The linear gradients temporally switched in the laboratory frame of reference are encoded by the Mellin transform during NMR filter response acquisition.

The tomographic slices form a canonical foliation consisting of projectively completed, symplectic affine planar leaves in the superencoded projective space. Selection of tomographic slices is achieved by using a frequency-selective pulse excitation. This pulse is applied in the presence of a computer-controlled longitudinal magnetic field gradient to resonate with the driving Larmor frequency via the Mellin transform and holding the coexistence of the foliation leaves along the bi-infinite stratigraphic time line $\mathbb{R}$. This procedure results in a variation in phase across the thickness of the tomographic slices, the gradient phase effects of which are to cause a large degree of NMR filter response cancellation. The cancellation drawback can be overcome by applying a spatial linear rewinder magnetic field gradient after the pulse excitation. This serves as the closest analogy to the refocusing procedure of diverging precession phases by pulse reflections in the synchronized frame of reference of rotating energetic coordinates, utilized in the course of the standard spin echo pulse sequence. The application of a linear magnetic field gradient of opposite polarity prior to the next following excitation is typically done by superimposing the phase encoding gradient in the reversed order along the bi-infinite stratigraphic time line $\mathbb{R}$. The purpose is to rewind the nonresonant Heisenberg helices the traces of which are encoded by the Mellin transformed phase encoding gradient.

Bloch and Purcell later shared the 1952 Nobel Prize in Physics in recognition of their pioneering achievements in NMR in condensed matter. During the next quarter of a century NMR spectroscopy flourished. More than 1,000 NMR units were manufactured, and according to whether a physicist spoke of nuclear magnetic induction or NMR absorption, one could decide whether he or she came from the West Coast or the East Coast. This influence became apparent in the original spin echo paper by Hahn in 1950 ([114], [223]). Hahn had taught radar and sonar and therefore was familiar with the duplex alternation of transmission and acquisition cycles. The spin echo technique had a dramatic impact on the development of both NMR spectroscopy and MRI scanner systems. Hahn's paper touched off a flurry of activity because it separated continuous-wave NMR from pulsed NMR spectroscopy and emphasized the wide-ranging importance of the spin echo interference patterns coherently excited by the reversed action along the stratigraphic time line $\mathbb{R}$. It was Varian's suggestion to Hahn to patent the spin echo technique for the commercial exploitation of NMR spectroscopy.

In the field of time-domain NMR, the term *spin echo* is not meant to imply a radar echo similiar to SAR high resolution imagery or an ultrasound pulse echo (Figure 2), but refers to the mirror image of reversed action, similar to the flow graph reversal and the bit-reversed ordering of input data arrays used in the FFT algorithms and their variants. In terms of photonic holography, the reflection principles or pancake flips, which fully exploit the sandwich symmetry offered by the coadjoint orbit visualization of G, have been summarized by Hahn as follows ([139], p. 408):

> In the time and frequency domain the delayed spin echo bears a resemblance to the recall of a holographic image. For weak input pulse shapes injected into a spin spectrum of much broader bandwidth than that of the pulse shape, the pulse shape can be stored with fidelity for a time T_2 and then recalled in "inverse shape order" as an echo after a short intense read-out π pulse. The stimulated echo clearly relies on a grating of x axis spin populations in $\Delta\omega$ space, prepared by two $\frac{\pi}{2}$ pulses for example. After a long time T less than relaxation times due to spin-lattice and diffusion, the pulse shape can then be recalled in "direct order" within a time T_2 as a stimulated echo after the application of a third $\frac{\pi}{2}$ pulse.

The geometrical analysis approach to quantum holography allows to make the relation between photonic holography and MRI more precise and to include the spin echo as a quantum teleportation effect, mathematically realized by the sandwich symmetry of the coadjoint orbit visualization of G. The bi-infiniteness of the stratigraphic time line $\mathbb{R}$ appears to indicate a violation of the second law of thermodynamics, which has been already observed by the pioneer of RF spectroscopy and chemical shift theory,

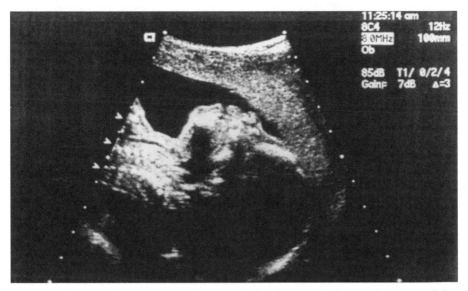

Figure 2. High resolution ultrasonic imaging study of a fetus in utero: The improved contrast resolution has been achieved by the inclusion of the phase. In contrast to fetal MRI, ultrasonography does not provide enough morphological details of the fetal cerebrum. Evaluation of the phase information is essential for quantum holography and clinical MRI. The phase information needs the field $\mathbb{C}$ of complex numbers for its mathematical treatment. The field $\mathbb{R}$ of real numbers, however, is not sufficient for a treatment of quantum holography and clinical MRI.

Norman Foster Ramsey, Jr., in 1956. Indeed, the concept of time reversal allows to prepare a nuclear spin system by means of a two-pulse sequence in such a way that, although it appears to be in an equilibrium state, at some later time its degree of order grows spontaneously from a previously negligible level. This would appear just as miraculous as a gas mixture separating of its own accord into its pure components. Spontaneous mixing of two gases cannot be reversed because it is impossible to reverse all the molecular velocities in a gas mixture to make the molecules retrace their previous paths. According to John S. Waugh of MIT, the idea of time reversal implicit in the idea of the spin echo refocusing and gradient rephasing challenges the validity of the second law. Because the spontaneous ordering is a spin echo, the second law of thermodynamics needs to add a proviso to make it reflect in the reality of spin echo phenomena by taking into account long transverse relaxation times ([362], p. 174):

> The spin echo is still striking to those who see it for the first time, as it probably was to Hahn. A nuclear magnetization, having disappeared in a free induction decay, spontaneously reappears as a giant fluctuation. While the phenomenon is easily understood from a mechanical point of view, it seems to verge on a violation of the second law of thermodynamics. It is this problem, about which Hahn and others have written, that we approach here again from what is at least partly a fresh perspective. Our point of view will be that echoes *do* violate the second law. After having defended this case we will discuss briefly how the problem can be avoided by appropriate statement of purely macroscopic thermodynamic principles.

In photonic terms, the generation of the spin echo interference patterns or quantum holograms critically depends upon the time delay of phase-coherent wavelets as well as on their *phase conjugate* copies to remove the dispersion component of the partial Fourier transform. The application of the principles of NMR spectroscopy to photonics played a dominant role in the work done by Bloembergen ([223], pp. 375–376):

> Many people aren't aware, but I certainly was, that all of these techniques—the theory of magnetic resonance—could be theoretically translated to what happens at optical frequencies. These frequencies are 10,000 times larger than the microwave frequencies, but they can all be described in the same language developed first to describe magnetic resonance.

Due to the massive parallelism inherent to photonics, it provides the fastest high resolution, two-dimensional FFT processor available, namely a magnifying *lens*. In retrospect, Hahn comments on NMR and MRI, and the analogy with photonic holography ([139], pp. 401–408):

> The technique of MRI developed following a period of years (1948–70) during which time the science of NMR matured as an analytic tool in the physical, chemical and biological sciences. The computerized pulsed NMR Fourier transform method of spectroscopy, initiated in the middle sixties by Ernst & Anderson, came into common usage, and set the stage for the pioneers of MRI to succeed.

> A good deal of MRI technique is common to both NMR and two-dimensional NMR spectroscopy ([88]). As an alternative view which involves Fourier transform spectroscopy, consider the method of holography. The image of an object in optical holography is stored in terms of a pattern of diffraction gratings formed by developed silver grains in a photographic emulsion. The pattern is a result of the interference between laser light scattered from the original object and a reference laser beam. The image of the object is recalled by viewing the superposition of read-out laser beam Bragg scattering off of the grating distribution $f(k_g)$. Each grating is characterized by a spatial frequency $k_g = 2\pi/\lambda_g$ where λ_g is of the order of the laser beam wavelength. Following the coherent scattering of a read-out laser beam into a restricted range of angles θ, the image is reconstructed from the Fourier transform of $f(k_g)$. If one neglects factors such as the granularity of the emulsion, λ stability of the laser, etc., the smallest resolvable image distance Δx is limited by the angular dispersion $\delta\theta \approx \lambda/\Delta x$. Although it is difficult to make a one-to-one comparison of holography with MRI, one notes that the MRI phase and frequency encoding of a spin slice is somewhat analogous to the diffraction grating pattern of holography; and the subsequent Fourier transform imaging "read-out" steps compare in each case where coherent optical scattering and coherent RF emission pertain to holography and MRI respectively.

The driving RF oscillator that Rabi used in his sophisticated molecular beam experiment by means of an adjustable resonance "sweet spot" was a technique suggested to him by Gorter in 1937. It was the first experiment to use NMR and earned Rabi the Nobel Prize in 1944.

The root of Gorter's fundamental idea is to employ in NMR spectroscopy the dynamical system

$$\mathbb{R} \lhd G \longrightarrow \mathbb{R} \oplus \mathbb{R}$$

at a *driving* oscillator frequency $\nu \neq 0$. The longitudinal line $\mathbb{R}$ can be identified with the one-dimensional center $C \hookrightarrow G$ of the three-dimensional two-step nilpotent Heisenberg Lie group G:

- In clinical MRI, the driving oscillator of central frequency $\nu \neq 0$ serves as the reference of quantum holography.
- The holographic transform $\mathcal{H}_\nu$ factors through the central character $\chi_\nu: C \ni z \leadsto e^{2\pi i \nu z}$ of G.

As a consequence, Gorter's idea of a driving oscillator suggests the consideration of G as a central *extension* by the line C. Then the transitive Hamiltonian action of G derives from the translations of the transversal symplectic affine plane $\mathbb{R} \oplus \mathbb{R}$ and hence from the transvections of its projective completion. The trajectory of the dynamical system is revealed to be the spin–relaxation weighted Heisenberg helix. The traces of the tuned-in Heisenberg helices are capable of encoding the phase and local frequency of the spin isochromats inside the selected, projectively immersed tomographic slice.

The driving oscillator and its *natural* global oscillation frequency ν of the magnetic resonance system impose onto the projectively immersed, flat coadjoint orbit

$$\mathbf{P}(\mathbb{R} \times \mathcal{O}_\nu) \hookrightarrow \mathbf{P}(\mathbb{R} \times \mathrm{Lie}(G)^\star)$$

the rotational curvature form

$$\omega_\nu = P_G(\nu)\,d\kappa \qquad (\nu \neq 0).$$

On the right-hand side, the contact one-form κ forms a section of the dual vector bundle

$$\mathrm{T}^\star(\mathrm{T}^\star(G))$$

so that the symplectic form ω_ν is well defined on the cotangent bundle $\mathrm{T}^\star(G)$. The important observation is that the transitive Hamiltonian action of G annihilates the alternating differential 2-form ω_ν on G. The coefficient of the symplectic form

$$d\kappa = dx \wedge dy$$

of the projectively immersed, generic coadjoint orbit $\mathbf{P}(\mathbb{R} \times \mathcal{O}_1) \hookrightarrow \mathbf{P}(\mathbb{R} \times \mathrm{Lie}(G)^\star)$ is given by the Pfaffian polynomial P_G. The polynomial P_G forms a measure for the volume growth. It is homogeneous of degree 1 along the dual of the one-dimensional center of the Heisenberg Lie algebra $\mathrm{Lie}(G)$. The traces of the nonresonant Heisenberg helices are parametrized by the symplectic affine coordinates

$$\left(t, \begin{pmatrix} x & -y \\ y & x \end{pmatrix}, 2\pi P_G(\nu) \right)$$

of the foliation leaves in the superencoded projective space $\mathbf{P}(\mathbb{R} \times \text{Lie}(G)^\star)$.

For most spectroscopy and imaging studies, the phase-coherent wavelets obtained of a single free induction decay are too weak to be distinguishable from noise. Because the quality of the spectroscopic data that are stored within the computer is ultimately determined by the signal-to-noise ratio, it is almost always necessary to improve the signal-to-noise ratio by collecting a large number of free induction decays and then storing the sum of these free induction decays. Finally, this idea gave rise to designing a modification of the standard spin echo pulse sequence, temporally switched along the bi-infinite stratigraphic time line $\mathbb{R}$. This spin echo refinement, which uses one $\frac{1}{2}\pi$ excitation pulse and one reflection $\vee$-pulse instead of two $\frac{1}{2}\pi$ pulses, was actually used by Hahn in explaining the spin echo technique ([223]) in terms of the rotating frame of reference. Now it is known as the Carr–Purcell–Meiboom–Gill pulse train of spin choreography ([107], [114]). It is interesting to note that the concept of spin echo needed nearly a decade to be developed in EPR spectroscopy. Today the concept of echo also appears in the very different area of photon echo.

The choice of time interval between consecutive RF pulses, incorporated into the MRI protocols along the stratigraphic time line $\mathbb{R}$, is influenced by the process of *saturation*. Here saturation means the progressive reduction of the NMR filter response that is associated to the (T_1, T_2) spin–relaxation decomposition of the contact one-form

$$\kappa = \underbrace{dz}_{(1)} + \underbrace{\frac{1}{2} \cdot (x\,dy - y\,dx)}_{(2)}.$$

The two components of the section κ of the dual vector bundle $T^\star(T^\star(G))$ are spin–relaxation weighted by (1) the incomplete spin-lattice, or T_1 relaxation time, and (2) the spin–spin relaxation time, or T_2 relaxation time:

- The longitudinal relaxation time T_1 is the measure of how fast the spins within a population achieve a net magnetization by aligning themselves parallel to and antiparallel to the external static magnetic field.

The superposition of spin-up and spin-down states represents an array of qubits. Considerable care has to be taken in selecting the value of the cycle or repetition periods T_R along the bi-infinite stratigraphic line $\mathbb{R}$, because any errors in the array of qubits can result in decoherences and hence in substantial losses in the signal-to-noise ratios:

- The transmission of RF pulse trains along the bi-infinite stratigraphic time line $\mathbb{R}$ for coherent excitation of spin echo interference patterns or quantum holograms reveals a basic operating principle of MRI: Visualization by means of repetitions.

These spin echo pulse trains, the transmission of which at the cycle or repetition periods T_R along the bi-infinite stratigraphic line $\mathbb{R}$ is temporally switched "on and off" by a gate, tend to give more accurate measurements of the spin–spin relaxation time T_2 than the standard spin echo pulse sequences:

- The transverse relaxation time T_2 is the measure of how fast a spin population loses its net magnetization after being excited by a RF field oscillating at the Larmor precession frequency of the spin isochromats.

To quote the original spin echo paper by Hahn ([114], p. 50):

In nuclear magnetic resonance phenomena the nuclear spin systems have relaxation times varying from a few microseconds to times greater than this by several orders of magnitude. Any continuous Larmor precession of the spin ensemble which take place in a static magnetic field is finally interrupted by field perturbations due to neighbors in the lattice. The time for which this precession maintains phase memory has been called the spin–spin or total relaxation time, and denoted by T_2. Since T_2 is in general large compared with the short response time of radiofrequency pulse techniques, a new method for obtaining nuclear induction becomes possible. If, at the resonance condition, the ensemble at thermal equilibrium is subjected to an intense r-f pulse which is short compared to T_2, the macroscopic magnetic moment due to the ensemble acquires a nonequilibrium orientation after the driving pulse is removed. On this basis Bloch has pointed out that a transient nuclear induction signal should be observed immediately following the pulse as the macroscopic magnetic moment precesses freely in the applied static magnetic field. The effect has already been reported and is closely related to another effect, given the name "spin echoes," which is under consideration in this investigation. These echoes refer to spontaneous nuclear induction signals which are observed to appear due to the constructive interference of precessing macroscopic moment vectors after more than one r-f pulse has been applied.

In quantum computing, the spin–spin relaxation time T_2 is known as the *decoherence* time. Since decoherence introduces errors into the intermediate results, it severely limits the time available for computation. The difficulty of isolating microscopic systems from their environment well enough to attain long decoherence times has proven to be one of the chief obstacles to implementing a true quantum computer. In contrast, the nuclear spins in a molecule are quite well isolated from its motional and electronic degrees of freedom and therefore have the capability to store quantum information.

One of the most remarkable features of the MRI modality is the extensive range of pulse trains, as well as user-friendly receiver and gradient coils that have been and continue to be designed, with a view to enhancing the quality and information content of spectra. The idea of spin echo and quantum hologram includes phase shifts and reflections in the synchronized RF pulse trains, temporally switched along the bi-infinite stratigraphic time line $\mathbb{R}$, to provide a powerful means of enhancement of wanted and suppression of unwanted signals by constructive and destructive *interference* of phase-coherent wavelets. The great advantage of the quantum holograms is that, because of the massive redundancy, environmental interactions only weakly perturb the MRI scanner's state.

In Fourier NMR spectroscopy, the RF radiation that is used for excitation of signals is applied in the form of computer-controlled pulses, the duration of which along the bi-infinite stratigraphic time line $\mathbb{R}$ may vary from a few microseconds to milliseconds. Denoting by $\theta \in [0, \pi]$ the flip angle, the (T_1, T_2) spin–relaxation decomposition of the contact one-form κ is implemented by the time evolution matrix of the tissue specific longitudinal and transverse spin–relaxation processes in Zeeman ordered samples:

$$\left(\begin{array}{ccc} \boxed{\begin{array}{cc} 0 & -e^{-\frac{|t|}{T_2}} \sin\theta \\ e^{-\frac{|t|}{T_2}} \sin\theta & 0 \end{array}} & \begin{array}{c} 0 \\ 0 \end{array} \\ \begin{array}{cc} 0 & \qquad 0 \end{array} & 1 - e^{-\frac{|t|}{T_1}}(1 - \cos\theta) \end{array} \right) \qquad (t \in \mathbb{R})$$

In the scaling matrix the longitudinal direction is aligned with the external magnetic flux density. According to the Bloch–Riccati equations, the entries formed by time evolving spin–relaxation weights display the rapid loss of the transverse components of the free induction decays responding via resonance to the magnetization perturbation displayed in the scale block $\square$. For any flip angle $\theta \in [0, \pi]$, the transverse spin–relaxation weighted matrices of phase-sensitive quadrature detection are infinitesimal generators of planar rotations which produce the tracial encoding of image contrast:

$$\square = \left(e^{-\frac{|t|}{T_2}} \sin\theta \right) \cdot J = \left(\begin{array}{cc} 0 & -e^{-\frac{|t|}{T_2}} \sin\theta \\ e^{-\frac{|t|}{T_2}} \sin\theta & 0 \end{array} \right) \qquad (t \in \mathbb{R})$$

The slower loss of the component in the longitudinal direction aligned with the external magnetic flux density is linearly superimposed by the slowly recovering spin–relaxation weight. Consequently the dissipative spin system approaches the equilibrium spin state of the sample as $|t| \to \infty$. Thus the time evolving, tissue specific spin–relaxation weights determine the distance of the dissipative spin system to equilibrium.

In practice, it is more convenient to use the spin–relaxation rates

$$\frac{1}{T_1} \leq \frac{1}{T_2}$$

as parameters of the T_k ($k \in \{1, 2\}$) spin–relaxation weighted MRI acquisitions. The spin–relaxation weights affect the encoding of image contrast via the additional, temporally switched external magnetic flux density of the RF excitation pulses. High soft tissue contrast, reproducibility of image quality, and good conspicuity of disease require the use of pulse trains that are robust and reliable and avoid artifacts. The development of new pulse trains has been a major theme of research in NMR for many years and has provided much of the basis for the continued progress in clinical MRI and NMR spectroscopy, not only for the visualization of specific clinico-morphological structures, but also for the investigation of tissue function and pathophysiology. The refinement of present pulse techniques is progressing so rapidly that it is likely that many up-to-date pulse sequences will be outdated by the near future.

On Fourier transformation, the spectrum of the free induction decay is obtained. Its characteristics depend upon a number of factors, including the biochemical composition of the spin sample. The inverse Fourier transform, or Fourier cotransform, of the block $\square$ at the frequency $\nu \neq 0$ can be computed by evaluation of the Fourier inversion integral. The residue theorem in conjunction with the inversion theorem for Fourier transforms yields, by closing the contour in the lower complex half-plane for $t > 0$ and in the upper complex half-plane for $t < 0$, the Lorentzian line profile of width $\frac{1}{T_2}$ at the optimum flip angle $\theta = \frac{1}{2}\pi$ for single pulse experiments. Let ν' denote the frequency of the rotating frame of reference, which may be different from the Larmor precession frequency ν of spin isochromats.

The trace filter sweep of quantum holography which is associated with the phase-sensitive quadrature detection of infinitesimal generator $2\pi\nu'J$ is denoted by

$$1_{\nu'} \oplus 1_{\nu'}.$$

Its absorption-mode spectrum is given by the real part of the free induction decay

$$\frac{\frac{1}{T_2}}{(\nu' - \nu)^2 + \left(\frac{1}{T_2}\right)^2}.$$

The dispersion-mode spectrum is given by the imaginary part of the free induction decay

$$\frac{\nu' - \nu}{(\nu' - \nu)^2 + \left(\frac{1}{T_2}\right)^2},$$

which is an odd, as opposed to an even, function of the frequency discrepancy $(\nu' - \nu)$.

The two components are proportional to the real and imaginary parts of a Fourier-transformed free induction decay. Thus the greater the spread in the frequency domain, the more rapidly the nuclear induction signal decays. If this causal process, which must be carefully distinguished from transverse relaxation (a random process), is allowed to progress too far, much of the NMR trace filter response is lost. It is not completely obvious how to overcome the problem of minimizing the dispersion component of the Fourier transform in order to exploit the richness of measurable characteristics inherent to the NMR trace filter response:

- The spin–relaxation weighted Heisenberg helices have to be refocused by a trace filter sweep in order to provide a phase-sensitive quadrature detectable NMR filter response of their traces inside the selected tomographic slice.

If the spectral spread were due to a field gradient, the gradient reversal would rewind the nonresonant Heisenberg helices, the so-called gradient echo technique. The dispersion process, however, is not under control. Nevertheless it can be reversed by the spin echo technique. It is based on the reflection $^\vee$ of the contact one-form κ of the improper block matrix of the purely real spectrum $\{-1, 1\}$:

$$\left(\begin{array}{cc|c} 1 & 0 & 0 \\ 0 & -1 & 0 \\ \hline 0 & 0 & -1 \end{array} \right)$$

The block $\square$ indicates the tracial reflection in the transversal symplectic affine plane $\mathbb{R} \oplus \mathbb{R}$ which is transformed into the reflection of the gradient echo technique by

$$J^2 = -\mathrm{id}_{\mathbb{R} \oplus \mathbb{R}}$$

of the block matrix

$$\left(\begin{array}{cc|c} -1 & 0 & 0 \\ 0 & -1 & 0 \\ \hline 0 & 0 & 1 \end{array} \right).$$

This is at the basis of the phase conjugate symmetry technique HASTE, or $\frac{1}{2}$ NEX. The $\frac{1}{2}$ NEX technique allows the radiodiagnostician to halve the number of phase encoding steps, not the number N_{EX} of coherent excitations. The transition via J^2 also indicates that, in a hybrid gradient and spin echo (GRASE) technique, the spin echo technique can be combined with the gradient echo technique.

After the time period

$$\tfrac{1}{2} T_E,$$

which is half of the *spin echo time*, an application of the reflection $^\vee$-pulse gives rise to the reverse trace filter sweep

$$1_{-\nu} \oplus 1_{-\nu}$$

associated with the reflected coadjoint orbit $\mathbf{P}(\mathbb{R} \times \mathcal{O}_{-\nu})$ of G. Due to the rephasing effect of its interference with spin isochromats, the reverse trace filter sweep globally compensates the spin–isochromat dephasing effect of temporally constant inhomogeneities associated with the external magnetic flux density. This major aspect of the spin echo technique is due to the additional magnetic flux density associated with the RF excitation pulses. It is stationary with respect to the rotating coordinate frame of reference revolving through the azimuth angle ϑ at the Larmor precession frequency $\nu = (1/2\pi)\dot{\vartheta}$. If T_R denotes the temporal repetition period of the spin echo pulse train, the spin–relaxation weight is given by

$$\underbrace{\left(1 - e^{-\frac{T_R}{T_1}}\right)}_{(1)} \underbrace{e^{-\frac{T_E}{T_2}}}_{(2)}.$$

The operator-controlled image protocol parameter of spin echo time T_E usually varies in the time interval from 10 to 160 ms whereas the protocol parameter of repetition period T_R varies in the interval from 20 to 5,000 ms:

- Short repetition period T_R (300 to 700 ms), in order not to eliminate the effect of T_1 spin–relaxation, and short spin echo time T_E (20 to 30 ms), in order to eliminate the effect of T_2 spin–relaxation, designate a T_1-weighted MRI scan. In contrast, long T_R (1,000 to 5,000 ms), in order to eliminate the effect of T_1 spin–relaxation, and long T_E (40 to 120 ms), in order not to eliminate the effect of T_2 relaxation, designate a T_2-weighted MRI scan. Balanced scans require a long T_R of 2,000 ms to eliminate the effect of T_1 spin–relaxation and a short T_E of 20 ms to eliminate the effect of T_2 spin–relaxation.

In the multiple spin echo technique, further echoes are obtained by repeating the reflection $^\vee$-pulses with not necessarily equidistant temporal distances during the spin–spin relaxation time T_2. The nth echo carries the attenuated spin–relaxation weight

$$\underbrace{\left(1 - e^{-\frac{T_R}{T_1}}\right)}_{(1)} \underbrace{e^{-n\frac{T_E}{T_2}}}_{(2)}$$

at time $t = nT_E$ of the stratigraphic time line $\mathbb{R}$. All n echoes of a pulse train are collected in multiple data lines with the same Mellin transformed phase encoding gradient. The whole pulse train can be repeated with the temporal repetition period T_R.

The only limit to the number n of echoes acquired after a single excitation pulse, the echo train length ETL, is the decay (2). In practice, the echo train length typically ranges from 4 to 16. The time interval between successive echoes, or between reflection $^\vee$-pulses, is called echo spacing. It is determined by the duration of the $^\vee$-pulses and the echo sampling time. To shorten the echo spacing, either the $^\vee$-pulses and/or the echo sampling time must be shortened or both. Typical echo spacings are in the range of 16 to 20 ms at typical bandwidths of ± 16 kHz.

The longitudinal part (1) corresponds to the spin–relaxation weight of the *partial saturation* pulse sequence. It consists of RF excitation pulses of flip angle $\theta = \frac{1}{2}\pi$ which are periodically repeated with a temporal interpulse interval T_R small enough *not* to allow complete recovery. Because the spin–relaxation weight

$$1 - e^{-\frac{T_R}{T_1}}$$

is independent of the spin–spin relaxation time T_2, the partial saturation pulse sequence is less flexible than the classical spin echo method. It requires accurate pulse flip angles $\theta = \frac{1}{2}\pi$, and its image contrast performance is not sufficient for the detection of many pathologies. For long repetition periods T_R the *saturation recovery* pulse sequence arises. Because external magnetic inhomogeneity becomes a problem, spin echo techniques are used to eliminate this problem.

The rephasing effect of the spin echo technique must be carefully distinguished from the spatial refocusing procedure of gradient echo techniques which is based on the inversion of in-plane linear gradients and their spatially encoding local magnetic flux densities with respect to the laboratory frame of reference in dissipative spin systems. Consequently image artifacts caused by inhomogeneities of the magnetic flux density may be more severe in the gradient field echo modality than in the spin echo technique. It follows that the simulation of spin isochromat manipulations in the gauge of a rotating coordinate frame of reference performed by transition to an in-plane linear gradient coordinate frame of reference via the symplectically invariant Weyl symbol isomorphism

$$\sigma : S'_{\mathbb{C}}(\mathbb{R} \oplus \mathbb{R}) \longrightarrow S'_{\mathbb{C}}(\mathbb{R} \oplus \mathbb{R})$$

can imply considerable practical disadvantages.

A major purpose of the spin echo technique is to acquire T_1 and T_2 spin–relaxation weighted scans. The spin echo pulse sequence has found wide applications in clinical imaging because most of the pathologies imply a prolongation of the tissue specific spin–spin relaxation time T_2. The introduction of the heavily T_2 spin–relaxation weighted spin echo pulse sequence into clinical practice in 1982 provided a very useful approach for disease detection based on differences in the T_2 relaxation time. This has since become the mainstay of clinical MRI diagnosis in the brain and spinal cord. The application of T_1 spin–relaxation weighted spin echo pulse sequences also provided a method for acquiring T_1 spin–relaxation weighted scans that were lower in contrast than *inversion recovery* pulse sequences but were quicker. As a result, there was less need for the inversion recovery sequence.

In contrast to the standard spin echo sequence, which still is the working horse of the day-to-day routine clinical MRI examinations, the basic form of the inversion recovery sequence is a three-pulse sequence. It was used in the first clinical MRI studies that showed an advantage of MRI over X-ray computerized tomography (CT). The sequence produced high contrast between normal and pathological tissues that had a prolonged T_1 relaxation time and was the single most effective imaging technique available from 1980 to early 1982.

The inversion recovery pulse sequence starts with a reflection $^\vee$-pulse of preparation. The purpose of this initial RF excitation pulse is to flip the lower spin-down state parallel to the main magnetic flux directon into the antiparallel state spin-up by interchanging the orientations of the counterpropagating rotating coordinate frames of reference. After the *inversion time* T_I a RF excitation pulse of flip angle $\theta = \frac{1}{2}\pi$ follows ([324]). The $\frac{1}{2}\pi$ pulse of the inversion recovery sequence is always slice selected. After waiting the repetition period T_R from the preparatory $^\vee$-pulse, another reflection $^\vee$-pulse follows. For single scans the $^\vee$-pulses need not to be slice selected. However, when the inversion recovery sequence is used to acquire an interleaved set of tomographic slices, the reflection $^\vee$-pulses must be slice selected. The additional timing parameter T_I determines the relaxation projection on the longitudinal direction. In view of the (T_1, T_2) relaxation decomposition of κ, the longitudinal spin–relaxation weight of the classical inversion recovery pulse sequence reads

$$\underbrace{1 - 2\,e^{-\frac{T_I}{T_1}}}_{(1)}.$$

Hence, the inversion recovery pulse sequence is a Fourier MRI method of producing T_1 spin–relaxation weighted images. The complete longitudinal spin–relaxation weight reads

$$\underbrace{\left(1 - 2\,e^{-\frac{T_I}{T_1}}\right)}_{(1)} \underbrace{\left(1 - e^{-\frac{T_R}{T_1}}\right)}_{(1)}.$$

A large temporal delay T_D is required between pulse sequences in order to complete longitudinal spin–relaxation. The inversion recovery pulse train is defined by applying additional $\vee$-pulses with temporal repetition period

$$T_R = T_I + T_E + T_D.$$

Because the application of $\vee$-pulse sequences and the *delay* time T_D in the range of $3\,T_I$ makes the technique time consuming if long inversion times T_I are chosen, the basic form of the inversion recovery pulse sequence is a less frequently used method of producing T_1 spin–relaxation weighted images in routine clinical MRI examinations ([43]). The superiority of inversion recovery pulse sequences over standard spin echo sequences for imaging myelination disorders ([347]) should be observed. The RARE (rapid acquisition with relaxation enhancement) sequence employs multiple differential phase encoding steps with repeated reflection $\vee$-pulses. The ultrafast EPI (echo planar imaging) technique typically acquires all the data for one scan in a single shot, with data acquired for 40 to 200 ms, and therefore represents an ultrafast imaging modality.

The differentiation between fat and water due to the different chemical shifts of these protons is an important issue in clinical MRI. The inversion recovery pulse sequence with medium inversion time T_I in the range of 250 to 700 ms shows high gray–white contrast in brain studies as well as strong sensitivity to pathology. An inversion recovery pulse sequence with a very short inversion time T_I in the range of 0 to 250 ms is called a short T_I inversion recovery (STIR) sequence ([366]). Because fat has a very short longitudinal spin–relaxation time T_1 of approximately 250 ms, water protons and lipid protons can be separately imaged. The STIR sequences with inversion times T_I in the range of 150 to 180 ms permit to suppress fat NMR filter response relative to water and provide high T_1 contrast. If the spin echo time T_E is chosen to provide very high lesion contrast, STIR is a useful technique in head, neck, and spine applications. The STIR techniques can be implemented with fast spin echo (FSE) sequences, where a $\vee$-pulse reflection and a RF excitation pulse of flip angle $\theta = \frac{1}{2}\pi$ are followed by multiple refocusing $\vee$-pulses to generate a train of echoes.

The concept of fat/water suppression by STIR sequences has been found to be useful for screening for pathology. In clinical ophthalmic imaging ([66], [311]), for instance, STIR scans prove an exceptional way to visualize orbital pathology against the background of orbital fat. The STIR modality is presently finding its way more and more into mainstream computerized pulsed Fourier MRI for such widespread applications as improved demonstration of tumors in fatty tissue regions like tumor metastases of the bone marrow in the musculoskeletal system ([34], [59], [329]), hepar neoplasms and focal hepatic and splenic lesions ([236], [312], [326]), the distinction of fatty cysts from aqueous cysts ([79], [210], [281]), the visualization of intramedullary spinal lesions ([323]), and the early noninvasive radiological diagnosis of femoral head necrosis ([34]). In MRI studies of avascular necrosis of the femoral head, the NMR filter response from the necrotic region is reduced due to a lengthening of the longitudinal spin–relaxation time T_1. In some cases one can also observe a halo of diminished NMR response intensity arising from a thickened joint cavity, synovial hypertrophy, or synovial effusion. In the inner pelvis FSE imaging has general applicability and is preferable to conventional body coil imaging with standard spin echo sequences for use in all nonmusculoskeletal applications in the pelvis ([162], [231], [284], [312]).

Similarly, fluid-attenuated inversion recovery (FLAIR) is an inversion recovery technique that allows to eliminate NMR filter response from cerebrospinal fluid (CSF) by choosing a long inversion time T_I in the range of 1,800 to 2,000 ms. For example, the FLAIR sequence is used in brain studies to suppress CSF to bring out the periventricular hyperintense lesions, such as plaques in multiple sclerosis (MS). Fast FLAIR is a relatively new pulse sequence that combines the FLAIR sequence with a fast imaging technique, such as FSE, to achieve CSF suppression in a fast manner. A repetition time $T_R = 10,000$ ms allows almost complete longitudinal recovery of CSF. When T_R is increased, the inversion time T_I to null CSF does not increase to the same degree. To increase the efficiency of the modality, the sequence takes advantage of the dead time $(T_R - T_I)$ to acquire a second multislice inversion read-out slab.

Both fluid suppression and fat or white matter suppression can be combined in the form of the *double-inversion recovery* (DIR) pulse sequence, which can be used, for example, to isolate the cerebral cortex.

Fast scanning, some manufacturers use the prefix *turbo* to denote fast scanning techniques, is a generic term used to describe rapid MRI acquisition techniques and is not meant to describe any particular manufacturer or application. Currently fast imaging techniques are undergoing progressive refinement and modification, and therefore no one strategy can be considered optimal for all applications. Either fast spin echo (FSE) imaging or turbo spin echo imaging is a commercial implementation of a fast imaging technique originally known as RARE. It is one of the most important recent advances in clinical MRI. FSE forms a very elegant way of manipulating the standard multiple spin echo technique to save time. It provides almost all the advantages of standard spin echo imaging at a faster speed.

Although the FSE pulse sequence superficially resembles a routine multiple spin echo sequence, the FSE technique is conceptually different. It changes the differential phase encoding gradient for each of these echoes, whereas the standard multiple spin echo sequence collects all echoes in a train with the same phase encoding gradient. As a result of changing the phase encoding gradient between echoes, multiple rows of the transient array of synchronously tuned Heisenberg helices, which collects the planar traces of the circular grating arrays of quantum holograms, can be acquired within a given repetition period T_R or one shot. The resulting image is therefore constructed from differential phase encoding steps having different spin echo times T_E. Denoting by N_P the radix-2 number of differential phase encoding steps, the number of shots is given by $(1/\text{ETL})N_P$. Therefore the image acquisition time for each pulse sequence is given as

$$T_A = T_R \cdot N_P \cdot N_{EX},$$

where N_{EX} is reduced by the number n of echoes acquired within a given repetition period T_R, hence by the ETL. In this way, FSE allows to significantly decrease the image acquisition time T_A compared to a standard spin echo pulse sequence with the same repetition period T_R, so that the FSE modality can be applied for faster scanning with less severe motion artifacts. Speed, the primary advantage of FSE, actually comes without the usual concomitant losses of signal-to-noise ratio.

Many fast MRI acquisition techniques use a repetition period T_R as short as 20 ms. This choice of T_R does not allow enough sampling time to acquire other planar tomographic slices during the time interval T_R. Typically these fast MRI scans acquire all the data on one selectively excited planar tomographic slice before going on the next one within the region of interest (ROI).

The bandwidths of the pulses have to be sufficiently large to excite spin isochromats within the required frequency range. Pulsed NMR has the great advantage that all signals can be excited simultaneously rather than one by one. In comparison with continuous-wave NMR, this approach produces a considerable improvement in spectroscopic sensitivity and faster data throughput.

The uses of pulses of RF fields were recognized early in the development of NMR, but pulsed NMR was little used in chemical analysis for many years. The award of the Nobel Prize in chemistry to Ernst in 1991 served to highlight the fact that the pulsed approach to high resolution NMR not only is an essential physical technique for alert chemists and biochemists but also offers a fascinating study of living systems critically dependent upon *noncommutative* Fourier analysis and *projective* geometrical analysis. Although Felix Bloch once commented that "when chemists enter a field it's time to get out," when physical chemist Ernst formulated the Fourier transform foundation for NMR spectroscopy from the system-theoretic perspective, he opened the window of MRI to mathematicians who recognized it as an exciting application of geometrical analysis, distributional kernel theory, and the FFT algorithms. However, at the time he did his NMR experiments he had no idea that computerized pulsed Fourier NMR spectroscopy and clinical MRI would become the big industries they are today.

It is sometimes claimed that the expansive development of NMR in chemistry, biology, and diagnostic radiology occurred after the introduction of computerized pulsed Fourier NMR spectroscopy in the late 1960s. The basic principles, however, had been known before, most of them from the research of Hahn. In his landmark paper with W. A. Anderson, Ernst summarized the application of Fourier NMR spectroscopy in 1966 as follows ([114], p. 84):

> It is well-known that the frequency response function and the unit impulse response of a linear system forms a Fourier transform pair. Both functions characterize the system entirely and thus contain exactly the same information. In magnetic resonance, the frequency response function is usually called the spectrum and the unit impulse is represented by the free induction decay. Although a spin system is not a linear system,

Irving J. Lowe and Richard E. Norberg (1957) have proved that under some very loose restrictions the spectrum and the free induction decay after a 90° pulse are Fourier transforms of each other. The proof can be generalized for arbitrary flip angles.

For complicated spin systems in solution, the spectrum contains the information in a more explicit form than does the free induction decay. Hence it is generally assumed that recording the impulse response does not give any advantages compared to direct spectral techniques. The present investigations show that the impulse response method can have significant advantages, especially if the method is generalized to a series of equidistant identical pulses instead of a single pulse. In order to interpret the result, it is usually necessary to go to a spectral representation by means of a Fourier transformation. The numerical transformation can conveniently be handled by a digital computer or by an analog Fourier analyzer.

The expansive development that led to the present importance of magnetic resonance in chemistry, biology, and medicine occurred after the introduction of Fourier spectroscopy in the late 1960s.

Here are some of the features of the pulse technique: (1) It is possible to obtain spectra in a much shorter time than with the conventional spectral sweep technique. (2) The achievable sensitivity of the pulse experiment is higher, providing the investigated spectrum possesses much fine structure (e.g., high resolution NMR spectroscopy). All spins with resonance frequencies within a certain region are simultaneously excited, increasing the information content of the experiment appreciably compared with the spectral sweep technique where only one resonance is observed at a time.

The idea of an initial impulse excitation in Bloch's dynamical approach establishes the linkage between temporal magnetic resonance organization and the Kepplerian phase-sensitive quadrature detection strategy for the study of time-dependent phenomena, such as spin–relaxation rates, chemical exchange, and molecular diffusion. It makes it possible to take advantage of the salient fact that in pulsed NMR experiments there is a temporal separation of the strongly nonlinear effects caused by short pulse train excitations and the free evolution of phase-coherent wavelets responding to the Larmor precession of spin isochromats. Here, the nonlinearity refers exclusively to the dependence of the NMR filter response on the pulse amplitude. The momenta of the selective pulses in the symplectic affine plane of incidence $\mathbb{R} \oplus \mathbb{R}$ are measured in accordance with the Kepplerian area law, and their tight control is exercised along the stratigraphic time line in accordance with the timing diagram of the NMR experiment protocol.

Two-dimensional spectroscopy is probably the most fruitful development that took place in NMR spectroscopy. The first proposal to introduce two-dimensional NMR spectroscopy was made by Jean Jeener of the Free University in Brussels in 1971. Its germ was implicit in the nuclear magnetic spin echo experiment ([87], [114], [223]) and critically depends upon the concepts of *direction* and associated directed quantities. Whereas in MMR spectroscopy the local frequency distribution associated with a given direction arises as a result of the different biochemical environments of the detected nuclei, in MRI it arises as a result of their differing spectral positions. These are detected by the directional derivative or linear magnetic field gradients of the *spectral localization* synthesis, a fundamental excitation procedure developed very early by Robert Gabillard in Paris, without having any perspective in 1951 that his efforts would have radiodiagnostic relevance.

The gradient phase effects excited by computer-controlled superposition of Mellin transformed linear magnetic field gradients along the stratigraphic time line $\mathbb{R}$, as well as the strategies to compensate for them, are perhaps among the least understood of MRI concepts; this may be because the pivotal method of spectral localization analysis is given inadequate attention in most treatments of basic NMR physics. Nevertheless, pulsed field gradients are now widely used as a device for purging undesirable phase effects.

Therefore, the idea of refocusing by time reversal via phase conjugation flip is implicit in both compensation strategies. The main difference between the spin echo and the gradient echo technique, however, is that due to the directional character of linear gradient superpositions, temporally switched in the laboratory frame of reference, the gradient echo does not refocus the dephasing effects of intrinsic magnetic flux inhomogeneities by means of a trace filter sweep. Gradient echo sequences, which may use an arbitrary flip angle for the acceleration of the acquisition of the data in the laboratory frame of reference, are therefore susceptible to inhomogeneities of the magnetic flux density. However, despite their favorable signal-to-noise ratio, conventional spin echo sequences have proven to be a failure for the dynamic examination of contrast behavior in pathological processes, due to their long acquisition times. They have now largely been discarded in favor of gradient echo sequences:

- The Heisenberg Lie group G is transvectionally coordinatized by the superposition of linear magnetic field gradients with respect to the laboratory frame of reference along the bi-infinite stratigraphic time line $\mathbb{R}$.

The phase directions within the tomographic slice are encoded by successively applying Mellin transformed phase encoding gradients. The linear magnetic field gradient excitations which are applied before, rather than during, the acquisition of data generate a phase shift in the acquired phase-coherent wavelet the magnitude of which reflects the spatial location of the excited spins within the tomographic slice. Of course, the application of just one phase encoding linear magnetic field gradient does not provide enough informatiom to the spectral localization analysis of the spin isochromats of two-dimensional Fourier NMR spectroscopy. The transvectional encoding needs a gradual stepping up of successive computer-controlled gradient excitations in order to acquire a line bundle within the tomographic slice. This line bundle is implemented as a circular grating array of energetic stratum coordinates. As a quantum hologram within the selected leaf from the canonical foliation of tomographic slices, it acts as a bank of matched filters which can be conceived as a multiresolution analysis.

Energetic coordinatization by superimposing linear magnetic field gradients with respect to the laboratory frame of reference perturbs the spin system. The modeling of computerized pulsed Fourier MRI by harmonic analysis of the Heisenberg Lie group G is justified by the fact that the geometrical *symmetries* inherent to the mathematical model offer *a posteriori* the tools for the compensation of the perturbations which are imparted by the coordinatization process.

Another virtue of computerized pulsed Fourier MRI is the ease with which the matched filter design is achieved inside the foliation leaves. Matched filter banks optimize the signal-to-noise ratio, but their effect is to double the linewidth. Therefore the spatial resolution is degraded by the matched filter bank design:

- The phase shifts of quantum holograms caused by the spectral localization synthesis along the bi-infinite stratigraphic time line $\mathbb{R}$ reveal another basic operating principle of MRI: visualization by means of differential phases.

In practice, the number of successive phase encoding steps is typically 256 or 512, in order to generate the spatial resolution in the phase encoding direction. The signal following successive pulses is then collected in the form of an echo in the presence of a read-out gradient along the local frequency encoding direction within the tomographic slice. An advantage of accumulating data in the form of a spin echo technique is that the acquisition of both halves of the echo trains provides an improvement in the signal-to-noise ratio.

Quadrature detection, in conjunction with phase-cycling and data-routing techniques, is now a routine feature of clinical MRI scanner design and SAR high resolution imagery ([365]). It has two main advantages over detection using a single phase-sensitive detector. First, noise is not folded about the reference frequency and, second, the reference frequency can be placed in the middle of the frequency window. This reduces bandwidth problems that may arise from the effects of finite pulse width.

Following the initial amplification steps, the phase-coherent wavelets enter the phase-sensitive detector. Quadrature detection is employed to determine the sense of the Larmor precession in a rotating coordinate frame of reference, which is synchronized to the transmitter frequency ([106]). The use of two phase-sensitive detectors in quadrature then allows the detection of the differences to the references which are endowed with the phase shift of $\frac{1}{2}\pi$. The outputs from the two phase-sensitive detectors, the free induction decay and the antidecay belonging to their space and antispace, respectively ([308]), differ in phase by $\frac{1}{2}\pi$. They are both filtered and amplified before being fed into two separate data channels of the digital computer. On Fourier transformation, the phase difference leads to the separation of positive and negative frequencies.

An important point of concern is that the *standard* bra–ket formalism of quantum mechanics does not imply an easy way of deducing the phase-coherent wavelet collapse as an instance of the deterministic Schrödinger evolution. By contradistinction with the standard procedures of quantum physics, however, the geometrical quantization procedure allows to deduce the coherent wavelet collapse phenomenon from the coadjoint orbit visualization of the unitary dual $\hat{G}$. It reflects a central *decomposition* of nilpotent Lie group representations implemented by the *spin echo* and *gradient echo* techniques. It is by the isometric *conjugation* reflections of the echo techniques, in conjunction with the central *disintegration* of nilpotent Lie group representations, that the spectral transform of the left-invariant sub-Laplacian differential operator

$\mathcal{L}_G$ unveils some of the mysteries of the phenomena of emergence occurring in the confocal observation plane.

Extending Lie(G) to its universal enveloping algebra, the associated differential operator is given by the left-invariant sub-Laplacian $\mathcal{L}_G$ of G. It is known from

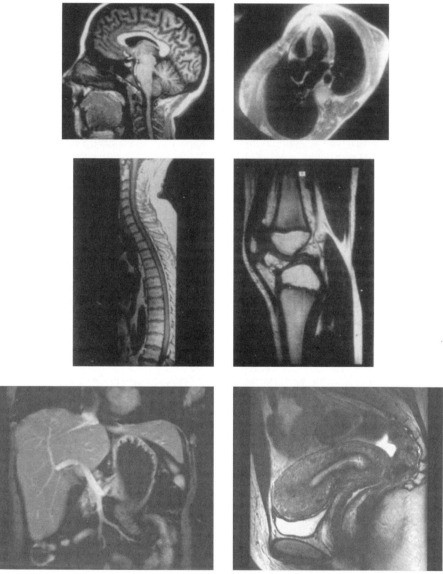

Figure 3. Radiologic pattern image gallery of clinical studies visualizing the typical morphological details that the MRI modality provides. For soft tissues, state-of-the-art MRI scanners provide a high contrast resolution of the final image. Artifacts by cerebrospinal (CSF) flow dynamics and motion can be compensated.

elliptic geometrical analysis that $\mathcal{L}_G$ is a positive self-adjoint differential operator with absolutely continuous central spectrum. The nomenclature is a little misleading since $\mathcal{L}_G$ is subelliptic. The spectral multiplicity of the differential operator $\mathcal{L}_G$ is uniform and given by $|P_G|$, and its spectral transform gives rise to a phase-locked, synchronized neural network representing the internal interference effects at the molecular level.

The square integrable, holomorphic/anti-holomorphic functional calculus of creation-annihilation operators of optical spectroscopy, implemented by the Bargmann–Fock model of G, allows to compute the Hilbert–Schmidt kernel of the central spectral transform of the analytic hypoelliptic differential operator $\mathcal{L}_G$. The ensuing Karhunen–Loève transform is matched to the collapse *statistics* as the optimum least-squares decorrelating transformation. The random signal theory of image compression establishes that the phase-coherent wavelet collapse phenomenon is of genuine quantum mechanical character and has no equivalent in classical physics.

Why is the transversally stratified Heisenberg Lie group G useful for the foundations of spin isochromat computing by NMR spectroscopy and clinical MRI? The reason is that the coadjoint orbit picture of $\hat{G}$ provides the key to quantum holography. Specifically, the energetic picture includes the *dichotomy* of coherent quantum deterministic resonance and stochastic resonance. The retrieval procedures of self-interference patterns by phase conjugation result from the geometrical quantization approach. The limitation of the amount of computational information that actually can be extracted from the resulting quantum states and then amplified to the macroscopic system level via coherent quantum stochastic resonance follows from the crossing of the energetic edge formed by the confocal observation plane (Figure 3).

In the confocal observation plane of emergence $\mathbf{P}(\mathbb{R} \times \mathcal{O}_\infty) \hookrightarrow \mathbf{P}(\mathbb{R} \times \mathrm{Lie}(G)^\star)$, the corresponding de Rham evaluation current takes the form

$$\omega_\infty = \varepsilon_{(\alpha,\beta)} \, d\alpha \wedge d\beta.$$

Due to the capability to implement the Weyl symbol map of pseudodifferential operators, the principle of "retrieving by reflection post-selection" represents a particularly fascinating aspect of the geometrical quantization approach performed by the transversally stratified Heisenberg Lie group G. In terms of the reversed linear magnetic field gradients superimposed in the laboratory coordinate frame of reference, it causes the rewinding of the nonresonant Heisenberg helices. Recently this principle has been verified also by experiments in neutron quantum optics, a discipline from which several of the pioneers of NMR spectroscopy started off.

Ein maschinelles Gefüge[1] *ist den Schichten zugewandt, reinen Intensitäten, die sie zirkulieren lassen, um die Selektion der "Konsistenzebene" zu sichern und den Subjekten zuordnet, welchen sie einen Namen nur als Spur einer Intensität läßt.*

—Gilles Deleuze and Félix Guattari (1992)

MR–*Scanner—Wunderwerke moderner Technologie.*

—Roland Felix (1994)

As part of a graduate course in medical imaging, I saw my first MR *image. It was a midline sagittal cut of the brain. I don't remember now if it was a* T_1 *or* T_2 *image, but what I do remember was how I just stared at that image. It looked like somebody had taken a knife, sliced a head in half and opened it up so we could see inside. I just couldn't believe you could get that kind of picture without using X-rays. That's when I knew that* MRI *would be my profession.*

—Moriel NessAiver (1997)

1.2 THE DEVELOPMENT OF COMPUTERIZED PULSED FOURIER NMR SPECTROSCOPY AND CLINICAL MRI: SECOND PART

The prime objective of an imaging system such as a SAR high resolution imager or a clinical MRI scanner system is to probe targets and perfectly *reconstruct* an image of the targets probed. The SAR imaging by airborne or spaceborne microwave radar systems is achieved by coherent processing of long echo data records *holographically* collected from the target's surface over wide bandwidths at shifting viewing angles presented during target probing. Clinical MRI is an adaption of NMR to probe the spin isochromats in the human body, and to characterize their chemical sites sufficiently to reconstruct diagnostically useful tomographic slices at carefully chosen angles and positions of the body.

Clinical MRI scanners reconstruct cross-sectional images of the human body through probing the magnetic moments of nuclei which are excited by the application of strong magnetic flux densities and weak magnetic flux densities associated with RF pulses (Figure 4). The spatial distribution of nuclear spin densities in tomographic slices is *holographically* recorded through the phase-coherent wavelet response of the stimulated nuclear spin isochromats derived from the free induction decay of protons associated with tissue water and, to a lesser extent, lipid molecules.

The discovery of frequency subbands of radiation in the electromagnetic spectrum which can penetrate human tissue to a sufficient depth culminated in the development of clinical MRI or NMR coherent tomography (Figure 5). The general term *tomography* refers to cross-sectional imaging of the whole human body by extracting the different images from either transmission or backscattering data of the planar array. The cross sections of the principal orientations are the central, coronal, and sagittal tomographic slices corresponding to yaw, roll, and pitch motions, respectively, in the inverse SAR (ISAR) detection mode (Figure 6).

The ISAR modification of the SAR high resolution image formation process is based on an *inversion* of the perspective. It can be used to reconstruct the high

---

[1] *"agencement"* in French

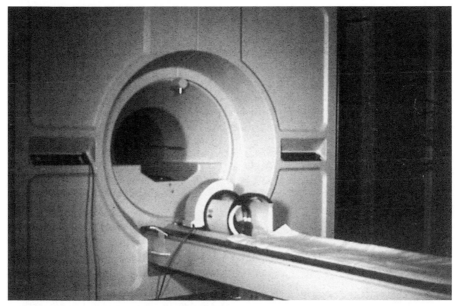

Figure 4. The center tube or bore of the magnet of a clinical MRI scanner at a magnetic flux density of 1.5 T for clinical examinations. More compact versions based on the short-bore technique have been installed on the promise that they will improve productivity while maintaining image quality on a par with conventional high magnetic flux systems. For routine clinical examinations the tendency is to lower the magnetic flux density. For MRI research and neurofunctional MRI experiments, however, the past few years have seen a tendency to higher magnetic flux densities.

resolution radar image of a moving target from either a stationary or a moving platform. The ISAR modality requires target motion, while uncompensated motion will degrade SAR images. Therefore ISAR needs the stroboscopic "freezing" of the target motion and local frequency adjustment in the presence of the gradient of Doppler frequencies prior to the holographic reconstruction procedure.

The process of NMR coherent tomography is based on perturbing the equilibrium magnetization of an object with a stimulating pulse train. The time-evolving phase-coherent wavelet responses resulting from resonances with the traces of the tuned Heisenberg helices are observed in a coil. Because, in terms of functional analysis, the image of the object generated by this noninvasive imaging procedure is *weakly* contained in the holographic data set recorded by the scanner, an approximation of the cross-sectional image can be retrieved by an application of the holographic reconstruction process to the received NMR trace filter response.

From the historical point of view, the advent of the NMR coherent tomography represents the most significant advance in the medical diagnostic image industry since the unexpected discovery of X-rays by Wilhelm Conrad Röntgen (1845–1923) in Würzburg, Bavaria, on November 8, 1895. To look into the body of a living patient without the use of a scalpel was a historical moment for the medical community. The exposure of the hand of his wife, Bertha Röntgen, was included with his paper

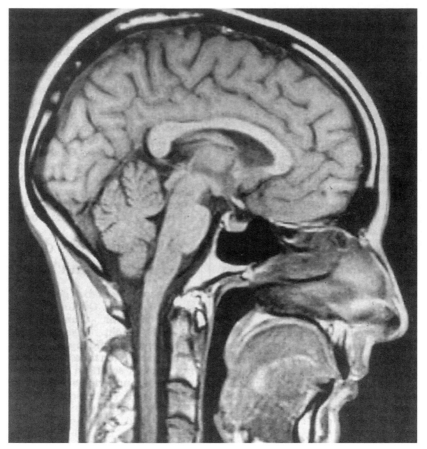

Figure 5. High resolution MRI study visualizing a sagittal tomographic cross-section of the cranium. This slice demonstrates the medial surface of the cerebral hemispheres. Note the cingulate cortex, which is apparent throughout its entire length. The corpus callosum provides the neurological guiding structure of the cerebrum. It is divided into genu, truncus, and splenium corporis callosi. The sulci and gyri of the medial surface are clearly visualized in this orientation. The precuneus is seen between the marginal branch of the sulcus cinguli and the sulcus parietoocciptalis. The cuneus is seen inferior to this, between the sulcus parietooccipitalis and the sulcus calcarinus.

announcing the sensational event that became known around the world in January 1896. Almost overnight, Röntgen was the focus of international praise, condemnation, and curiosity. Although Röntgen lived 27 years longer, the only public demonstration given by him took place in Würzburg on January 23, 1896, when he made the exposure of the hand of the famed anatomist and Privy Councillor Albert von Kölliker (1817–1905) before the physics society. The induction coil and transformer that produced the strong electrical currents of high voltage used by·Röntgen in his X-ray experiments are based on the principle of electromagnetic induction.

To the shifted time line of many physicists, Röntgen's revolutionary discovery and first crude demonstration marks the beginning of the twentieth century. The rays

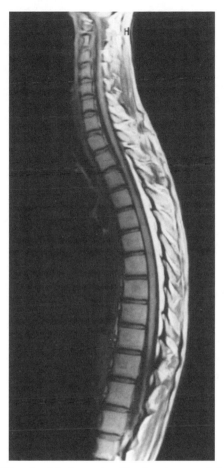

Figure 6. Phased array MRI study of the long spine. The phased array technique has been suggested by synthetic aperture radar (SAR) imaging to generate high resolution views in a noninvasive manner. MRI is superior in the evaluation of the patient with congenital/developmental cerebral or spinal pathology.

he designated as "X," for lack of a better term, to capture the unknown character of the "new type of rays," known in Germany at von Kölliker's suggestion by their discoverer's name as "Röntgen rays," ushered in not only a new era in physics but also a new era in medicine. Purcell's published announcement of his extension of Rabi's molecular beam experiment to solid, condensed matter was submitted to the publisher just four days less than a half-century after Röntgen's. Then 82 years elapsed between Röntgen's X-ray and Damadian's NMR free induction decay response. Not only are the diagnostic benefits for soft tissues worlds apart, the X-rays also contain much higher energy than the RF pulse excitation needed for NMR. Indeed, even a soft X-ray photon contains over 10^{12} times the energy of one RF photon in clinical MRI.

The spread of the epochal discovery and the clinical use of diagnostic X-radiographs had already begun on January 13, 1896, at Birmingham, England, and on

January 20, 1896, at Dartmouth College in Hanover, New Hampshire. It touched off a flurry of activity in the clinical application of X-radiographs. Already in May 1896 the first technical periodicals reported the many experiments and results with X-rays. And by July 1896 the X-ray units were developed to the point that high enough voltages were available to make exposures of the human skull possible. On November 27, 1896, Röntgen wrote to the manufacturer of the vacuum tubes (Source: Original handwritten correspondence of W.C. Röntgen):

> Ihre Röhren sind in der That sehr gut, aber für meine Verhältnisse zu teuer.... Ich möchte mir deshalb die Frage erlauben, ob Sie mir die Röhren nicht zu M. 20 statt zu M. 30 liefern könnten.

Today, the clinical utility of MRI has been established to such an extent that MRI scanners at $2 million plus are being sold to and used by most major medical centers throughout the world.

At the time of Röntgen's breakthrough, it took only one year to see more than a thousand X-ray systems operating throughout the world. Even around 1900 a mobile X-ray system named a "Röntgen cabinet" was part of the equipment in a physician's consultation room. Hence Röntgen's discovery ranks as one of the fastest ever published and clinically applied at all medical centers. Although he clearly envisioned the radiodiagnostic value of his experiments as did Damadian about 80 years after him, Röntgen persistently refused to enter into any contract with the beginning diagnostic imaging industry to commercially exploit his landmark discovery. Moreover, he bequeathed the prize money of the first Nobel Award for Physics in 1901 to the University of Würzburg.

For clinical X-ray examinations about one hundred years ago, the exposure time to radiation took between 10 and 120 min so some patients and early practitioners of diagnostic radiography, unaware of the safety hazards, suffered severe radiation burns. Harvey Cushing (1869–1939), commonly recognized as the father of modern neurosurgery, reported in 1897 and in 1925 again that in 1896 a first clinical X-ray examination of the cervical spine required an average exposure time of 35 min, as did several attempts at Johns Hopkins Hospital to produce the final image of a hematomyelia. Nevertheless, only six months after the discovery of X-rays, Francis H. Williams presented a live demonstration of skeletal imaging to a Boston medical society.

Never before had a scientific breakthrough caused such excitement in the contemporary health care environment than Röntgen's initially unforeseen extension of the human visual system perception which took place 36 years after the discovery of cathode rays and 2 years after development of the first cathode-ray tube—a display device called a Lenard's tube. As an undesired side effect, the current plain film-based X-ray radiography practice forms a significant bottleneck for efficient data presentation and display.

In 1896, following Röntgen's landmark observation, the first detailed reports of harmful biological effects and tissue damage of the skin caused by X-rays appeared in the medical literature which already comprised more than thousand publications dealing with the new kind of radiation and its impact on diagnostics. Numerous pioneers of X-radiology became victims of the new technology. The mistake was to assume that the harmful effects of radiation would be visible soon after an X-ray exam was performed, but in reality the effects are often only seen 20, 30, 40, or even 50 years later. As great a boon to diagnostic medicine as X-ray imaging became shortly after its discovery, MRI promises to make X-rays obsolete in radiodiagnostics.

As a result of continuing experience with ionizing radiation, the genotoxic and oncogenic effects of clinical X-ray examinations revealed not to be negligible even with dedicated X-ray tubes. Although the statistical risk is well known within the health care environment, many X-ray examinations are still ordered because of so-called medicolegal considerations. The assessment of one study is that up to 30% of the total X-ray examinations ordered are related to physician concern for potential malpractice threats and are not primarily designed to assist the patient. This should remind the referring physicians that the radiologists' responsibility is to aid in the diagnosis and treatment of patients, not simply in providing clinical images.

Throughout the total range of the electromagnetic spectrum, from soft X-rays to ultraviolet, and visible light to microwaves, as used in SAR high resolution imagery, the strong attenuation of probe and response radiation in the human body prevents clinical imaging. Only at very great wavelengths, that is, in the short-wave RF subbands of the electromagnetic spectrum, does the depth of the electromagnetic radiation's penetration into the tissue increase to an adequate degree. Compared with X-rays and radioisotopes, the energy of the electromagnetic radiation in the short-wave RF subband is, according to the Einstein relation, at least nine orders of magnitude (approximately one billion times) less than the energy of X-rays and radioisotopes. The subbands of the electromagnetic spectrum used in the RF imaging technology in general are not known to cause any harmful biological effects. It should be observed, however, that the frequencies employed in computerized pulsed Fourier NMR spectroscopy and clinical MRI at the same range as used for radio transmission do *not* imply that the NMR phenomenon uses radio waves. Clinical MRI scanner systems perform the calculations using quantum parallelism of phase-locked, synchronized neural networks at the molecular level and then amplify the results of coherent stimulus-evoked resonance to the macroscopic level via classical parallelism.

In electroencephalography (EEG) based brain research, such coherent stimulus-evoked resonances have been taken to be indicative of a neural network organization linking or temporally coordinating the distributed intracortical spectral representation of stimuli by frequencies lying in the gamma band ([18]). The synchronization has been approved between neurons in different cortical areas, and even between the two cerebral hemispheres across the falx cerebri, the interhemispheric fissure.

The major use of digital computer technology in clinical medicine is to ascertain images for diagnostic evaluation. The medical discipline of radiodiagnostics exists today only because of the hardware and software designs of computer technology and the discovery of frequency subbands of radiation in the electromagnetic spectrum which can penetrate human tissue to a sufficient depth and thus can be exploited by signal processing techniques for probing clinical imaging targets *in vivo*.

Digital computer technology offers a wide range of controlling, storing, processing, and postprocessing applications to radiodiagnostics. Imaging system design is moving away from isolated devices and toward integration into hospital information networks. Automated clinical radiodiagnostic imaging systems can support a distributed array of microprocessor-based workstation-style user interfaces operating as remote image retrieval and display platforms with their own high-speed memories and digital-to-analog converters (DACs). Such imaging systems are operating either directly via local-area networks (LANs) and wide-area networks (WANs) or as part of a computer-intensive hospital picture and archiving system (PACS). In areas such as neuroradiagnostics, where an MRI study might include 300 to 400 scans, the clinical demand of the semantically interpreting expert agents for rapid access to clinicomorphological and functional scans has accelerated the trend toward a completely digital, filmless environment as offered by large-scale modular and distributed PACS networks.

After the image dataset is generated, it is usually stored on a revolving magnetic disk. From there, it may be retrieved for display or transferred to an archival medium such as magnetic tape or optical disk. Magnetic resonance images are usually formatted as a quadratic matrix of $N_P \times N_P$ pixels, where $N_P \in \{256, 512\}$ denotes the radix-2 number of differential phase encoding steps. Presently formatting as 512×512 imaging matrix size with up to 16 bits of gray scale information per pixel has become standard. The pixel data are mapped into the available contrast and brightness ranges of the display device by scaling and offsetting the pixel data. The scanning MRI technologist can continuously adjust the contrast and brightness of the image for display or filming.

Because a clinical radiodiagnostic imaging system is capable of acquiring a large number of high resolution images in a short period of time, the display device may include tiled multi-image displays, the rapid sequential display of multiple images in a cine loop, multiplanar reformatting of stacks of two-dimensional images, and synthesized three-dimensional renderings of surfaces and volumes to convert the vast amounts of information available into clinically relevant presentations. Some of these techniques are computationally intensive and may require dedicated electronic hardware to be diagnostically useful in a clinical setting.

Radiology information systems such as PACS promise to cut health care costs by providing external and internal teleradiology features. A combined telepathology and teleradiology option includes the capability to post medical images on a server to be accessed by remote hospitals or the departments within one site in a cost-effective manner. A discussion mode allows widely spaced diagnostic radiologists and clinicians with the proper security clearances to interact upon the same scan ([165]).

The trend is going toward development of multimedia patient radiology reports using images, sound, and text as medical instrument industry taps into the increasing availability of inexpensive and powerful workstation systems. As these computer platforms become more powerul, they are able to more fully support three-dimensional image processing, graphic display, and parameters and multimodality data integration. The MRI scans are unique in that, to understand the semantic content, many of the details and image parameters used in formation of the image must be considered. The converse of this is also true. In order to receive diagnostically useful information from a patient imaging study, the appropriate parameters and imaging procedures must be selected and organized. The NMR spectroscopic and neurofunctional MRI studies for brain functional localization exploit the richness of the underlying principles of MRI. A thorough knowledge of the principles of MRI is necessary in order to understand these advanced techniques.

The data files must be converted from analog to digital format before they can be transmitted over a PACS network. After conversion, the files can be sent over the Internet, or intranets, in which usage is limited to within the facility's network. Concerns over patient privacy and data encryption could slow the development of this technology. However, projects like MIRIAM in the Hospital of Paris establish that even a large-scale PACS has moved beyond the pilot project stage to become an everyday component of clinical radiology which is able to present and display the tremendous amount of infomation now being produced from the digital imaging modalities ([165]).

The PACS network handles all diagnostic image information in the form of digital electronic signals. It involves image acquisition, archiving, communication, retrieval, display, processing, and postprocessing. The growth of large-scale PACSs was slow in the 1980s, because of high start-up costs, the requirements of comprehensive interfacing with radiological modalities and existing administrative information systems, a lack of standardized methods of mass storage and image transmission, and the high sensitivity to system failures. It was an unfortunate obstacle to the timely development of the PACS concept that conventional plain film radiography, which accounted for more than 70% of the total number of diagnostic imaging procedures to be digitized, did not exist in digital format. Presently very effective flat-panel digital detectors based on amorphous silicon and converters based on charge-coupled device (CCD) technology are available. Modular PACS growth therefore appears to be poised for rapid expansion in the 1990s because computer hardware costs for remote image retrieval and display workstations have dropped dramatically while the performance has increased. The PACS networks built upon a scalable hardware architecture using multiple RISC processor-based workstations which are linked within a client–server networking environment offer a promising solution of the cost–benefit problem. Integration of postprocessing improvement capabilities such as fuzzy-logic-based segmentation algorithms increases acceptance by clinicians.

The standards for Digital Imaging and Communication in Medicine (DICOM) enjoy widespread support from scanner equipment manufacturers ([29]), and DICOM image management software has eliminated the causes of slower than expected PACS growth. Today's greatest hindrance, however, still is that software engineering concepts dealing with the interfacing issues required to run centralized PACS in a medical network environment have not kept pace with the rapid hardware development ([165]). Nevertheless, even a less ambitious, medium-scale PACS-supported environment will have a much stronger impact on work flow within the clinical radiological departments than first assumed. It is not difficult to foresee that PACS networks will shift the balance of power in hospitals toward radiologists by casting them in the role of information managers.

Traditionally, clinical radiodiagnostic imaging systems have been run by an isolated digital computer combined with one or more attached consoles and one or more monitors for displaying images and text information. The console is the primary device for operator input of the clinical MRI protocol. It allows interactive control by its keyboard, computer mouse, or trackball over the automated procedures for tuning the scanning parameters and procedural setups. The mouse-controlled screen utilizes icons for quick access to system functions and postprocessing capabilities. With LANs and WANs becoming reliable, attention of the medical community is being given to using networks in a hospital environment and attaching arrays of display workstations to these networks. In analogy to the wavelet-based imaging algorithms used in SAR data processing ([128]), new image compression algorithms ([209]) permit the transmission of image data lines with minimal loss of spatial and contrast resolution, making teleradiology a more practical technique of telemedicine where equipment from different vendors is able to communicate with each other.

Some radiology departments are exploring use of the World Wide Web (WWW) technology to allow referring physicians to access digital radiology reports which integrate MRI scans with digital data from a PACS. One such system is in place at the University of Pennsylvania Medical Center in Philadelphia, Pennsylvania, where the integrated radiology reports are stored on a Web server and from there can be transmitted to either the emergency room or the intensive care unit.

At the Laurie Imaging Center in New Brunswick, New Jersey, clinicians can use the Web to access patients' radiology reports as well as MRI scans from their office, home, or hospital using the semantically interpreting expert agents' Web browser. Though physician access to patient data on the Laurie site is password protected, sample reports are available for viewing by any visitor. Additions to future report software packages that are riding on the Web will include audio enhancements as well as cine studies.

Magnetic resonance imaging has been called the most important development in medical radiodiagnosis since the discovery of the X-ray one hundred years ago. Due to the superficial resemblances of MRI scans to X-ray CT scans, the imaging modalities are often confused. However, their physical foundation and hence their mathematical modeling are completely different, and there are only few thematic similarities. The change of geometry under the influence of a strong magnetic field, from the flat Euclidean space to the left-invariant metric geometry of the sub-Riemannian manifold G, has no counterpart in X-ray CT. As a result, in interventional radiology, the accuracy of tumor localization and monitoring the therapeutic effect by MRI are superior to X-ray CT (Figure 7).

The MRI modality was introduced into clinical radiodiagnostics in the mid-1980s, although the practicality of MRI in obtaining clinical images and studying the metabolic basis of disease *in vivo* by means of NMR was initially doubted. Thus clinical MRI is a remarkably recent technological development. Its clinical realization surprised even the pioneers of NMR. The discoverer of pulsed NMR spectroscopy, Erwin Louis Hahn, for example, stated in 1990 ([139], pp. 403):

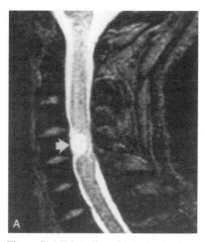
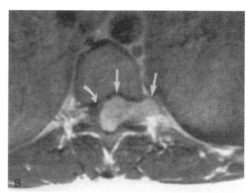

Figure 7. MRI studies of intradural extramedullary nerve sheath tumors: Neurofibromatosis (A). The medulla spinalis is compressed (*arrow*). Schwannoma (B) that deviates the spinal cord (*curved arrow*) to the right-hand side and extends into the left foramen intervertebrale. When compared with X-ray CT, pathology involving the compartments of the spinal canal such as extradural, intradural extramedullary, and intramedullary spinal disease, are best evaluated by MRI.

I have never practised magnetic resonance imaging (MRI) nor designed anything intended for MRI. I take the opportunity to apologize to MRI pioneers because I never believed MRI would work, like Rutherford, who said that anyone who believed nuclear radioactivity would be useful "is talking moonshine." However, I was only one of many unbelievers. Another infidel in particular was Anatole Abragam, a distinguished French physics researcher in magnetic resonance. The French Society of Radiology wanted to award Abragam a medal in spite of the fact that he told them he hadn't contributed to MRI and didn't believe it would work.

As a nonpractitioner perhaps I would be preententious to make predictions about MRI when I do not live with its problems or shortcomings. But as a patient who has been scanned several times my guess is that the speed of scanning will be greatly improved to accommodate motion due to breathing, heartbeat, peristaltsis, and so on. The onset of prostate cancer will probably be routinely detected, along with other cancers that may be manifested by more sensitive chemical-shift scans that expose biochemical imbalances. High-temperature superconductivity may develop to a point where magnets are cheaper to build and to maintain, using liquid nitrogen only.

The preceding description states that NMR spectrocopy pervades the MRI methodology so a distinction of these modalities is not very helpful. The historical origins of a complex subject such as clinical MRI are frequently difficult to trace. It is, however, well documented that the window to diagnostic applications of two-dimensional NMR spectroscopy as a noninvasive means of obtaining clinical scans and of monitoring the state of tissue metabolism *in vivo* at any given time was opened by the nephrologist Raymond Vahan Damadian. As a medical scientist engaged in basic research, Damadians's research work was not performed at the bedside of a patient but rather at the side of a laboratory bench. He audited a quantum physics course taught by Purcell at Harvard University where he was introduced to NMR spectroscopy. The detection and recording of tune signals were virtually unknown during Damadian's undergraduate studies of mathematics at the University of Wisconsin.

In 1969 Damadian wrote one of the first documents in which he mentioned his vital idea for extending the concept of relaxation rates as a technique for differentiating between normal and pathological tissue for the purpose of medical diagnosis ([223] Appendix Chapter 8, A3):

> I will make every effort myself and through collaborators, to establish that all tumors can be recognized by their potassium relaxation times or H_2O–proton spectra and proceed with the development on instrumentation and probes that can be used to scan the human body externally for early signs of malignancy.

In 1971 he reported his successful 1970 experiments proving that implanted tumors in experimental animals did indeed display differences in their magnetic resonance properties from noncancerous tissue and that even normal tissues could be differentiated from one another by their relaxation rates. His *in vitro* measurements of relaxation rates exerted a strong stimulus in the development of clinical MRI for the *in vivo* study of malignant tumors. Having Damadian's approach in mind, Lauterbur wrote the following observation under the title "Spatially Resolved Nuclear Magnetic Resonance Experiments" ([223], p. 714):

> The distribution of magnetic nuclei, such as protons, and their relaxation times and diffusion coefficients, may be obtained by imposing magnetic field gradients (ideally, a complete set of orthogonal spherical harmonics) on a sample, such as an organism or a manufactured object, and measuring the intensities and relaxation behavior of the resonance as functions of the applied magnetic field. Additional spatial discrimination may be achieved by the application of time-dependent gradient patterns so as to distinguish, for example, protons that lie at the intersection of the zero-field (relative to the main magnetic field) lines of three linear gradients.

> The experiments proposed above can be done most conveniently and accurately by measurements of the Fourier transform of the pulse response of the system. They should be capable of providing a detailed three-dimensional map of the distributions of particular classes of nuclei (classified by nuclear species and relaxation times) within a living organism. For example, the distribution of mobile protons in tissues, and the differences in relaxation times that appear to be characteristic of malignant tumors, should be measurable in an intact organism.

In a patent application submitted in 1972, Damadian showed a representation of a man standing in a magnet with NMR transmitter and receiver coils mounted on a helical track which spiraled around him. Here, the idea of acquiring information sequentially from various parts of the body in order to detect malignancy is clearly present. The patent was issued in 1974. By midnight of July 2, 1977, the world's first whole-body scanner, the prototype MRI scanner, dubbed "Indomitable" to capture the spirit of its construction, was ready ([223]). After completing a seven-year construction, comparable with Keppler's "struggle" against the "indomitable Mars," the world of radiodiagnostic imaging was irrevocably altered. The Indomitable is now located at the Smithsonian Institute of Technology in Washington, D.C.

The first whole-body transaxial scan took 4 h 45 min to produce by analog means. During the scanning procedure, the patient had to be physically moved 106 times on a trambler to accomplish spatial excitation at the resonance "sweet spot," or "focus" in Keppler's terminology. The proton density weighted tomographic slice image showed the thoracic spine of Larry Minkoff, who built the Indomitable scanner with Damadian and Michael Goldsmith. Damadian's "amazing detail" claim of the roughly delineated body wall, the right and left lungs, and the heart including the right atrium and one of its ventricles seems amusing when compared with the quality of images MRI scanners routinely produce today, but the first whole-body MRI scans were far ahead of the images generated by the first X-ray CT scanners only a few years earlier. Damadian expected far less than what actually showed up on the first scan generated by the FONAR (field-focused nuclear magnetic resonance) technique, because the first X-ray CT scans required that specialists explain to the radiologists what they were viewing.

The Indomitable's resonant window, or sweet spot, approach to accomplish a point-by-point scan was analogous to the spectral sweep technique employed in early NMR spectroscopy. Prior to the computerized pulsed Fourier transform technique of NMR spectroscopy, frequency spectra were acquired using a point-by-point sweep of the magnetic field. The amplitude of the signal at each setting of the magnetic field was recorded sequentially to create the frequency spectrum. The pulse technique, however, is faster and of higher spectroscopic sensitivity. It requires computer hardware to evaluate the confocal plane *in silicio* by dedicated fast Fourier transform (FFT) processors and sophisticated computer software to electronically address the spectral locations within the selected cross section. Damadian's patented sweet spot technique of spatial localization was later set aside in favor of the spin warp method developed by the Aberdeen University group and which is now mainly used commercially. Starting in 1981, the Aberdeen University group published several reports indicating the ability of NMR to differentiate malignant from benign tissue and its superiority over ultrasound and radionuclide liver scan for the diagnosis of a wide spectrum of hepatic diseases.

In the same year, a group at Hammersmith Hospital in London showed that NMR was superior to X-ray CT scanning for the demonstration of small areas of demyelination in patients with MS and for depicting the posterior fossa and its contents. Nonetheless, it was the analog sweet spot technique of Damadian's original patent that provided an approach simple enough to acquire the first MRI scan of the human body *in vivo*. The magnet was initially exceedingly heavy (one commercially available 0.3-T magnet weighted 100 tons) and hospital installations needed magnetic shielding for hospital suites that were developed for top-secret military electronics installations because of environmental RF interference and the influence of stray magnetic fields. Nevertheless, the performance of the FONAR technique was able to convince the medical community that radiodiagnostic MRI scanning of normal and diseased soft tissue exhibiting different relaxation rates was, in fact, a reality ([223], p. 689, completed by oral communication, Ruhr-Universität Bochum, 1997):

MRI combines such an extraordinary constellation of beneficial properties so uniquely suitable for medicine its progenitor may almost be divine. It is noninvasive, thereby freeing medicine of the hazardous radiations of other diagnostic technologies. This characteristic alone qualifies it for repeated use in the care of patients as the need arises and as the medical situation might demand. It is not a transmission technology in the same sense as other diagnostic modalities, so the location of the image-generating nuclear spins can be known with precision. This confers a high degree of spatial resolution on the magnetic resonance image. And the nuclear spin is so profoundly sensitive to its local environment that both the frequency and relaxation rate of the nuclear spin signal change dramatically with small changes in the local environment, such as those created by disease processes.

In the years since the first image of two 1-mm capillary tubes was reconstructed from four projections independently by Lauterbur in 1973, the conversion of temporal magnetic resonance into full *spatiotemporal* magnetic resonance and the development of NMR coherent tomography have constituted one of the great success stories of this century. Given the implicit role of the nuclear spin position in determining the Larmor precession spectrum under the influence of phase encoding affine linear magnetic field gradients described by Gabillard on the one hand and Herman Y. Carr and Purcell in 1954 on the other hand, it is remarkable that 23 years elapsed after Hahn's original nuclear magnetic spin echo experiment in 1950 before Lauterbur used this spatial signature in MRI to perform spectral localization analysis in order to acquire clinico-morphological structural information from a heterogeneous sample ([223]).

Thus the idea of applying affine linear magnetic field gradients in NMR spectroscopy is almost as old as NMR itself. The main advantage of the Lauterbur spectral localization procedure of MRI over the superposition of a saddle-shaped nonuniform magnetic field, chosen by Damadian for his prototype whole-body MRI scanner, is the affine linearity of the magnetic field gradients superimposed in the laboratory coordinate frame of reference. This linear system approach captures the spirit of Keppler's ingenious stratification strategy of addressing the spatial location of the planets on their orbits by a projectively immersed bundle of parallel lines, whereas the resonance sweet spot technique of Damadian's FONAR toolkit depends upon the minimum inhomogeneity of the main magnetic field and therefore is of a nonlinear character. In references to a "transmitter probe with beam focusing mechanism" a basic misunderstanding of magnetic fields is present.

Due to its inherent slowness, Lauterbur's original method of reconstructive tomography is not currently used on clinical MRI scanner systems. The back projection approach performed by rotating the frequency gradient combines gradient localization with X-ray CT imaging principles. It lacks Keppler's phase-sensitive quadrature detection technique. Because the reconstruction from X-ray CT data is an ill-posed problem, Lauterbur's original approach does not exploit the full advantages of NMR spectroscopy over other transmission technologies and makes MRI prone to image artifacts.

As linear magnetic field gradients are superimposed on the stationary magnetic flux density over time, local frequency encoding changes and traces a trajectory through the quantum hologram. These trajectories are records of the time history of gradient superpositions during NMR filter response acquisition. Specifically, they are precise records of the polarity, duration, and direction of the applied linear magnetic field gradients. In this way, the primary axis is no longer a time scale, but the polarity of differential phase encoding gradients, sequentially applied with respect to the laboratory frame of reference:

- The sequence of differential phase encoding gradients controls the direction of a projectively immersed bundle of parallel lines.
- One line of the bundle is selected by the polarity and duration of the differential phase encoding gradient pulse.
- A pure absorption-mode spectrum of the free induction decay is generated by reversing the polarity of the sequence of differential phase encoding gradients.
- The FFT algorithm decodes the variables involved in the linear gradient coordinatization of the selected tomographic slice.

The spatial deployment of the temporal magnetic resonance phenomenon by the Lauterbur linear gradient encoding technique, however, has finally motivated the application of the spatiotemporal quantization strategy of quantum holography to clinical MRI. Its implementation by the transitive Hamiltonian action of the Heisenberg group G, which designs the symplectic reconstructive analysis–synthesis filter bank by coherent wavelet multichannels, is mathematically performed by the decomposition of transvections into computer-controlled dilations.

From 1956 onward, the studies of V. Kudravcev at the National Institutes of Health of the NMR absorption mode allowed to determine the projection of a quail egg with embryo and to display its hydrogen distribution by use of a surface coil on a television screen. Following the imaging of dead chicken legs in 1974, the first human MR image of a live finger was reported by Peter Mansfield in Heidelberg in 1976. This was followed by a cross-sectional magnetic resonance image of a mouse chest by Damadian in 1976, the first cross-sectional magnetic resonance images of the thorax of a live human by Damadian in 1977, an abdomen by Mansfield in 1978, the differences between a carcinoma and surrounding normal tissue in a mastectomy specimen imaged in a whole-body scanner by Mansfield and co-workers in 1979, an intracranial pathology by Brian S. Worthington in 1980, NMR chemical shift imaging by Kâmil Uğurbil in 1982, imaging of all organ systems by Lawrence E. Crooks in 1982, a placenta within the first trimester of pregnancy by the Aberdeen University group in 1983, a fetus and maternal anatomy in the final trimester of pregnancy by a Nottingham group in 1984, the breasts of a long series of female patients by Werner A. Kaiser in 1984, and the application of clinical MRI to blood flow imaging by William G. Bradley and Gustav K. von Schulthess in 1985. Thus, to appreciate the beginnings of NMR coherent tomography, as well as the various subspecialities of clinical MRI, such as magnetic resonance angiography and NMR spectroscopic imaging, requires the account of many historic firsts.

The pioneering work of Raymond V. Damadian, Paul C. Lauterbur, and Sir Peter Mansfield was performed independently of radar remote sensing imaging technology.

Actually, Mansfield was close to the holographic processing of SAR images in the superencoded projective space, because his approach applied the optical diffractive principle to excite holographically in-plane encoded images by a far field superposition of coherent spin echo phases ([219]). The work of the pioneers triggered an enormous activity in the application of NMR coherent tomography to clinical diagnostics. It made believers of the sceptics as the lab configuration of a programmable NMR spectrometer was being scaled up from a size designed to study samples in test tubes to a size capable of accommodating the whole body. It made possible the imaging of cross sections of the human body by spatiotemporal magnetic resonance combined with advanced computer technology, a situation facilitated by the increased availability of clinical MRI scanners of improved design. Since then, a veritable explosion of interest in this powerful and highly sophisticated imaging technique has taken place, outstripping the rate of development of any other clinical imaging technique. The more than 20,000 papers on clinical MRI currently published yearly is a testimony to the increasing interest in this area of computer-assisted medicine.

The MRI process is based on physical principles which are by far more subtle and completely different from those associated with the more familiar imaging techniques of clinical diagnostics. The underlying subband image encoding method and hardwired coherent lock-in detection technique are particularly sophisticated, so that a deeper understanding of the high resolution image processing specific to the MRI modality is intellectually and esthetically stimulating. In addition, a thorough mathematical understanding of the magnetic resonance image formation process is of great theoretical significance because it is essential to good diagnostic practice and practical advice to the scanning MRI technologist, particularly when image artifacts occur. Prominent examples of controllable artifacts in clinical MRI include image foldover, aliasing in the phase encoding direction, and magic angle spinning artifacts. These may lead to severe misinterpretations of the end results in the case reading room.

Because MRI employs probe radiation in the RF subband, it opens the final window in the electromagnetic spectrum for probing medical imaging targets, with no radiation risk to the patient. In the MRI process, it is the nucleus that provides the phase-coherent wavelet used in creating *in vivo* images with a soft tissue discrimination which are unrivaled in the contour and contrast resolutions of any other clinical imaging technique. In fact, the magnetic resonance image formation exploits the resonance interaction of electrodynamic radiation with dissipative nuclear spin systems. The analysis of the Larmor precession spectrum of the underlying spatiotemporal signals represents a semiclassical subspeciality of quantum electrodynamics which provides insight into the quantum physical structure of the nuclear spin systems:

- Despite the strong nonlinearity of dissipative nuclear spin systems, the symplectic linear response theory of coherent tomography holds exactly in MRI processing.
- In view of the symplectic linear response theory of coherent tomography, the tomographic slices $\mathbf{P}\left(\mathbb{R} \times \mathcal{O}_\nu\right) \hookrightarrow \mathbf{P}\left(\mathbb{R} \times \mathrm{Lie}(G)^\star\right)$ of G form substrates for

the spatial encoding in the symplectic affine leaves at center frequencies $\nu \neq 0$ of the Larmor precession spectrum.

Due to the time evolution of nuclear spin systems, MRI differs from conventional clinical radiodiagnostics in which the electrons are responsible for the imaging signal and image formation process. With the history of nuclear magnetic resonance spectroscopy in physicochemistry and solid state physics, NMR, as an analytical technique for the study of inter- and intramolecular interactions, swept across the disciplines of analytical and structural chemistry to biochemistry and physiology and then on to medical radiodiagnostics, where it serves as a measurement and visualization technique for the noninvasive probing of the morphology of macrolevel targets (Figure 8). Much of the excitement generated by NMR coherent tomography has been about the clinical applications of MRI to radiodiagnostics:

- Clinical MRI scanners are basically computer-controlled, automated imaging systems to perform coherent tomography by circular grating arrays. In contrast to

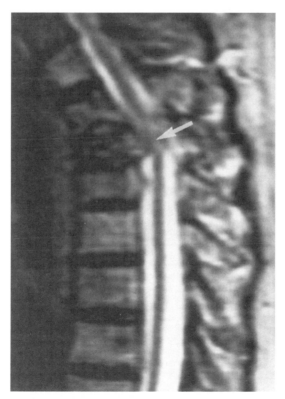

Figure 8. Sagittal MRI study of spinal cord compression from vertebral tumor: A fracture of an upper corpus vertebrae thoracicae (*arrow*) severely compresses the thoracic spinal cord. The lesion and the pathologic feature of the bone marrow are caused by a prostate carcinoma which is the primary tumor.

the X-ray CT modality of radiodiagnostic imaging, NMR coherent tomography preserves phase as well as amplitude rather than intensity information in scan planes of any tomographic slice orientation.

- Unlike X-ray scattering, NMR scattering is highly selective by virtue of the different gyromagnetic ratios of different spin species.

- Magnetic resonance imaging is not a transmission technique. Like SAR high resolution imagery it is a phase-coherent radar-type tomographic imaging modality of cross-sectional targets in the superencoded projective space. Due to the spatiotemporal strategy of quantum holography, the cross-sectional targets actively form contrast-manipulated, computer-controlled, backscattering grating arrays in projective space.

Essential to diagnosis by any clinical imaging system are detectability and capability to localize. It was the symbiosis of computer science with quantum electrodynamics which opened a whole new vista of detectability and capability to localize for the areas of radiodiagnostic imaging, mental imagery, and interventional medicine. Magnetic resonance imaging is a coherent tomography modality which basically requires the following:

 (i) a stable homogeneous magnetic flux density over the desired imaging volume for proton spin polarization;

 (ii) the transmission of wavelets within the RF window for computer-controlled choreography of spin isochromats;

 (iii) the temporal discrimination of the spatial location of polarized proton spins obtained by superimposing *linear magnetic field gradients* onto the time-invariant baseline magnetic flux density in the laboratory coordinate frame in a way analogous to the frequency linear gradient associated with the target-induced local Doppler frequency shift in SAR high resolution imagery;

 (iv) the procedures to correct for phase incoherence caused by RF pulse flipping, as well as for magnetic field inhomogeneities imposed by the frequency modulating linear magnetic field gradients; and

 (v) the in-plane acquisition of quantum holograms excited by the emitted phase-coherent wavelets, plus efficient numerical hologram evaluation, raw dataset analysis, and external postprocessing of the reconstructed image.

- In SAR high resolution imagery, ISAR is the radar analog to the synchronized rotating coordinate frame of reference of the MRI modality. It generates contiguous subband multichannels at local frequencies of the NMR filter response wavelets.

- The ISAR approach explains the subband narrowing phenomenon called the magic angle spinning effect. Physically spinning the sample at the magic angle narrows the broad spectral lines in solid state NMR.

It follows that a real understanding of the symplectic linear response theory of coherent tomography applied to the MRI formation process requires a study of those wavelets of quantum electrodynamics which are at the heart of the MRI coherent tomography modality. Motivated by the perceptual features of the human visual system and emulated by computer vision and pattern recognition, affine wavelet algorithms have been successfully applied to digital image processing for image compression purposes ([346], [349]) and contrast enhancement ([194]), both of importance for clinical imaging. In comparison to windowed Fourier transforms, which have a fixed resolution in the spatiotemporal domain, the resolution of a wavelet transform varies with a scale parameter, decomposing an image by the subband coding technique into a set of contiguous local frequency channels of constant bandwidth ([4]). The improved flexibility due to this scale variation enables a wavelet transform to zoom into the discontinuities of image presentations and to characterize them locally by the multiresolution signal decomposition. Because some of the most beautiful and useful properties of the inverse wavelet transform, such as the interference property, are lost under digitization, it is not this multiresolution level of affine wavelet applications which is appropriate for the MRI technology, but the computer-controlled generation of quantum holograms by hybrid MRI scanner architecture as an analog to SAR and ISAR high resolution imagery. Nevertheless, the property of extracting features of the wavelet transform can be used for the purposes of postprocessing MRI scans in order to improve soft tissue contrast resolution.

The concept of multiresolution analysis leads to subband decompositions of input signals and to perfect reconstruction analysis–synthesis subband filter banks. Similarly, quantum holography gives rise to subband decompositions at the local frequency levels of the excitation–response wavelets which are compatible with the uncertainty principle of quantum physics as well as the symplectically formatted reconstruction analysis–synthesis subband filter banks:

- Adopting the signal processing point of view, the central concept of multichannel reconstruction analysis–synthesis filter bank brings out the link underlying both the multiresolution signal decomposition and the subband coding of the quantum holographic analog image presentation.

The mathematical approach to magnetic resonance imagery reveals that a clinical MRI scanner architecture implements a multichannel reconstruction analysis–synthesis filter bank inside the foliation leaves and actually acts as a hybrid quantum computer using a spatiotemporal encoding principle for establishing synchronized connections for corticomorphic processing. In this sense, the *synchronized* timing recorded by the stratigraphic time line $\mathbb{R}$ is everything in MRI. The mathematical approach to clinical MRI is based on noncommutative geometrical analysis. It will be articulated in terms of Lie groups of dilation-controlled transvections, in terms of the associated Lie group representations in a complex Hilbert space, and in terms of the Kepplerian spatiotemporal quadrature and stroboscopic procedure of phase history triangulation for eccentric circular orbits with respect to the synchronized rotating coordinate frame of reference. For an in-depth understanding of the underlying quantum electrodynamics, the extraordinary sensitivity to the presence and the precise location of lesions and neural activities, no less than the richness, versatility, and elegance of the MRI coherent tomography, require more advanced and sophisticated mathematical tools:

- sub-Riemannian geometry,
- projective geometry, and
- noncommutative Fourier analysis.

Due to the intrinsic subtlety of the MRI processing, a thorough mathematical treatment requires a step-by-step approach, passing from the spectral localization aspects of noncommutative Fourier analysis to projective geometrical analysis. Modeling the intricate physical principles on which the mathematical syntax of the various imaging modalities is based allows one to approach the spectral analysis and synthesis of spatiotemporal signals involved in radiodiagnostic medicine.

The need for improved mathematical understanding of the clinical image formation and reconstruction processes which includes the subjective conscious experience of the semantic interpretation of observational contexts is particularly intense in the case of NMR tomography. A leading musculoskeletal MRI diagnostician states: "I don't feel you have to know basic physics or MR physics in depth to interpret images; and I don't know any physics." This does not seem to provide a very convincing argument to stopping short of a description of clinical MRI in a hands-on fashion. If clinical MRI scanner systems are to further improve the quality, efficiency, and economics of diagnostic imaging practice, a new breed of experts must be sired, a breed of clinicians, mathematicians, physicists, engineers, and computer and imaging scientists who, on the one hand, grow up and live with the clinical practice and, on the other hand, can set proper examples and develop meaningful communication with the medical diagnostic imaging industry.

The mature *analog* computation art of Fourier optical processing of SAR high resolution imagery serving as the symplectically formatted model and the mathematical discipline of noncommutative geometrical analysis provide a deep insight into the intricacy of the spatiotemporal signal analysis which underlies clinical MR processing, as well as the computer-controlled multiparameter contrast dependence of this sophisticated noninvasive imaging technique. Specifically, projective geometrical analysis establishes the implementation of multichannel coherent wavelet filter banks via the symplectic linear response theory of NMR coherent tomography applied to MRI scanner architectures. Therefore the bulk of signal processing in the digital world of the hybrid MRI scanner architecture consists of a cascade of FFTs. With sampling time intervals of about

$$5 \,\mu\text{s} \leq t_\text{s} \leq 20 \,\mu\text{s},$$

the FFT algorithms are performed by a phased array processor which generates the images from the digitized data line bundle in the spatiotemporal domain under the tight control exercised by the host computer.

The data acquisition presents instantaneous dynamic range demands of up to 80 dB. Analog-to-digital converters (ADCs) of 14 to 16 bits per data channel, overseen by the pulse programmer, are used to digitize the data lines. In order to free up the general-purpose host computer bus for other functions, the ADC can be connected directly to a dedicated input port of the phased array processor.

Two-dimensional spectroscopy measurements in NMR experiments always require a finite period of time to establish the differences between energy levels, during which the nuclear spin system continues to evolve and during which the linear magnetic field gradients of the MRI experiment can be changed. Due to this delay, the data acquisition for MRI formation is intrinsically a slow process. It was this intrinsic slowness which misled sceptics to believe that it would represent a major physical barrier to achieve scan speeds in clinical MRI comparable to those in X-ray CT and that speed therefore would limit the widespread clinical use and dissemination of the MRI modality. Nevertheless, MRI burst onto the clinical scene as a diagnostic imaging tool with even more intensity than the X-ray CT modality in the 1970s. Although greatly advanced beyond plain film radiography, CT still uses harmful X-rays and is therefore destined for obsolescence, while MRI continues to grow.

Multiple slice imaging mitigates the problem of slow data acquisition by making effective use of the dead time following data acquisition for excitation of neighboring tomographic slices. Beyond fast imaging techniques, *fast* imaging modalities such as the ultrafast high speed echo-planar imaging and several high resolution imaging variants have been developed by referring to the analogy between the MRI process and coherent optical processing. Fast MRI techniques need even shorter sampling time intervals to produce snapshot images than conventional MRI processing. By virtue of improvements in signal-to-noise ratio, which is a crucial factor in producing good image quality and diagnostically useful information, these techniques have gained credibility over the last few years.

The average data throughput of the data acquisition system must keep up with sustained data rates of up to about 800 kilobytes/s. For two-dimensional multislice and three-dimensional acquisition techniques, the total volume of spatiotemporal data may exceed 4 megabytes/s. The MRI scanner systems employing multiple surface coils, placed parallel to the magnetic axis as a receiver for improved sensitivity due to improvement in signal-to-noise ratio, will multiply the data rate and data size requirements by the number of surface coils. In clinical MRI scanners which are equipped with twin self-shielded gradient coils, a gradient coil set performs normal work load, while a supplementary gradient coil provides small field-of-view (FOV) imaging of quadratic pixel size

$$\left(\frac{FOV}{N_P} \right)^2 .$$

The analog operations of the hybrid MRI scanner architecture include linear magnetic field gradient and RF power amplifiers. Two principal data streams are flowing across the interface between the digital and the analog worlds. Timing and amplitude information for tight control over linear magnetic field gradients and RF spin excitation pulse trains acting as filter bank input along the stratigraphic time line are directed from the digital to the analog world of the MRI scanner architecture. Conversely, a spatiotemporal NMR data stream is flowing in the direction from the receiver coils to the digital world for data processing.

Based on a stable reference clock, in order to exercise tight control over the pulse repetition frequencies by a tuned circuit with a crystal, the pulse generator must generate at least 4 independent parallel trains of pulses. Three pulse trains serve to control the gradient power supplies and one to shape the RF transmitter output. Even with a single image formation technique, several timing and amplitude parameters need to be controlled in order to select the desired pulse repetition rates, echo times, and field of view. Typical MRI pulse generators will allow adjustment of the relative timing of any pulse sequence feature in steps of 100 ns. To avoid the loss of signal and the generation of image artifacts, it is necessary to generate programmed pulse trains acting as filter bank input with stable and replicable timing and amplitude characteristics. For shaped pulses, sufficient dynamic range is required to avoid digitization artifacts in low-amplitude pulses. Twelve- to 16-bit DACs are currently employed in state-of-the-art MRI scanner architectures.

Clinical MRI scanners need a number of built-in pulse sequences to handle routine scanning protocols as imaging systems. Automated procedures tune the scanning parameters. Due to the intrinsically slow data acquisition process, MRI would not be clinically practical without the multiple slice imaging technique. Standard clinical scanning usually employs a selective pulse sequence design which acquires up to about 20 tomographic slices at a time in an interleaved procedure by modulating the wavelets. Three-dimensional sequences acquire data from an entire volume at once and excite images of a higher signal-to-noise ratio, at the cost of a more time consuming data processing.

Patient motion such as breathing, cardiac-cycle-induced motion, respiratory-related motion, peristalsis, pulsatile blood flow, gross patient movement, and various other kinds of motion can generate image artifacts in clinical MRI scans, principally by interfering with the phase of the acquired wavelet. Whereas motion is the solution and the problem simultaneously in remote sensing SAR, voluntary and involuntary motion is a severe problem in clinical MRI. Gating to cardiac or pulmonary motion can be employed to synchronize data acquisition and reduce these distortions at the cost of losing tight control over the timing of the spin sensitization pulse sequences. The record of physiological information during scan is used to correct phase changes during data processing.

Barely 15 years have passed since the introduction of clinical systems; yet MRI is established as a routine radiodiagnostic technique the power, utility, and importance of which have been amply demonstrated in most hospitals. Just as in the clinical application of X-ray CT to intracranial scans, NMR coherent tomography started with cerebral scans as a clinical modality about 10 years after CT had become an established radiodiagnostic tool. Magnetic resonance imaging has the potential of *totally* replacing CT (Figures 9 and 10). The only circumstance under which X-ray CT still plays a role in cranial imaging is if the pathology is suspected of being located in the human eye or within the bony orbit ([247], [248]). Nevertheless, it is the historical merit of X-ray CT that it started an awakening of the potential of computer applications to the field of diagnostic imaging. Due to the fact that clinical MRI is a valuable

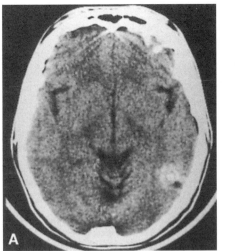
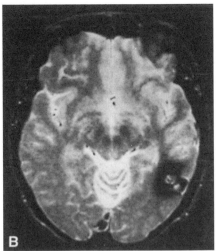

Figure 9. Left temporal cavernous hemangioma: X-ray CT imaging (A) and morphological MRI study (B). In these studies, the lesion is easily visualized on both X-ray CT and MRI scans.

imaging modality for cranial and spinal studies as well as musculoskeletal studies, radiologists currently pursue subspecialization in neurological and nonneurological imaging.

In neurodiagnostic imaging the problem of discriminating intracerebral tumors from surrounding edema and the difficulty in detecting small meningiomas, the

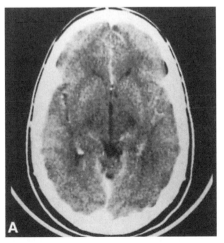
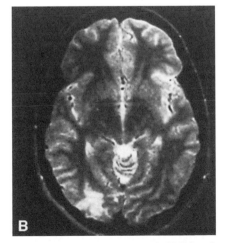

Figure 10. Right occipital lobe astrocytoma: X-ray CT imaging (A) versus a morphological MRI study. This infiltrating glioma could *not* be visualized by an X-ray CT study alone. Clinical MRI is superior to X-ray CT imaging in detecting cerebral and spinal lesions. The patient is seizure free 5 years after tumor resection.

most common primary nonglial intracranial neoplasm, have represented initially severe limitations to the acceptance of clinical MRI, but these were bypassed with the introduction of intravascular paramagnetic contrast agents ([10]). Although still early in the decade of the brain (the 1990s), MRI has become firmly established as the premier radiodiagnostic modality for the head, covering the diseases encountered in the clinical practice of today's health care environment. Specifically, clinical MRI is the technique of choice in the subacute and chronic stage of neurological disease evaluation as a result of its capability to construct images in any plane. Who in 1996 would have the courage to bypass MRI in cases of parietal epilepsy, intracranial hypertension, and isolated cranial nerve palsy or diagnose monosymptomatic MS or intramedullary tumor without first confirming or rejecting the clinical hypothesis by MRI findings?

The clinical role of MRI has been expanded step by step from neurodiagnostic studies of the central nervous system (CNS) to the disorders affecting other parts of the human body:

• Currently about 70% of the volume of clinical MRI examinations are concerned with the CNS.

Nonneurological clinical MRI examinations are concerned with the musculoskeletal system ([100]), including body imaging of the spine and major joints, the chest and cardiovascular system, the abdomen, and the male and female pelvis ([41], [79], [82], [152], [213]). It is exceptionally well suited for study of the female pelvis, and it is gaining acceptance as an integral part of the gynecologic imaging armamentarium, particularly because it can, in many instances, be cost-effective ([101]). Finally the neurofunctional MRI examination based on the hemodynamics upon neuroactivation forms its own speciality. The early scepticism of neurosurgeons and orthopedic surgeons has been so thoroughly overcome that hardly any lesion or trauma of the brain, spine, joints, and muscles in the human body are diagnosed today without the help of MRI processing. The initial promise of MRI has come to fruition to an extent that could hardly have been anticipated.

Although in the beginning MRI was identified with neurodiagnostic studies of the CNS, its applications to disorders of the musculoskeletal system have revitalized the radiodiagnostic subspeciality. The magnetic resonance evaluation of ligaments, tendons, muscles, vessels, and nerves is now commonplace in clinical radiodiagnostics ([82]). The applications of clinical MRI to disorders of the musculoskeletal system ([100]) equaled and even surpassed in clinical importance its application to disorders of the CNS. In the fields of neuroradiology and musculoskeletal imaging, at least, clinical MRI is firmly established as a core diagnostic tool.

Until a few decades ago, detection of soft tissue tumors usually did not take place until late in the course of disease. This resulted from their low incidence and nonspecific clinical findings and from the poor sensitivity of conventional plain film radiography, which was the only imaging modality available. Many of these problems were solved by the introduction of clinical MRI ([67]). Today, a correct assessment of disorders of bones, joints, or musculoskeletal soft tissues is unimaginable without clinical MRI. Its excellent spatial and contrast resolution and its ability to separate hematopoietic from fatty bone marrow make it ideal for marrow evaluation. It is extensively used for the evaluation of musculoskeletal neoplasms in adults and children. The primary goals of clinical MRI in a patient with a suspected soft tissue tumor are to define the margins of the lesion, assess its relationship to major vessels and organs, and determine whether the lesion invades adjacent bones or joints. Abnormal bone marrow signal is a sensitive indicator of bone invasion. When the lesion involves both soft tissue and bone, it may be difficult to be certain of its tissue of origin. Adequate evaluation can often be accomplished by performing standard spin echo pulse sequences in at least two orthogonal tomographic slices. During and after completion of therapy, which usually consists of chemotherapy and radiation or both, or surgical resection with wide margins, clinical MRI is the primary method of detecting locally recurrent disease.

The number of papers published on the application of MRI to choliangiography and pancreatography in the past two years reflects a growing excitement about the potential of these techniques to dramatically improve clinical MRI of the areas of the biliary tract and the pancreas, which have been historically difficult areas for MRI to have a clinical impact ([262], [263]). The speed of its growth is a testimony to the clinical significance of the technique.

The proliferation of clinical MRI into other parenchymal morphologies of the human body is rapidly advancing and includes the examination of the chest and cardiovascular system, mediastinum, retroperitoneum, liver, spleen, pancreas, and gastrointestinal tract. Hepatic MRI faces major change when the next generation of contrast enhancing agents, composed of a crystalline magnetic core and therefore extensively different from the Gd chelates, is used routinely. The primary clinical application of the superparamagnetic nanoparticles is the detection of lesions in a neoplastic context, where it is necessary to distinguish between the detection of metastases in a patient who is likely to require surgical resection and the detection of a hepatocellular carcinoma in a patient presenting with liver cirrhosis.

In the clinical radiodiagnostic evaluation of the heart, clinical MRI excels in the area of ischemic heart disease, congenital heart disease, and abnormalities involving the pericardium. The pericardium defines the outer margin of a cone-shaped space that contains the heart and the proximal part of the aorta and pulmonary artery. Clinical MRI provides excellent visualization of the normal and abnormal pericardium and plays an ancillary role when echocardiography fails to resolve a clinical question because clinical MRI possesses the advantages of echocardiography but not its limitations ([370]). Because MRI is the only essentially three-dimensional imaging method among the existing imaging modalities, a closely related technique, the subspeciality of magnetic resonance angiography (MRA), has become an effective radiodiagnostic method capable of obtaining high resolution clinico-morphological and physiological vascular information throughout the human body ([27], [149]).

The intense enthusiasm and the rapid introduction of MRI into the clinical environment stem from the abundance of diagnostic information present in MRI scans and the potential offered for physiological images. The pathological information it provides about diseases has led to earlier treatment, thus increasing the likelihood of recovery.

Therefore, NMR coherent tomography has assumed a role of unparalleled importance in medical high technology, diagnostic radiology, and cognitive neuroscience during a relatively brief period of time and experience. As in all clinical imaging modalities, understanding the normal development of morphological anatomy is a fundamental step to recognizing the abnormal clinico-morphological structures through imaging:

- Up to the present stage of technological development, the prime goal of routine clinical MRI is to confirm normal clinico-morphological anatomy of the internal organs in the human body and to define the abnormal morphology associated with pathological changes and congenital defects, with a strong perspective to the functional implementation as routine clinical MRI protocols of the future.

The MRI modality does not expose the patient or physician to ionizing radiation or iodinated contrast media. Recent statistical evaluations have provided evidence that persistent exposure to ionizing radiation is capable of significantly increasing the rate of mamma carcinoma in female flight attendants. Because its sensitivity is proved by biopsy, surgical histology, or clinical follow-up results to be close to 100%, MRI is one of the most prominent imaging methods in clinical examinations among the noninvasive procedures for the diagnosis of breast cancer (Figure 11). Due to the intrinsic soft tissue contrast and the capability of MRI to depict thin contiguous

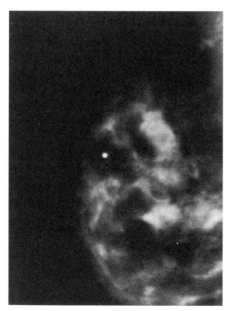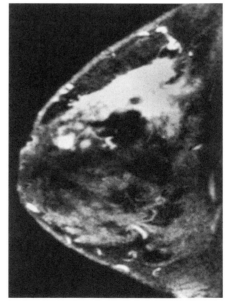

Figure 11. The conventional mammogram indicates a palpable lesion whereas MRI mammography performed of the same patient displays more details. MRI of the mamma offers more soft tissue contrast than other imaging techniques predominantly mamography and ultrasonic imaging. MRI mammography allows investigations to devise new techniques to enhance lesions of the female breast and to help patients avoid biopsy.

tomographic slices throughout the entire breast, contrast-enhanced MRI is able to identify breast lesions occult to X-ray mammography ([27], [63], [122], [149]). In fact, magnetic resonance mammography (MRM) is the only modality which allows for reliable detection of multifocality in breast cancer.

In view of the fact that the radiation risk of X-ray mammography appears to be higher than previously assumed ([264]), breast MRI processing represents a promising development to achieve decreased patient morbidity, a reduced number of biopsies by means of the intravenous application of paramagnetic contrast-enhancing agents, and high resolution fast imaging techniques with dedicated surface coils for an improved signal-to-noise ratio ([150], [171], [210]). Of all breast masses referred for biopsy following palpation and X-ray mammography, only 20 to 30% are malignant and therefore many patients undergo unnecessary biopsy. Magnetic resonance mammography as a valuable complementary examination procedure in cases where neither X-ray mammography nor ultrasound are able to provide an unequivocal result ([151]) can greatly improve this situation.

Although cancer of the breast is the second leading cause of mortality from cancer among women, and early detection is a key ingredient of any strategy designed to reduce breast cancer mortality, the high sensitivity of contrast-enhanced breast MRI for the detection of mamma carcinoma is not fully exploited. In selected patients, however, MRI is superior to X-ray mammography ([194]) in detecting malignant breast lesions. Nevertheless, breast imaging is still one of the most controversial domains in MRI because significant overlap of benign and malignant tissues has been encountered so that in an emotion-charged medical scenario there exists disagreement regarding the appropriate indications and clinical imaging protocol for this modality. The MRI-guided biopsy can confirm the MRI-detected abnormality in order to improve the specificity of breast MRI. Presently, MRI-guided nonferromagnetic fine needle localizations assume a role in the minimally invasive evaluation and management of breast disease. The future development of improved specificity of noninvasive magnetic resonance mammography appears to be extraordinarily promising.

The diagnostician is not about to be replaced by an expert system. The most advanced and fastest growing clinical imaging modality requires radiologists who are primarily competent MRI diagnosticians, not narrow-minded clinical pixelists and voxelists. The physicians who fare best in dealing with the rapid changes in medical imaging caused by the progress of computer science and can take fullest advantage of them will understand the basics of the science and revolutionary technologies that underlie them.

In today's health care environment, with its limited resources, it is critical to select the proper imaging modality and to understand its proper utilization for the clinical evaluation of pathology. Less than a decade after the advent of X-ray CT, the MRI modality was thought to provide the radiologist with a unique high technology window through which to visualize human anatomy *in vivo*. It has become one of the major new tools of radiology, now being applied to virtually every part of the human body to detect the clinico-morphological alterations of anatomic structures caused by a wide range of pathological conditions. Therefore, knowledge of the clinico-morphological anatomy of the internal organs is no longer the preserve of the anatomist or required only in medical school. *Bedside* knowledge of anatomy is needed in order to diagnose and treat patients appropriately.

It is worthwhile to observe that, for the therapeutic benefit of the patients, the theoretical developments and clinical applications of computerized pulsed Fourier MRI are still proceeding at a rapid pace. Magnetic resonance imaging has a strong tendency to revolutionize *interventional* medicine by its application to the field of image-guided, minimally invasive therapy.

As an example of an MRI-guided, minimally invasive procedure, the recently developed laser-induced interstitial thermotherapy should be mentioned ([354]). Magnetic resonance imaging guidance has proved to be the clinical instrument of choice for this technique of local tumor destruction within solid organs. It is the ideal tool for the exact positioning of thin optical fibers in the pathologically altered parenchyma. Through the fibers, a semiconductor diode laser focuses light energy. Photon absorption and heat conduction result in coagulative and hyperthermic effects. The real-time monitoring of the hyperthermic effects and subsequent evaluation of the locoregional extent of coagulative necrosis are essential parts of MRI-guided interstitial laser photocoagulation therapy.

Initial experiments applying a laser burn to mamma carcinoma were made using ultrasound and X-ray CT to define the tumor size and monitor the effect of treatment. However, neither of these techniques could accurately map the tumor or monitor the therapeutic effect. The MRI-guided *minimally invasive* interventional technique is now being used in routine clinical practice for ablating some solid tumors, including liver metastases, head and neck tumors, and mamma carcinoma. In selected patients it offers a result superior to surgical excision. The laser therapy follow-up is then monitored by MRI scanning.

Another example of a powerful combination of laser technology with the clinical MRI modality is the laser-polarized inert-gas-enhanced MRI for visualization of lung anatomy and function with acute respiratory distress syndrome. Inert-gas-enhanced MRI is based on the fact that nuclei in the gas phase that are hyperpolarized by laser light yield very high wavelet signals *in vivo*. Once inhaled, an enhancement of a factor of 10^5 with a dramatic increase of spatial resolution can be achieved. In particular, ventilated regions of the lungs can be systematically mapped by this technique with much higher resolution than nuclear ventilation scintigrams ([12]). In fact, multislice imaging can be performed with spatial resolution comparable to that of proton MRI because the enhanced spin polarization in the airways has a sufficiently long half-life. Thus the application of the ^{3}He MRI method to the thorax establishes an alternative diagnostic imaging system of the human respiratory system to established nuclear medicine techniques without ionizing radiation. The MRI scans obtained in a breath-hold are particularly striking in patients with obstructive pulmonary disease and bronchiectasis. In this way, the previously impenetrable black holes of lung air-filled spaces are finally yielding their secrets to MRI.

Currently, diagnostic imaging of the lungs is mainly performed by means of standard X-ray chest radiography and X-ray CT. Neither technique, however, allows for direct evaluation of airway ventilation. Up to now, ventilation imaging studies could only be performed with radioactive gases or ultrasonically generated technetium-tagged aerosols. However, these techniques of nuclear medicine lack the spatial resolution and visualization of the cross-sectional anatomy of the internal organs in the human body routinely acquired by MRI scanner systems. The MRI of inhaled hyperpolarized ^{129}Xe or ^{3}He gas allows for an elegant visualization of air-filled spaces in the human body. It promises scans which give new insights into pulmonary anatomy and function and has applications in the earlier detection of lung diseases and presurgical workup of candidates for lung transplantation.

Due to its extraordinary sensitivity, high soft tissue contrast with multiparameter dependence of wavelets originating from tissue voxels, that is, detectability, and flexibility of tomographic slice sectioning together with high contrast and spatial resolution, clinical MRI has displaced the time-honored diagnostic capabilities of X-ray CT, plain film radiographs, diagnostic arthrography, myelography and post-myelography CT, and even angiography as the noninvasive imaging study of choice for a preponderant list of diseases. The weighting between MRI an X-ray CT is illustrated by the fact that the Johns Hopkins Medical Institutions with their large outpatient center currently works with five MRI scanner systems and one helical X-ray CT imager. Nothing, however, indicates the strong tendency toward the MRI modality as the superior clinical tool in a more impressive manner than the fact that atlases which originally used X-ray CT in conjunction with MRI to display human cross-sectional clinico-morphological anatomy finally completely eliminated X-ray CT. After having abandoned X-ray CT as the primary way to evaluate soft tissue and paraspinal masses as well as joint abnormalities, MRI was used exclusively as the imaging modality to visualize the clinico-morphological anatomy of the internal organs in the human body ([82]).

The appearance of clinico-morphological structures on CT scans depends upon the differential degree of attenuation of the X-ray beam by the different tissue types. Adipose, for instance, causes very little attenuation of X-rays and therefore appears dark on CT scans. Bone structures, which are very dense, on the other hand, attenuate a considerable portion of the X-ray beam and appear white on the CT scans ([44], [133], [276]). This forms the standard scale for X-ray CT absorption in Hounsfield units, ranging from $-1,000$ allocated to air, 0 allocated to water, and $+1,000$ allocated to bone, on which the scanning CT technologist simply falls back. In the era of X-ray CT of the brainstem, for example, a lesion was invisible unless it was large enough to distort the fourth ventricle or had enough contrast by virtue of calcification or enhancement to be seen through the dense interpetrous beam-hardening effect.

The diagnostic advantage and difficulty of clinical MRI is that there is nothing like a universal gray scale as in X-ray CT, and Hounsfield units completely lack importance in MRI. Due to the capability of computer-controlled multiparameter contrast resolution, the advent of MRI, for instance, revolutionized imaging of the truncus encephali. It is now possible to visualize lesions 2 to 3 mm in diameter on routine clincal MRI scans and relate them to recognizable large brainstem structures and to several readily identifiable tracts running the length of the truncus encephali. Knowing the relationships of the key tracts to known clinico-morphological landmark structures greatly improves diagnostic capabilities in this important anatomic structure. Due to its main radiodiagnostic advantages of multiplanarity without the need of repositioning the patient, superb soft tissue discrimination, and superior contrast and spatial resolution, which facilitate the recognition of disease in relationship to normal parenchyma, MRI is the imaging modality of choice for the morphology of the CNS, including the cross-sectional clinico-morphological anatomy of head, neck, and spine.

Frequently, MRI is the definitive examination modality, providing invaluable information to help the surgeon not only to improve understanding of the underlying pathoanatomy but also to generate a *road map* and to make the critical decision regarding surgical intervention. In orthopedics, for instance, very few top surgeons will operate without having such a road map available:

- Rarely, a clinical MRI evaluation may have to be supplemented by an X-ray CT study. Conversely, if CT is the first study, chances are considerably higher that a supplementary MRI examination will need to be done.

There has continued to be significant improvement in MRI instrumentation hardware as well as software. In particular, receiver coil design and selective pulse sequence development continue unabated. The design of surface coils, pioneered by the work of Kudravcev in 1960, was initially deemed a marginal scientific curiosity. However, only since the development of surface coils has routine clinical MRI of the spine been practical. A surface coil can image only in localized ROIs, typically covering only the cervicothoracic region containing 7 vertebrae, the thoracic spine consisting of 12 vertebral bodies, or the lumbar spine with 5 vertebral bodies, in any given acquisition. Prior to this, spine imaging was performed with the whole body coil, which provides uniformity and coverage but lacks sufficient resolution and signal-to-noise ratio for accurate detailed diagnosis. Whereas long spine tomographic imaging is not accessible to the X-ray CT modality, a quadrature phased array multicoil MRI receiver enables the acquisition of large volumes with the signal-to-noise ratio of small surface coils. Each coil of the quadrature phased array receiver is linked to a separate receiver channel consisting of a low noise preamplifier, demodulator, and data acquisition system. In this way, the cost of the electronic hardware increases considerably.

Proposed MRI scanner architectures would employ more than a dozen parallel surface coils to receive the image of the spinal cord, extending from the medulla oblongata to the apex of the conus medullaris, with improved sensitivity due to higher signal-to-noise ratio. The quadrature phased array multicoil MRI receiver of the spine increases the dataset handling requirements to unwieldy proportions unless digital computational hardware is employed. Hence clinical MRI follows the same tendency to digital electronic hardware as does SAR high resolution imagery. In particular, dedicated computer hardware is needed near the front of the signal processing chain to compress the data going to later stages. It will help to reduce costs and enhance the flexibility of the MRI scanner system:

- Clinical MRI is the procedure of choice for evaluation of the vertebral column and spinal cord. In fact, MRI has become established as the only modality that directly images the parenchymal morphology of the medulla spinalis. It is unique since no other invasive or noninvasive imaging technique possesses this capability and allows visualization of thecal and spinal cord compression, protrusion and herniation of degenerate disks, syrinxes, hemorrhage, metastatic deposits in the vertebral bodies, spinal inflammatory diseases, marrow disorders, and congenital malformations.

Of all areas of spinal pathology, it was on the diagnosis of neoplastic diseases of the spinal cord that clinical MRI has had the greatest impact ([204]). Using the traditional spinal lesion parlance, spinal tumors are categorized as extradural, intradural extramedullary, or intramedullary. This categorization is not strict because neoplasia may reside in two compartments simultaneously, and two lesions with identical pathology may occur in different compartments. For example, spinal neurofibromas, which together with neurinomas belong to the most common intraspinal tumors to arise from the nerve root sheats, may extend into both the extradural and the intradural extramedullary space and may even occur in any of the three compartments, including the intramedullary space. Intramedullary lesions include astrocytomas, which are most frequently located in the cervical and thoracic regions; the ependymomas, which are glial neoplasms with a propensity for the conus medullaris and the filium terminale located at the apex of the conus; and the hemanglioblastomas, which may involve the cervical and thoracic regions. Extramedullary intradural lesions include meningiomas usually located in the thoracic region; neurinomas or schwannomas and neurofibromas, which are benign nerve sheath tumors; and lipomas, which are most common in the thoracic region but can be seen throughout the spine.

The vertebral bodies are the most frequent site of metastatic disease to the spine. Different primary tumors appear to have a propensity to metastasize to different sites. The vast majority of metastases begin in the vertebral body and subsequently grow into the region of the pedicle. Metastases can deposit on the dura, pia-arachnoid region, and the medulla spinalis itself. Almost immediately after its inception, even with the poor contrast resolution of the early scans, the potential of clinical MRI in the evaluation of suspected neoplasms of the medulla spinalis was recognized. With the availability of surface coils to improve the signal-to-noise ratio, the superiority of MRI over myelography and postmyelography CT in the assessment of intramedullary tumors was established. Clinical MRI also proved to be as efficacious as the traditional imaging modalities in the evaluation of suspected extradural tumor impingement on the thecal sac and is a noninvasive radiodiagnostic modality.

No imaging modality other than clinical MRI has been able to faithfully visualize the changes of internal architecture of the spinal cord and ligaments as a result of trauma. Most of the diagnostic information in spinal trauma is derived from sagittal tomographic slices. The ligamentous structures that are identified on routine sagittal scans of the spine include the anterior and longitudinal ligaments running along the anterior and posterior aspect of the vertebral bodies, respectively, the ligamentum flavum situated in the posterolateral aspect of the spinal canal connecting the lamina of adjacent vertebrae throughout the spine, and the interspinous ligaments between two adjacent spinous processes. Failure of either ligament at any spinal level is indicative of spinal instability. Because sagittal scans depict most of the soft tissue abnormalities including ligamentous injury, disk herniation, spinal cord edema and hemorrhage, cord contusion, nerve root avulsions, and epidural fluid collections, clinical MRI has the greatest impact on spinal traumatology in the clinical management of cord injuries of patients with persistent neurological deficit.

Another important use of clinical MRI in respect to the traumatology of the spine is in the detection of posttraumatic cyst formation. Development and expansion of such cysts may be catastrophic in patients with permanent neurological deficits. These cysts may occur either above or below the original site of the cord trauma and are readily detected by MRI.

Because the CNS has higher incidence of congenital malformations, clinical MRI has a major impact on the diagnosis of developmental anomalies:

- Due to the excellent visualization of the posterior cranial fossa structures and the regions around the foramen magnum and craniocervical junction, clinical MRI provides the definitive study of diagnosing anomalies of the metencephalon such as the various types of Chiari malformations.

Magnetic resonance imaging opened a new window to the pediatric CNS and has proved to be a modality in unraveling some of the mysteries of normal brain maturation. Noninvasive diagnostics of congenital and perinatal malformations is of particular significance for sequential studies in pediatric neuroimaging and cerebrovascular diseases in neonates, infants, and children ([15], [16], [195]). Clinical MRI is the imaging study of choice in most children with complex congenital anomalies of the hindbrain; holoprosencephaly, which is characterized by hypoplasia or aplasia of the rostral brain and of the premaxillary segment of the face; congenital malformations of the spine such as spinal and occult dysraphisms as well as caudal spinal anomalies and ensuing neurological disorders. To be more specific, the disorders of dorsal induction or neurulation include the Chiari II malformation, anencephaly, cebocephaly, encephaloceles, meningoceles, spinal cord tethering, and thoracic and lumbar diastematomyelia ([10], [49], [79], [238], [344]), which all are accessible to clinical MRI studies.

Only on very few occasions is myelography indicated in the pediatric patient because most clinical problems may be solved with MRI. Due to the ability to excite images in any plane, clinical MRI has revolutionized pediatric neuroimaging by assessing the state of myelination *in vivo* of a child's normal and abnormal brain development and detecting small areas of dysplastic cerebral cortex and regions of heterotopic gray matter in the cerebral parenchymal morphology ([10], [15]–[17], [30], [49], [79], [188], [276], [287], [289], [347], [372]). Obviously, modifications of scan techniques from those used with adults are required due to patient size and the intrinsic differences in imaging parameters ([328], [331]).

In neurodiagnostic imaging, MRI represents a significant advance for the detection of diseases involving cerebral white matter, and in many instances it is the only acceptable imaging modality of white matter pathology, even when it is compared with the new fourth-generation X-ray CT scanners, with a fan beam consisting of an X-ray tube rotating about the patient and an opposing stationary array of individual X-ray detectors. As with fourth-generation X-ray CT scanners, the fifth-generation X-ray CT scanners have a fixed array of X-ray detectors and a radically new design, mechanically fixed but electronically movable X-ray source. Both X-ray CT and clinical MRI show gross morphological changes in the maturing brain parenchyma, but only the high contrast resolution of MRI permits highly sensitive assessment of cerebral gray and white matter changes and differentiation of cerebral cortex versus basal ganglia.

Several of the long-standing problems with standard dynamical X-ray CT were overcome with the introduction of spiral X-ray CT scanning in 1990. However, the difficulties with the filtered back projection algorithm needed for X-ray CT data processing and the limited intrinsic contrast and spatial resolution remained, and the invasiveness of the ionizing radiation even increased. As a result, clinical MRI is superior to rapid image acquisition by spiral X-ray CT with iodinated contrast enhancing material in definitely demonstrating or excluding, for example, pancreatic neoplasm.

Experience with ionizing radiation has shown that the absorption rate of a spinal examination with a modern X-ray CT scanner is about 20 times the absorption rate of a plain radiograph and a cranial neuroanatomic X-ray CT examination needs about 30 times the absorption rate of a highly sensitive X-ray film. Therefore intracranial X-ray CT examinations should be restricted to the radiodiagnostic evaluation of emergency patients with acute cranial trauma ([289]).

In the area of neurodiagnostic imaging cerebral conditions, MRI has made tremendous strides in understanding the pathophysiology of cerebral white matter diseases in the past decade. White matter diseases can be divided into two major categories, demyelinating and dysmyelinating diseases. By far the most common demyelinating disease is MS ([175]). As a chronic inflammatory disease of the entire neuraxis, MS was described for the first time 175 years ago by the most prominent neurologist of the nineteenth century, Jean Marie Charcot, termed as *sclérose en plaques*. In MS, the oligodendroglia cells are destroyed and the axons spared. The normally myelinated regions of the human brain are replaced by plaques, which consist of reactive astrocytes, lymphocytes, and macrophages ([347]). Patients experience a variety of disabling neurological symptoms related to the disruption of normal conduction of neural pulses. Dysmyelination involves the abnormal development or maintenance of myelin. The rapid increase in data in genetics and molecular biology as well as in MRI of cerebral white matter diseases has given a new approach to the cerebral myeloarchitecture and the myelin disorders:

- The radiodiagnosis of MS can be made when spatiotemporal separated CNS lesions are documented. Because with X-ray CT it is possible to visualize lesions in about 35% of the MS patients, CT studies are rarely used in the radiodiagnostics and follow-up of MS. In contrast, MRI scans displaying lesions at the callosal-septal interface admit a degree of sensitivity of 93% and specificity of 98% in differentiating MS from vascular disease.

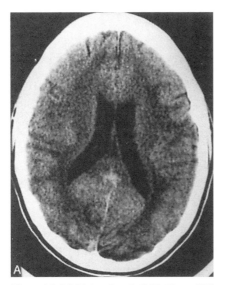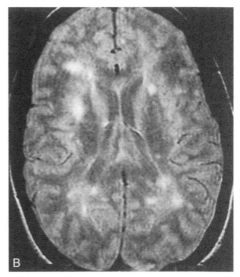

Figure 12. Multiple sclerosis (MS): X-ray CT imaging (A) versus a morphological MRI study of the same patient one day later. The X-ray CT scan displays a single focus of enhancement whereas the MRI scan reveals numerous MS plaques. Clinical MRI forms the imaging modality of choice for the diagnosis of MS. Contrast enhancement of MS plaques identified on prior unenhanced MRI studies indicates active disease in the inflammatory phase. Nonenhancement of MS plaques, on the other hand, represents quiescent demyelinative disease. Such observations will influence patient therapy.

The general policy today is that, if a clinical imaging modality is used in the search for demyelinating plaques and follow-up, it should be MRI. Depending on the MRI scanner equipment, it reveals foci of demyelination in 71 to 100% of patients with MS.

Clinical MRI is the only modality that allows direct visualization of spinal cord demyelinating plaques (Figure 12). In a series of 15 demyelinative brainstem lesions seen on MRI scans in 35 patients, none was demonstrated by X-ray CT ([179]). Clinical MRI forms the neuroimaging procedure of choice in the evaluation of patients presenting with developmental anomalies, infarcts and ischemia, infections such as encephalitis and acquired immunodeficiency syndrome (AIDS), inflammations, subarachnoid, subdural, and intraparenchymal hematomas and other vascular abnormalities, hydrocephalus which may be associated to Chiari I but is not mandatory for the diagnosis of Chiari I malformation, CNS tumors, and primary CNS lymphoma in the AIDS population. The intensity patterns of MRI scans are extremely varied in focal intracerebral lymphoma, particularly in AIDS patients. Progressive multifocal leukoencephalopathy and AIDS encephalomalacia affect the cerebral white matter ([10], [37], [79], [152], [276], [289]):

- The cerebral myeloarchitecture with the corpus callosum, the largest interhemispheric commisure, as a clinico-morphological landmark structure in the human brain is evaluated far more accurately by a clinical MRI examination than by an

　　　X-ray CT study. Agenesis of the corpus callosum causes characteristic anatomic
　　　brain abnormalities that are easily seen on midline sagittal MRI scans.

　　　Recently, initial research in neurofunctional MRI has demonstrated that human
brain function, together with reliable clinico-morphological information, can be noninvasively mapped by MRI sensitized to regional changes in blood oxygenation upon
neuroactivation of the cerebral cortex ([55], [140], [149]). Especially at high baseline
magnetic flux density, which implies an improved signal-to-noise ratio, functional
images of high contrast and high intrinsic spatial resolution depicting neuroactivated
cortical gray matter areas can be acquired. In this way, neurofunctional MRI has
shown great promise as a modality of regional human brain activity with strong
impact on cognitive neuroscience.

　　　The spatial localization of human brain function using neurofunctional MRI techniques hold great promise for an improved understanding of the neuronal cooperativity among various cerebral regions in mental imagery ([48]), visual, speech,
and memory organization principles ([189], [221]), and motor processing ([121],
[149]). Because many disease processes do not have a clear anatomic correlate, functional MRI can support the diagnostic performance of neuroanatomic MRI. Such
disease entities include acute cerebral ischemia and infarction in the study of stroke
and cerebrovascular pathological conditions ([134], [372]), focal seizures and sub-
clinical or interictal events in the investigation of human symptomatic epilepsies
([196]), and dementing disorders which reveal progressive cerebral cortical atrophy
such as morbus Alzheimer ([120], [287]) and subacute spongiform encephalopathy or
Creutzfeldt-Jakob syndrome ([289]), of which the potential relation to bovine spongiform encephalopathy (BSE) is presently discussed in an emotion-charged scenario.
Finally, neurofunctional MRI is frequently helpful in tumor characterization ([27],
[149]), preoperative neurosurgical trajectory planning, and stereotactic neurological interventions ([169]). A combination of conventional MRI, which provides the
best neuroanatomic detail, with other noninvasive techniques of localizing cerebral
regions such as magnetoencephalography opens up promising applications to mental mapping which refine the time-honored invasive recording of stimulus-evoked
potentials ([253]).

　　　In the past, the diagnosis of the causes of an epileptic attack was extremely difficult *in vivo*, and only neurosurgery or postmortem neuropathology could reveal the
epileptogenic lesion. The advent of NMR coherent tomography completely changed
the study of epilepsy, leading to *in vivo* diagnosis of epileptic attacks. Excitement
was kindled by MRI when epileptologists first realized that they could actually see
the amygdala and the hippocampus during life. It is safe to predict that no single
force since the discovery of human EEG by Hans Berger in 1929 and the computer
analysis of EEG bank filters ([18]), which opened a window on the physiology of
epilepsy, will do more to push clinical epilepsy research forward over the forthcom-
ing years than the MRI modality ([192]). Simultaneous neurofunctional MRI and
electrophysiolocal recording ([164]) seems to be a particularly promising technique.

　　　The rapidly developing field of neurofunctional MRI techniques, which provides
a way of noninvasive mapping of human brain function in real time, together with

reliable anatomical information has important applications to neurosurgery. The significant morbidity associated with surgical procedures that involve the cerebral cortex can result from a disruption of primary sensory and motor cortical areas. Neurosurgeons who attempt to preseve these primary areas during therapeutic operations are handicapped by variations in the normal organization of these areas and by the reorganization that may follow neurological disease, particularly in pediatric neurosurgery. To bypass this difficulty, intraoperative cortical mapping in the awake patient can be used in an attempt to define the extent of a primary area in an individual cerebrum and allow the neurosurgeon to search a decision that balances therapeutic need against potential functional impairment. A routine noninvasive procedure to identify the primary area, such as that afforded by neurofunctional MRI, is valuable in clinical management.

Despite the commonly cited delineation between clinico-morphological MRI and functional MRI, the terms are not exclusive. Due to individual morphological variability and the sophisticated variation of neuroanatomic scanning incidence, imaging of the normal brain in order to identify and trace the exact location and orientation of the bewildering variety of sulci, gyri, lobes, sublobes, and subcortical structures of the telencephalon and cerebellum at the global morphological level is difficult. The permanent tension between neuroanatomic constants and individual variation is even stronger in the neuropathological and traumatic state of the human brain as well as at the functional level. Certainly a mass lesion or infarction demonstrated in gross morphology by a cerebral MRI scan explains localized neurological dysfunction. There is nothing, however, as compelling to the understanding of a neurological disease as being able to directly reconstruct and visualize the neuropathological state of the brain activity. Hence, the singular merit of high resolution MRI is that it has permitted to create a new medical discipline, human neuroanatomy *in vivo*, which came to replace most of the postmortem studies at the autopsy table ([168], [338]).

Beyond the neurofunctional brain mapping of regions of neuronal activity and of clinical seizure disorders, the use of functional MRI for the purposes of interventional medicine is very promising. The most important interventional applications include image-guided frameless stereotactic methods for an optimal surgical approach, MRI-guided biopsy, endoscopy, and arthroscopy and real-time intraoperative imaging during minimally invasive procedures such as laser-induced interstitial thermotherapy. Like functional brain imaging, interventional functional MRI has an enormous potential, but this potential will take time to develop and mature.

This inexorable progress is part of the excitement that clinical MRI exerts on anybody who is interested in the interplay between coherent photonics and computer-assisted clinical medicine. The mathematics of geometrical quantization provides an approach to both of these MRI-guided high technology fields.

Redundanz hat zwei Formen, Frequenz und Resonanz, *wobei die erste die Signifikanz der Information betrifft und die zweite die Subjektivität der Kommunikation.*

—Gilles Deleuze und Félix Guattari (1992)

Magnetic resonance (MR)—*with its multiplanar imaging capability, high sensitivity to pathologic processes, and excellent anatomic detail—has had a major impact on routine clinical care over the past decade. Our knowledge base with regard to normal and pathologic brain processes has also been substantially increased. The future of* MR *continues to be bright.*

—Val M. Runge (1994)

Cherchez la lésion!

—Robert I. Grossman (1994)

1.3   THE NMR AND MRI METHODOLOGIES CONTINUED

The speed with which the clinical technology of MRI spread throughout the world was phenomenal. In 1980, the first commercial MRI scanner ever sold in the United States, a permanent magnet scanner, was placed in a private diagnostic imaging center in Cleveland, Ohio, and at the end of 1981 there were only three working clinical imagers available in the United States which showed modest contrast resolution performance. The scan time they needed suggested that MRI would probably not be a clinically practical imaging modality. At the time of the inception of clinical MRI, the performance that fast and ultrafast MRI techniques, like HASTE and EPI, opened up was unforeseen.

Today, MRI is a basic clinical tool in noninvasive medical diagnostics available in every clinical center in the United States, Japan, and Western Europe. At the time of writing, there are worldwide approximately 12,000 clinical MRI scanners working. Presently about one-third of the total number of clinical MRI scanners work in the United States. There are about 700 clinical MRI scanners in Germany to visualize the cross-sectional clinico-morphological anatomy of the human body, leaving virtually no internal organ system unprobed. A simple amplification of the phase-coherent wavelet response to the required output level would yield an output that is swamped by noise. The widespread availability of NMR technology is due to the fact that the electronic instrumentation for the NMR trace filtering of response wavelets originating from a background of tuned-in Heisenberg helices superimposed by thermal fluctuations and other noise has enjoyed an explosive development during the last 10 years, perhaps more than any other field of technology ([158]). The development of commercial MRI systems reflects this through continuing trends toward market stratification and specialization.

The applications of NMR systems are extensive and diverse. For example, some of the systems are being used for spectroscopic studies of human metabolism, while smaller scale instruments are suitable for more basic spectroscopic research studies in biomedical magnetic resonance on biopsy specimens, body fluids, cultured cells, isolated tissues, and small animals. Early MRI systems closely followed the advancement of the art, which generally meant employing systems of the highest magnetic flux density and the most capabilities. Current systems are increasingly tailored toward more specific applications, economic structures, and siting requirements. The MRI systems with specific implementations for neurological, cardiac, interventional, extremity, and spectroscopic studies will likely become more available.

Notwithstanding the limitations of medical charges for high technology diagnostic procedures, even radiology groups in private practice enthusiastically acquired the noninvasive scanning systems because of the unique type of diagnostic information and distinguishing features they provide and the continuing revolution in medical technology they represent. The diagnostic performance of clinical MRI due to its unparalleled capability for contrast and spatial resolution justifies the immense enthusiasm for this exciting, clinically invaluable, and ever-changing field of research (Figure 13). New and emerging techniques and a wide spectrum of new pulse sequences for fast imaging as well as standard clinical applications are becoming incorporated into protocols.

The protocols of NMR spectroscopy experiments and clinical MRI studies basically distinguish four periods of ensemble quantum computation that are recorded by

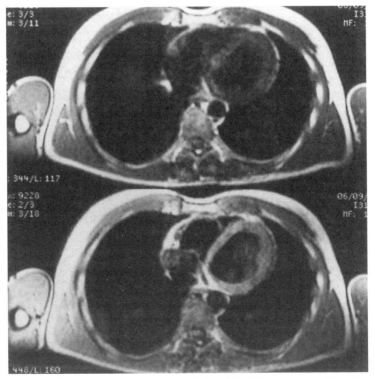

Figure 13. Effect of cardiac gating on image quality: Gating of the MRI scanner provides an improvement of the contrast resolution of internal cardiac morphology. Due to the synchonization of the data acquisition with the cardiac cycle, the myocardium is much better seen in the lower scan than in the ungated MRI study.

the stratigraphic time line $\mathbb{R}$ of the superencoded projective space $\mathbf{P}\left(\mathbb{R} \times \mathrm{Lie}(G)^{\star}\right)$. Stepping through the four relevant periods of the timing diagram allows to implement the geometrical patterns in the leaves of the canonical foliation $\mathbf{P}(\mathbb{R} \times \mathcal{O}_{\nu})$ and to read them out via the confocal observation plane of emergence $\mathbf{P}(\mathbb{R} \times \mathcal{O}_{\infty})$:

- *The Preparation Period.* In the course of the creation process of quantum coherence, single preparation pulses and coherent pulse trains are used to select the tomographic slices and excite the spin isochromats, respectively.
- *The Period of Coherent Evolution.* In the course of the evolution process of the phase-locked synchronized neural network, the precession of the spin isochromats evolves in time within the selected tomographic slices. As central spectral transforms, synchronized sequences of linear magnetic field gradients tracially encode the spectral localization information in the geometrical substrate. In order to maintain the coexistence of the geometrical substrates, the spin system is not observed during the evolution period.
- *The Quantum Holographic Mixing Period.* In the course of the holographic process, the spin system is perturbed by use of computer-controlled pulse trains and synchronized linear magnetic field gradients to remove the dispersion components in the spectra. In this way, the ensemble quantum computation of the Weyl symbol is performed by a time reversal or polarity reflection, respectively.
- *The Phase-Sensitive Detection Period.* In the course of this procedure, the wide-band RF scanning signal is measured while the spin system is in the free precession state. The symplectic Fourier transform reconstruction of the steady state absorption spectrum then amplifies the result from the observation plane of wavelet collapses to the macroscopic system level via coherent quantum resonance.

After having performed the calibrations during the prescan period, the coherences are prepared from an initial high temperature equilibrium state and evolve under Schrödinger propagators. After holographic mixing by the mixing propagators, the observation of the spin system is restricted to the detection period.

In the conventional NMR spectroscopy experiment, the four periods correspond to

- excitation,
- encoding,
- refocusing, and
- read-out.

The problem is to model the emergence of the geometrical patterns through the preparation periods. Due to the hardware and software developments of NMR technology during the last 10 years, clinical MRI has become the mainstay of radiodiagnostic imaging modalities for nearly all diseases, with residual exceptions most often due to practical aspects of health care delivery in a limited resource environment, rather than because of either technical issues or clinical aspects of disease. It establishes a sophisticated high resolution mirror for the clinical radiodiagnostic evaluation of both gross and microscopic pathology. Indeed, whereas clinical MRI scanning is concerned with clinico-morphological imagery, NMR microscopy has the capability to excite images with spatial resolution similar to histologic sections and has even depicted single cells ([254]). As an example, *in vivo* NMR microscopy allows probing of the microarchitecture of the human skin. Preoperative staging and postoperative follow-up of skin tumors, which account for a third of all human tumors, demonstrate that the high contrast provided by MRI for soft tissues makes NMR microscopy superior over imaging of the dermis by high frequency ultrasound.

As with any radiodiagnostic imaging technique, the basis of clinical MRI is the excitation of the living tissue by a suitable external energy source. In conventional radiographic examinations, an X-ray tube generates high energy waves that penetrate the tissue and subsequently interact in a very specific way: A position-dependent fraction of the X-ray radiation is absorbed and scattered by the tissues. Because the photon *intensity* of the X-ray diffraction is recorded, implying that the phase information is lost, a direct reconstruction of the image is not possible. The tissue characteristic that is displayed in clinical MRI scans is fundamentally different since the external energy source is a transmitter of electromagnetic waves at RFs and since the full *phase* information in-plane encoded by quantum holography is retained.

The differential phase and local frequency information of the Heisenberg helices of spin isochromats is *traced* as planar excitation profiles and stored as circular grating arrays. After elimination of the dispersive components of the Larmor precession spectra implemented by the ray traces of the Heisenberg helices, the quantum holograms are amenable to the linear response theory of NMR coherent tomography. Specifically the spatial information of water and lipid proton densities is acquired via the encoding of differential phase and local frequency of the Heisenberg helices of spin isochromats *traced* inside the selected tomographic slice. The spectral localization is performed by sequences of linear magnetic field gradients which are imposed on the main magnetic field.

From the geometrical point of view, the linear magnetic field gradients generate transvections which are computer controlled by affine dilations. As spectral transforms lifted to G, the gradient matrices act on the projectively completed tomographic slices $\mathbf{P}(\mathbb{R} \times O_\nu), (\nu \neq 0)$. The directions of the linear gradients coordinatize the quantum holograms in the laboratory frame of reference which are excited by the RF pulse responses and are recorded with respect to the rotating coordinate frame of reference.

The spatial information inherent to the quantum holograms provides the receiver, via coherent quantum stochastic resonance, projective geometry, and symplectic Fourier transform, a precise anatomic and topographic depiction of the lesion inside the confocal observation plane at infinity. Fortunately, the principles useful in the design of a high quality receiver of the linear pulse responses are of considerable assistance in the design of the transmitter.

The concurrent development of clinical MRI was influential in that the Lauterbur encoding technique which defines subbands by linear magnetic field gradients, ran counter to a widespread dogma that meaningful NMR spectra could not be obtained from complex heterogeneous organizations such as living tissues. Apart from the ability to span a wide range of contrast resolutions, MRI processing showed that it has more to offer both in the medical sense, especially when combined with *in vivo* NMR spectroscopic imaging ([117], [123]), and also in a wide range of nonbiological applications. In fact, biochemistry, geology, mineralogy, and enzymology have all been further opened up by the magic wand of the NMR phenomena.

For the most part, the NMR phenomenon is viewed as opposed to the EPR phenomenon. When certain types of paramagnetic ions, such as Fe^{3+} or Cr^{3+}, are placed in a crystal lattice such as aluminum oxide, the energy levels of the electron spin system vary strongly with magnetic field. Because the electron's Larmor precession frequency is higher than that of nuclei, EPR spectroscopy is based on microwave technology. Despite the difficulty in finding suitable paramagnetic electron species capable of participating in the resonance process, EPR is inherently more sensitive than NMR spectroscopy. Microwave radiation in the 3-cm region of the X-band passing from a klystron master oscillator down a waveguide into a resonant cavity containing the magnetic sample can induce transitions between the energy levels. In EPR spectroscopy, the energy absorption by the magnetic ions is detected.

In the dichotomy of nuclear spin versus electron spin, clinical MRI, with its various subspecialties, has its foundation in NMR spectroscopy. Nuclear spin, or, more precisely, *nuclear spin angular momentum*, represents one of the external characteristics of atomic nuclei. Because different configurations of local molecular electrons cause different shielding effects, the coherently measured value of the nuclear spin angular momenta depends on the precise atomic composition. Therefore NMR spectroscopy can be used as a powerful and versatile tool of macroscopic physics for the study of molecular structures and reaction mechanisms in the various branches of chemistry. As a topic, NMR spectroscopy is similar to EPR spectroscopy, except that the magnetic momenta of nuclear spins are typically 1000 times smaller and more difficult to detect than those of electron intrinsic spins. However, in the ENDOR detection experiment, an additional nuclear frequency in the range of 5 to 30 MHz is applied to the sample to stimulate nuclear resonances. By slowly sweeping through the nuclear resonance frequencies, it is possible to enhance the detection of the resonances of the nuclei that are near to, and strongly coupled with, the electron intrinsic spins.

Less spectacular than high resolution MRI, but also of enormous importance and explosive expansion, is the application of NMR spectroscopy for biochemical assay ([123]). Because NMR spectroscopy is one of the very few methods that provides information on the structure of molecules in solution at low concentrations, it allows for detecting the ratios of a wide range of metabolites *in vivo* and noninvasively and is used to study the way in which those ratios alter when disorders or diseases are present. Among the metabolites of interest are choline, lactate, alanine, phosphocreatine, and *N*-acetylaspartate. The signal detected from lactate can provide information about abnormal glycolyte metabolism, for instance, in malignant tumors of the human brain, and cerebrovascular pathology. Patients with MS present a decrease in *N*-acetylaspartate signal, which is interpreted in terms of axonal loss or damage. In patients with intractable temporal lobe epilepsy, it has been shown that a high portion of spectra obtained from the medial region of the temporal lobe, ipsilateral to the seizure focus, reveal markedly decreased N-acetylaspartate signals relative to other metabolite signals. Specifically, N-acetylaspartate can serve as a noninvasive marker for neurons ([116]).

The future of *in vivo* NMR spectroscopy for the diagnosis and biochemical assessment of brain disease appears to be promising. In conjunction with other clinical tests, such as clinico-morphological MRI, evoked potential tests, and immunological assays, NMR spectroscopy could provide a means for monitoring MS during clinical trials ([116], [152], [282]).

The major difference between clinical MRI and its foundation, NMR spectroscopy, is that the two studies use local frequency to encode different types of information. In MRI, the local frequency is determined by spatial position as in the Kepplerian dynamics, whereas in NMR spectroscopy the frequency is determined by the chemical content of the tissue scanned. In clinical MRI, protocols of temporally switched linear combinations of linear magnetic field gradients, which are used to tracially encode spectral localization, suppress the biochemical information. In *in vivo* NMR spectroscopic imaging, repositioning these gradients within the pulse sequence permits encoding of both spatial and biochemical information from many different regions simultaneously.

The original concept of the nuclear magnetic spin echo method required relatively large bandwidths and proved to be unsuitable for high resolution NMR purposes and continuous-wave methods with balancing devices continued in use. However, with the advent of very large scale integrated (VLSI) microcircuitry and sophisticated electronic hardware components interfacing analog and digital computing, used in conjunction with elaborate digital computer software technologies, the practice of NMR spectroscopy was completely transformed. These developments made possible previously undreamt of stability of the ratio of the applied external time-invariant baseline magnetic flux density to the RF and of the differential phase and local frequency, so that nuclear magnetic spin echo measurements could be performed in which a virtually unlimited number of shots could be applied and superimposed for improvement of the signal-to-noise ratio. The result of these hardware advances was a series of significant refinements to the two-dimensional Fourier transform techniques for the study of Larmor spectra in NMR spectroscopy ([86], [87], [123], [127]).

The nuclear magnetic spin echo method represents an excellent example of what was initially a purely academic idea of nuclear magnetic resonance spectroscopy, which the development of Fourier MRI transformed into a technique for the benefit of humankind. Specifically the application of two-dimensional Fourier transform methods to proton NMR spectroscopy has had a major impact on the development of the MRI modality for high resolution *in vivo* studies. The key move is to relate the two-dimensional Fourier transform to *noncommutative* projective geometry. Although commutativity, as opposed to noncommutativity, is typically thought of as contributing to simplicity, the rationale here is to deal with proton NMR spectroscopy in terms of quantum physics and to take full advantage of the structural richness and flexibility of Lie group theory that is embedded in the mathematical framework of geometrical quantization:

- The MRI modality offers a case study of the process of acquiring images by resonant intralevel interactions and controlling them by the spectral transform of linear magnetic field gradients.
- The intralevel interactions are due to an energy exchange between external magnetic fields and spin isochromats.
- The reconstruction via the symplectic linear response theory of coherent tomography is performed by stochastic resonance.

At the foundation of the quantized calculus is the three-dimensional Heisenberg two-step nilpotent real Lie group G. Up to isomorphy, G represents the unique connected, simply connected, three-dimensional, non-Abelian, nilpotent Lie group:

- The Lie group G admits a realization by a faithful matrix representation $G \longrightarrow$ $\mathbf{SL}(3, \mathbb{R})$.
- There is a faithful matrix representation $G \longrightarrow \mathbf{Sp}(4, \mathbb{R})$ such that the image group realizes G as a group extension and arises via matrix multiplication.

Under its *polarized* or dual pairing presentation, the Heisenberg group G is considered to be embedded into the real linear group $\mathbf{SL}(3, \mathbb{R})$. Under its *isotropic* or basic presentation, G is considered to be embedded into the symplectic group $\mathbf{Sp}(4, \mathbb{R})$.

More general, the Pfaffian polynomial function

$$\nu \rightsquigarrow P_G(\nu)$$

of the $(2n + 1)$–dimensional real Heisenberg group G, which dilates the rotational *curvature* form $\omega_\nu = P_G(\nu).d\kappa$ of the cotangent bundle

$$\mathrm{T}^\star(G/\text{center}),$$

is homogeneous of degree n.

- The volume growth of the $(2n+1)$–dimensional Heisenberg nilpotent Lie groups is polynomially.

It follows that P_G is *linear* only for $n = 1$. Hence only the *lowest* real dimension of the Heisenberg groups under their natural sub-Riemannian geometry provides a *linearization* of the Pfaffian. Therefore, according to the three-dimensional Heisenberg group model, the tomographic slice selection can be performed by superposition of *affine linear* magnetic field gradients.

The spectral localization by superposition of affine linear magnetic field gradients in the laboratory coordinate frame of reference is based on the fact that the *transvections* implementing the Hamiltonian action of the three-dimensional Heisenberg group G admit a factorization into affine *dilations*. The continuous affine wavelet transform, applied to transvections, lifts the radial trace to a central spectral transform in the rotating coordinate frame of reference. The central spectral transform diagonalizes the weak action of the left-invariant sub-Laplacian differential operator $\mathcal{L}_G$ of the natural left-invariant metric of the sub-Riemannian manifold G on the *symplectic* Fourier transform in the rotating coordinate frame of reference. The symplectic Fourier transform itself acts as a phase-sensitive average, sweeping over the spin isochromats to generate purely absorption-mode spectra for spectral localization purposes. The Karhunen-Loève expansion of the Ornstein–Uhlenbeck kernel associated with the central spectral transform verifies that clinical MRI scanner systems perform the calculations of weak site identification by using quantum parallelism of phase-locked, synchronized neural networks at the spin isochromat level. The scanner system amplifies the relaxation-weighted results from the plane of emergence to the macroscopic system level. The emergence of geometrical patterns arises by coherent quantum stochastic resonance. As a form of classical visualization parallelism, it displays the depth information of the clinical MRI scan in the bit plane:

- The essence of spin isochromat computation by pulsed Fourier MRI is the gauged synergy of the wavelet spectra and the coexistence of their geometrical substrates, recorded and rearranged within response data holograms along the bi-infinite stratigraphic time line.

Another key consequence of the geometrical quantization approach to clinical MRI is the fact that in the "tunnel" within which the patient is placed, or the center tube or bore of the superconducting magnet, the sub-Riemannian geometry of the Heisenberg group G replaces the geometry of the flat Euclidean space. The solutions of the system of Hamilton-Jacobi equations reveal the Heisenberg helices as the *geodesic* trajectories of the left-invariant sub-Riemannian metric of G.

The Pfaffian P_G represents the central spectral density of G in the longitudinal direction of the Heisenberg helices. This direction is transversal to the tangent bundle $T(G/\text{center})$. The bundle $T^\star(G/\text{center})$ is dual to $T(G/\text{center})$. Therefore P_G should be considered as a density with respect to the differential form $d\nu$ along the *affine* line of the longitudinal direction determined by the dual of the one-dimensional center of the Heisenberg Lie algebra

$$\text{Lie}(G) = \log_{\text{Lie}(G)} G.$$

In the MRI encoding process, P_G indicates the longitudinal direction of the affine linear magnetic field gradients applied for tomographic slice selection of those spin isochromats which are on speaking terms. Then another way of expressing the Larmor frequency equation for the precession dispersion in terms of P_G is that the pitch of the Heisenberg helices is inversely proportional to the polarity of the slice-select linear magnetic field gradients:

- In terms of the geodesic trajectories of the sub-Riemannian geometry of G, the Heisenberg helices of the free induction decay are losing energy due to the transverse relaxation effect and are gaining energy due to the longitudinal relaxation effect.

The mapping $\log_{\mathrm{Lie}(G)}$ allows a transformation of the holographic mixing process into coherent superposition. The logarithm of the real line $\mathbb{R}$ extends to a homomorphism of the affine linear group $\mathbf{GA}(\mathbb{R})$ onto the additive group of transvections implementing the Hamiltonian action of G. The extension of $\log_{\mathbb{R}}$ transports the gradient matrices onto the translations by the gradient polarities which realize the laboratory coordinate frame of reference of G in terms of coexistent transvections.

The pair (P_G, ω_ν), consisting of the longitudinal central spectral density P_G and the rotational curvature form ω_ν, defines the transversal stratification over G/center performed by resonance. The Heisenberg helices defined off resonance by the Pfaffian P_G encode radial traces in the rotating coordinate frame of reference of the symplectic affine cross section G/center.

Due to the thermal motion inherent in living tissue, the visualization of cross-sectional anatomy by clinical MRI scanners is performed with a noisy background. To bypass this problem by the resonance phenomenon, the scans are holographically encoded in quadrature format by imposing a phase difference of $\frac{1}{2}\pi$. Then signal wavelets embedded in a noisy environment are coherently lock-in detected in the confocal observation plane $\mathbf{P}(\mathbb{R} \times \mathcal{O}_\infty) \hookrightarrow \mathbf{P}\left(\mathbb{R} \times \mathrm{Lie}(G)^\star\right)$ of the equation

$$\nu = 0$$

from the hierarchical fibration of contiguously excited, adjacently decoupled, energetic strata

$$\{\mathbf{P}(\mathbb{R} \times \mathcal{O}_\nu) \mid \nu \in \mathbb{R},\, \nu \neq 0\}$$

in the complement of $\mathbf{P}(\mathbb{R} \times \mathcal{O}_\infty)$ inside the real projective space $\mathbf{P}\left(\mathbb{R} \times \mathrm{Lie}(G)^\star\right)$. It is this hierarchical fibration of energetic strata which represents the basic organizational principles of clinical MRI scanner systems for phase-coherent wavelet reconstruction via the symplectic linear response theory of NMR coherent tomography. To serve as a substrate for the tracial encoding process, the strata need to be equipped with the specific structure of a symplectic affine plane. This can be performed by the geometrical quantization strategy which gives rise to the quantized calculus.

Quadrature detection consisting of a four-phase demodulation cycle is a classical phase-coherent procedure for the evaluation of NMR experiments. In the presence of an external time-invariant homogeneous *baseline* magnetic flux density, a mathematical model of the demodulation process is given by the quadrature pair

$$(U^\nu, V^\nu) \qquad (\nu \neq 0)$$

of isomorphic irreducible unitary linear representations of the Heisenberg group G. It is diffeomorphic to $\mathbb{R}^3$, hence a connected, simply connected Lie group. The Lie group $\mathbf{SL}(3, \mathbb{R})$ is generated by the transvections of the real vector space $\mathbb{R}^3$. Due to this embedding, the natural diffeomorphism

$$G \longrightarrow \mathbb{R}^3$$

allows for transportation of the sub-Riemannian geometry onto the flat real vector space $\mathbb{R}^3$, which is *different* from its standard Euclidean geometry. Indeed, the Heisenberg helix as an analogue of a geodesic curve might serve as a paradigm for the sub-Riemannian geometry of G. The embedding of G under its basic presentation

$$G \hookrightarrow \mathbf{Sp}(4, \mathbb{R})$$

displays the symplectic structure associated to G. The symplectic structure of G inherited from $\mathbf{Sp}(4, \mathbb{R})$ is of central importance for the application to quantum holography and Fourier MRI.

Recall that the functor $\mathrm{Lie}(\cdot)$ from the category of connected, simply connected Lie groups to the category of Lie algebras is an equivalence of categories:

- The Heisenberg group G implements the Heisenberg canonical commutation relations of quantum physics in terms of the Jacobi bracket $[\cdot, \cdot]$ of the Heisenberg nilpotent Lie algebra $\mathrm{Lie}(G)$, which consists of the infinitesimal generators of G.
- Transition to the vector fields of directional derivatives presents the canonical commutation relations in terms of the Poisson bracket $\{\cdot, \cdot\}$ on the real vector space $C^\infty(G)$.

Thus the Heisenberg group G is the basic Lie group of the geometrical quantization strategy. Because Fourier analysis of G implements the transactional interpretation of quantum mechanics ([56]), the geometrical quantization strategy does *not* require a revision of the mathematical formalism of quantum mechanics. However, Fourier analysis of G is a geometrical adaption of the mathematical formalism of quantum mechanics appropriate to fuse quantum physics and principles of information organization in terms of geometrical quantization. This fusion, indicated by the bracket transition

$$[\cdot, \cdot] \rightsquigarrow \{\cdot, \cdot\}$$

from Jacobi to Poisson, is of particular importance for the structure-function problem of clinical MRI because it provides the Hamiltonian action of G which gives rise to the trace filter encoding of quantum holography.

- A diffeomorphism of the symplectic affine cross section G/center preserves the Poisson bracket $\{\cdot, \cdot\}$ if and only if it preserves the system of Hamilton-Jacobi equations.

Choosing the principal symbol of the left-invariant sub-Laplacian differential operator $\mathcal{L}_G$ as Hamiltonian operator, the group of isometries of the sub-Riemannian manifold G allows to tune in the Heisenberg helices.

On the other hand, geometrical quantization is closely related to the isomorphy classes of unitary linear representations of G. Because the irreducible unitary linear representations of G allow for a stratification of the tuned-in Heisenberg helices by the coadjoint orbit visualization, it is no surprise that the quantum holographic organization of the clinical MRI modality can be modeled by transition to the unitary dual $\hat{G}$ of the basic Lie group G. The punchline is that the transition from the cotangent bundle $T^\star(G)$ to $\hat{G}$ allows the filtering of the differential phase and local frequency encoded by the circular grating arrays of the traces of the Heisenberg helices which form the quantum holograms:

- The quadrature format which is obtained by imposing a phase difference of $\frac{1}{2}\pi$ corresponds to the corner turn mapping. This isomorphism acts as a nonlocal Fourier transform intertwiner at the level of the unitary dual $\hat{G}$ of G.

The pair (U^ν, V^ν) of irreducible unitary linear representations is induced from one-dimensional representations of closed normal subgroups of G:

- In Lie group representation theory, the coadjoint action in the real vector space dual $\mathrm{Lie}(G)^\star$ of $\mathrm{Lie}(G)$ is contragredient to the adjoint action of G in $\mathrm{Lie}(G)$.
- The projectively completed coadjoint orbits $\{\mathbf{P}(\mathbb{R} \times \mathcal{O}_\nu) \mid \nu \in \mathbb{R}\}$ immersed into the real projective space $\mathbf{P}\left(\mathbb{R} \times \mathrm{Lie}(G)^\star\right)$ which is canonically associated with the dual vector space $\mathrm{Lie}(G)^\star$ are used as an organizational principle of affine geometry to classify, up to isomorphy, and categorize all the irreducible unitary linear representations of the Heisenberg group G.

It is this organizational capability of the coadjoint orbit method, foreshadowed by the work of Harish-Chandra, which plays a crucial role in the structure–function problem of Fourier MRI. The fact that the coadjoint orbit picture allows the implementation of *geometrical pattern* emergence and its semantic interpretation makes it attractive for fusing quantum physics and the principles of the organization of information in terms of geometrical quantization.

Because the semantic filter bank interpretation leads to the philosophical relevance of the coadjoint orbit method, this seems to be a reasonable place to note some of the interactions beyond physics. Indeed, if philosophy is conceived from the point of view of constructivism, the coadjoint orbit picture exhibits an organizational principle more fundamental than quantum physics. It allows the deployment of complementary but basically different aspects. In terms of time ordering, the stratigraphic time scale $\mathbb{R}$ visualizes the plane of immanence which, endowed with its rotational curvature, implements the coexistence of *conceptual* structures. The changing connections implemented by the slice are acting as a kind of filter bank. According to this line of constructive reasoning, the stratigraphic time replaces correspondences by a manifold of resonances which are immersed into the superencoded space ([64], [65], [91], [92], [358]).

The read-out procedure of photonic holograms suggests the identification of the confocal observation plane of equation $\nu = 0$ with the projective plane at infinity

$\mathbf{P}\left(\mathbb{R} \times \mathcal{O}_\infty\right)$ of the projective completion $\mathbf{P}\left(\mathbb{R} \times \mathrm{Lie}(G)^\star\right)$. Because the complement of $\mathbf{P}\left(\mathbb{R} \times \mathcal{O}_\infty\right)$ in the projective space $\mathbf{P}\left(\mathbb{R} \times \mathrm{Lie}(G)^\star\right)$ has the structure of a linear affine variety, the projectively completed coadjoint orbit $\mathbf{P}\left(\mathbb{R} \times \mathcal{O}_\nu\right) (\nu \neq 0)$ can be immersed into the superencoded projective space $\mathbf{P}\left(\mathbb{R} \times \mathrm{Lie}(G)^\star\right)$.

The pair (U^ν, V^ν) is associated with the energetic stratum $\mathbf{P}\left(\mathbb{R} \times \mathcal{O}_\nu\right)$ of the MRI hierarchical system labeled by the center frequency level $\nu \neq 0$ of the Larmor spectrum. The corner turn mapping, which transforms the generic infinite-dimensional unitary linear representation U^1 of G into its *swapped* copy V^1, represents the dynamical symmetry of the generic symplectic affine plane $\mathcal{O}_1$. The smallest eigenvalue of the corresponding Pauli spin matrix is $\frac{1}{2}$ rather than zero; this is interpreted in quantum mechanics as the uncertainty principle, in quantum electrodynamics as the zero-point energy or energy of the vacuum, and in the dynamics of physical astronomy and NMR spectroscopy as the rationale for the quadrature format design of the Kepplerian spatiotemporal phase-sensitive detection strategy:

- The decoding by the symplectically formatted Fourier transform is performed by averaging with respect to the phase-sensitive point measures $\varepsilon_{(x,y)}$ over the confocal observation plane $\nu = 0$.

Application of the symplectic Fourier transform allows the reconstruction of the accumulated phase histories encoded in the contiguous channels of the quantum hologram within the plane of incidence. The symplectic linear response of NMR coherent tomography applied to the quantum holograms gives rise to the Larmor spectra in the observational contexts chemists are used to interpreting. Protocols for temporally switched linear combinations of magnetic field gradients make possible the spatial encoding, while the application of the Kepplerian strategy for the dynamics of physical astronomy to the NMR technique accomplishes holographic processing in quadrature format within projectively immersed, symplectic affine planes $\{\mathbf{P}\left(\mathbb{R} \times \mathcal{O}_\nu\right) \mid \nu \neq 0\}$ of resonant intralevel interactions:

- The resonant intralevel interactions are encoded in quadrature format. The reconstruction is performed in conjunction with the tomographic slice selection process operating on the hierarchical fibration of contiguously excited, adjacently decoupled, energetic strata $\{\mathbf{P}\left(\mathbb{R} \times \mathcal{O}_\nu\right) \mid \nu \neq 0\}$.
- The interlevel reconstruction, via the symplectic linear response theory of coherent tomography in the confocal projective observation plane at infinity $\mathbf{P}\left(\mathbb{R} \times \mathcal{O}_\infty\right)$ of the superencoded projective space $\mathbf{P}\left(\mathbb{R} \times \mathrm{Lie}(G)^\star\right)$, represents the Fourier MRI modality.

The change from the geometrical aspect to the spectral domain makes the computational treatment of the magnetic environment of protons in soft tissues possible. The use of the Fourier transform technique results in proton densities of the tomographic slice selected from the hierarchical fibration:

- Use of the nonlocal Fourier transform reconstruction for the read-out precludes the ability to directly relate NMR response wavelet intensities to the number of excited nuclear spins in the selected and projectively completed, symplectic affine plane $\{\mathbf{P}(\mathbb{R} \times \mathcal{O}_\nu) \mid \nu \neq 0\}$.

- Direct projection of the energetic stratum $\mathbf{P}(\mathbb{R} \times \mathcal{O}_\nu) \hookrightarrow \mathbf{P}\left(\mathbb{R} \times \mathrm{Lie}(G)^\star\right)$ ($\nu \neq 0$) onto the confocal observation plane $\mathbf{P}(\mathbb{R} \times \mathcal{O}_\infty) \hookrightarrow \mathbf{P}\left(\mathbb{R} \times \mathrm{Lie}(G)^\star\right)$ relates signal wavelet intensities to the number of locally excited nuclear spins in the selected tomographic slice $\mathbf{P}(\mathbb{R} \times \mathcal{O}_\nu)$.

Therefore, like any important imaging technique, the clinical MRI modality brings with it the need for a mathematical understanding of the underlying wavelet signal theory and of its reconstructive procedures via the symplectic linear response theory of coherent tomography. The signal theory represents a blend of analog and digital techniques which admit, at least at the analog level, a quantum physical meaning. The emerging discipline is called *quantum holography*:

- In quantum holography, the projectively completed coadjoint orbits $\mathbf{P}(\mathbb{R} \times \mathcal{O}_\nu) \hookrightarrow \mathbf{P}\left(\mathbb{R} \times \mathrm{Lie}(G)^\star\right)$ ($\nu \neq 0$) are interpreted as a hierarchical system of energetic strata, and the stationary plane $\mathbf{P}(\mathbb{R} \times \mathcal{O}_\infty)$ consisting of focal points is interpreted as the observation plane.

- The hierarchical fibration of contiguously excited, adjacently decoupled, energetic strata $\mathbf{P}(\mathbb{R} \times \mathcal{O}_\nu) \hookrightarrow \mathbf{P}\left(\mathbb{R} \times \mathrm{Lie}(G)^\star\right)$ ($\nu \neq 0$) establishes the underlying substrate for the tracial encoding of the semantic filter bank which represents the quantum holograms.

- The confocal observation plane at infinity $\mathbf{P}(\mathbb{R} \times \mathcal{O}_\infty)$ allows for the reconstruction of the quantum holograms from the hierarchical fibration of energetic strata $\mathbf{P}(\mathbb{R} \times \mathcal{O}_\nu) \hookrightarrow \mathbf{P}\left(\mathbb{R} \times \mathrm{Lie}(G)^\star\right)$ ($\nu \neq 0$) via the reproducing kernel of the symplectic linear response theory of coherent tomography.

The problem of reconstruction is an important feature common to all quantum physical systems which are based on the mathematical syntax consisting of noncommutative projective geometry ([112]). By switching from the microphenomenon to the macrolevel, the mature Johann Keppler observed, in the *Epitome Astronomiae Copernicanae* of 1618, that a major problem of physical astronomy is the reconstruction of planetary motions from geometrical hypotheses ([327]). The reconstruction procedure of quantum holography applies to both of these cases. In terms of the *spatiotemporal quantization* of quantum holography, the reconstruction from the hierarchical fibration of contiguously excited, adjacently decoupled, energetic strata $\mathbf{P}(\mathbb{R} \times \mathcal{O}_\nu) \hookrightarrow \mathbf{P}\left(\mathbb{R} \times \mathrm{Lie}(G)^\star\right)$ ($\nu \neq 0$) is accomplished by an application of the symbolic calculus of *pseudodifferential operators* associated with the Heisenberg group G. By its duality, $G \hookrightarrow \mathbf{Sp}(4, \mathbb{R})$ designs the quantum holgrams acting as symplectically formatted multichannel reconstruction analysis–synthesis filter banks.

The mature analog computation art of Fourier optical processing in synthetic aperture radar (SAR) high resolution imagery, and its digital implementation serves as the *leitmotiv* for the quantum holographic approach to the following procedures of the symplectically formatted Fourier transform MRI modality:

- intralevel in-plane encoding procedure, and
- interlevel reconstruction procedure.

These topics are relevant since images appear naturally as the final representation of the scanned data input in both SAR and Fourier MRI.

The Kepplerian spatiotemporal quadrature phase-sensitive detection strategy is quite flexible. It penetrates clinical MRI in complete analogy to the holographic viewpoint of range Doppler frame radar imagery and in particular SAR and inverse synthetic aperture radar (ISAR) high resolution imagery. Although these technologies are closely related, they have, like most well-developed disciplines, their own vocabularies which are created by the mathematical language:

- The mathematics common to SAR and clinical MRI is the duality of the Heisenberg group $G \hookrightarrow \mathbf{Sp}(4, \mathbb{R})$ expressed in terms of the spatiotemporal quantization strategy of quantum holography.

After reconstruction in the confocal observation plane of emergence, the variables deployed by the clinical MRI scanner for the coordinatization of the planar tomographic slices require a semantic interpretation in the contexts of observation. A thorough grasp of clinico-morphological anatomy of the internal organs in the human body, pathology, and the clinical aspects of disease is the key to this interpretation. This is particularly so for neuroanatomy and neuropathology. Neuroradiologists and head and neck radiologists agree that MRI is the modality of choice in patients with cranial and spinal neuropathies. The subspeciality of magnetic resonance angiography (MRA) requires knowledge of neurovascular anatomy. For the reader's convenience, the terminology used for the semantic interpretation of clinical MRI scans is a compromise between current radiological and anatomic vocabulary and the commonly used nomenclature following *Nomina Anatomica* ([24], [62], [148]).

Its proper basis is to be formed in the spatiotemporal quantization strategy of quantum holography ([293], [294]). This philosophy has recently found its way beyond the range of mathematical physics, photonics, and optical engineering. In fact, the quantum holographic conception has recently become of interest for an Apollo astronaut's approach to the problem of conscious awareness ([237]). This is due to the fact that the unitary invariances of the spatiotemporal quantization are determined by the action of the metaplectic group $\mathbf{Mp}(2, \mathbb{R})$. Notice that $\mathbf{Mp}(2, \mathbb{R})$ forms the twofold covering group of the special linear group $\mathbf{SL}(2, \mathbb{R})$ consisting of all the automorphisms

$$\tau : \mathbb{R} \oplus \mathbb{R} \longrightarrow \mathbb{R} \oplus \mathbb{R}$$

which satisfy the area condition

$$\det \tau = 1 .$$

The invariance of the spatiotemporal quantization under the action of $\mathbf{Mp}(2, \mathbb{R})$ rather than $\mathbf{SL}(2, \mathbb{R})$ itself implies the zero-point energy, that is, the energy of the vacuum of quantum electrodynamics:

- Quantum holography incorporates coherent wavelet theory into quantum physics by means of the spatiotemporal quantization strategy.
- The symplectic linear response theory of coherent tomography gives rise to a reconstruction procedure for the symplectically formatted multichannel filter bank.
- Perfect interlevel reconstruction from the subband channels of the filter bank can be achieved even when the constraints of relaxation attenuation and linear magnetic field gradient control are imposed on the phase-coherent wavelets in quadrature format.

A major technique for constructing representations of Lie groups is by the inducing mechanism. In the case of the Heisenberg group G, it is sufficient to induce one-dimensional representations from maximal Abelian, connected subgroups. A convenient vehicle to link the geometrical interpretation of the inducing mechanism to the spatiotemporal quantization strategy of quantum holography is the notion of a Hilbert bundle.

An exciting atmosphere of anticipation pervades the field of clinical MRI which has not yet become classical. The area is vast, and the territory is largely unexplored. The reward for those mathematically inclined readers who simply press forward will be to recognize how the coherence transferring dynamical symmetries lead to a noncommutative structure, the three-dimensional Heisenberg group G with one-dimensional center C and its various realizations via faithful matrix representations. The direction of C is along the external, time-invariant, homogeneous baseline magnetic flux density, generated inside the clinical MRI scanner, and therefore it plays a *pivotal* role in the quantized calculus approach to Fourier MRI. By factoring out the center

$$C \hookrightarrow G,$$

which is also the commutator subgroup or derived group

$$C = [G, G]$$

of G, this configuration allows to consider G as a nonsplit central group extension

$$C \lhd G \longrightarrow G/C$$

which is isomorphic to the polarized symplectic realization

$$\mathbb{R} \lhd G \longrightarrow \mathbb{R} \oplus \mathbb{R}$$

and the isotropic complex realization

$$\mathbb{R}.i \lhd G \longrightarrow \mathbb{C}.$$

In the spatiotemporal quantization approach to the structure-function problem of clinical MRI, other realizations corresponding to compact cross sections G/C from the polarized symplectic and the isotropic complex cross section are of equal interest.

According to the duality theory of the nilpotent Lie groups, the unitary dual $\hat{G}$ of G is embedded into the real vector space dual $\mathrm{Lie}(G)^{\star}$. It represents the spatiotemporal quantization strategy of quantum holography. Due to the fact that G is a nilpotent Lie group, it has the property that every finite-dimensional unitary linear representation is trivial on C and thus factors through to a representation of the quotient $\mathbb{R} \oplus \mathbb{R} \cong \mathbb{C}$:

- The finite-dimensional unitary linear representations, whose isomorphy classes belong to $\hat{G}$, do not distinguish all the elements of the set G.

Realization of the infinite-dimensional part of $\hat{G}$ by the isomorphy class of the linear Schrödinger representations U^{ν} ($\nu \neq 0$) of G demonstrates the *signal-theoretic* aspects of the spatiotemporal quantization strategy. The associated noncommutative convolution structure of tempered distributions on the cross section G/C and the reconstructing quantized calculus in the theory of pseudodifferential operators admit a phase-coherent wavelet implementation of bank filters by means of the least-squares filter design. This implementation is achieved by feeding phase-coherent wavelets into delay circuits and spin-labeled multipliers and finally by summation in an adder chip ([158]):

- The geometrical property of flatness of the projectively completed, symplectic affine planes $\mathbf{P}(\mathbb{R} \times \mathcal{O}_{\nu}) \hookrightarrow \mathbf{P}(\mathbb{R} \times \mathrm{Lie}(G)^{\star})$ is equivalent to the square integrability mod C of the associated linear Schrödinger representations U^{ν} ($\nu \neq 0$) of G and therefore implies the discrete series trace formula for the holographic transform $\mathcal{H}_{\nu}$.
- The flatness of the projectively completed, symplectic affine planes $\mathbf{P}(\mathbb{R} \times \mathcal{O}_{\nu}) \hookrightarrow \mathbf{P}(\mathbb{R} \times \mathrm{Lie}(G)^{\star})$ implies a factorization of the skew-adjoint Schrödinger operators of trace class into the product of a Hilbert-Schmidt operator and a unitary rotational operator.
- The pseudodifferential operators defined by means of Schwartz kernel symbols of the kernel distributions on the cross section G/C can be expressed in terms of Toeplitz operators acting on square integrable holomorphic functions on the open unit disk of the complex plane $\mathbb{C}$.
- The transition is accomplished by switching from the polarized symplectic realization $\mathbb{R} \lhd G \longrightarrow \mathbb{R} \oplus \mathbb{R}$ to the isotropic complex realization $\mathbb{R}i \lhd G \longrightarrow \mathbb{C}$ and the subsequent orthogonal projection.

The crucial role of Toeplitz operators is well known in the field of matched bank filter design and medical image reconstruction ([208], [283]). Actually, the discipline of matched filter bank design exerts considerable impact on clinical research and cognitive neuroscience applications and has a long track record in the history of science. Because, in many ways, the surface of the knowledge obtainable via MRI has been barely scratched, clinical MRI and neurofunctional MRI techniques will continue to be refined, and as computer software and key hardware capabilities improve, additional clinico-morphological and neurofunctional imaging capabilities will become practical ([185]). The responsibility for their continuously evolving growth and application rests in the hands of both research scientists and clinicians who seek to avoid ionizing radiation.

Although the principal years of discovery in the area of Fourier optical processors for mapping the radar cross-sectional distribution by SAR or ISAR high resolution imaging systems appeared to be well in the past, the advent of the clinical MRI modality revitalized the interest in these elegant and intriguing analog image processors. Because SAR high resolution imaging systems supply a flexible multichannel coherent wavelet filter bank implementation, they represent a powerful analog to the truly striking high technological development of MRI in clinical radiodiagnostics. With the advent of routine second and subsecond imaging anticipated with the next generation of clinical MRI scanner systems, neurofunctional MRI of cortical activation masked by conventional MRI of the cerebral parenchyma will have a major impact on cognitive neuroscience, and MRI-guided therapy will have an impact on monitoring interventional procedures.

The MRI coherent tomography modality can provide the best neuroanatomic detail, such as exquisite visualization of the 12 cranial nerves I to XII ([202], [247], [248]). Specifically, MRI is the modality of choice for imaging the normal anatomy and pathology of the olfactory (cranial nerve I), optic (II), oculomotor (III), trochlear (IV), trigeminal (V), and abducens (VI) nerves. Moreover, MRI will take the lead in performing microvascular dynamical topographic neuroimaging of cognitive processing.

The final goal of cognitive neuroscience is to study the mechanisms that relate brain and cognition. Therefore, cognitive neuroscience has to describe the mechanisms that drive structural neural elements into the physiological activity that results in perception, cognition, and even conscious awareness. The main objective of using clinical MRI in the field of cognitive neuroscience is the localization of cerebral activation. The neuroimaging capabilities of MRI at high temporal resolution enables accurate tracing of stimulus-induced response changes. This extension of clinico-morphological MRI has been first exemplified by the primary visual cortex located along the sulcus calcarinus along the midline of the lobus occipitalis and clinico-morphologically acquired by coronal craniocerebral MRI scans ([24], [62], [265]). The organization of the primary visual cortex is generated by the projections of spatial retinal coordinates and iso-orientation onto the human striate cortex under the retinotopic mapping. Dynamical topographic MRI studies allow for localization of neurofunctional activity areas of the cerebrum associated with specific visual stimulation ([189], [261], [265]).

A key role in brain control over motor function is occupied by the motor cortex, located in the gyrus precentralis of the cerebral cortex, in front of the sulcus centralis ([24], [62]). The motor cortex provides major outputs to the spinal cord and the truncus encephali and is interconnected with the major subcortical structures, the cerebellum, and the basal ganglia. An approach to the problem of how the motor cortex performs its function has been given by neurofunctional MRI at high magnetic flux densities of 4.0 T producing scans of high contrast resolution and spatial resolution of less than 0.7 mm in the observation plane ([121], [261]). The world's first clinical 8.0-T MRI scanner installed at the Ohio State University in Columbus, Ohio, is nearly twice as powerful as the 4.2-T MRI scanner that operates at Columbia University and the 4.1-T MRI unit responsible for neurofunctional MRI and NMR spectroscopy at the University of Minnesota.

Recently the dynamical topographic neuroimaging studies of visual imagery have been extended to complex cognitive processing to create reliable mental images by neurofunctional MRI. As a result, the neurofunctional MRI studies provide abundant cerebral physiological evidence that the mental operations involved in creating mental imagery are carried out in localized neuroanatomic areas of the human brain but different mental operations may be carried out in widely different cerebral areas. An increase in temporal resolution raises the prospect of deeper insight in the underlying physiological mechanisms and the investigation of influences of physiological noise like respiration or heart beat. Therefore neuroradiologists are the beneficiaries of a most remarkable revolution in noninvasive techniques for studying the cerebrovascular morphology and pathology *in vivo*, as well as neurofunctional activity of the human brain, while preserving anatomic specificity.

In numerous cases, the signs and symptoms cannot be completely explained by clinico-morphological imaging methods. Functional disturbances can precede detectable parenchymal morphological damage. Only functional imaging permits early assessment of biochemical damage that precedes parenchymal morphological damage, correlation of functional alterations, and clinical symptoms in the absence of detectable morphological damage. Specifically, neurofunctional MRI studies can help to explain symptoms due to abnormalities that occur in areas proximal and remote from the primary lesion, due to neuronal deafferentiation. In numerous cases, it is only the integration of parenchymal clinico-morphological and functional information that leads to a full understanding of the nature and extent of the damage that produces clinical symptoms. In this way, neurofunctional MRI improves the lesioning method.

Stroke is diagnosed approximately 400,000 times per year in the United States and contributes to approximately 150,000 deaths per year. The role of neurofunctional MRI in the evaluation of acute stroke is best understood when placed in the context of cerebral hemodynamics and ischemia. The key finding in the relationship between cerebral blood and neuronal dysfunction is that there is a level of cerebral blood flow at which neurons stop functioning without having undergone cell death, and therefore the damage from ischemia may be reversible. This fact has led to the concept of an ischemic penumbra. Since the pathophysiology of the penumbra is still incompletely understood, one of the goals of neurofunctional MRI is to visualize this penumbra and ideally identify the difference between salvageable, nonsalvageable, and undamaged cerebral parenchyma.

The clinical MRI modality is an intrinsically slow imaging technique, the processing of which is characterized by cycling schemes:

- The acquisition of MRI data sets and their accumulation in the memory of the host computer, the implementation of programmed pulse sequences acting as filter bank input, the realization of linear magnetic field gradient switching protocols, as well as the read-out procedure of the quantum holograms require long cycles of repetitions.

- In accordance with the timing diagram of the NMR experiment, the tight control over the repetitions of changing cycle lengths along the stratigraphic time line is exercised by the word bus running from the pulse programmer to the scanner hardware components.

In view of these intrinsic process prolongations, a mathematical treatment of phase-coherent wavelets in fast and ultrafast MRI procedures by compact realizations of the cross section G/C is of particular importance. These techniques are particularly helpful in cardiac and abdominal MRI. Moreover, ultrafast MRI techniques have attained an accepted preeminent role in the application of neurofunctional MRI modalities to cognitive neuroscience. They allow to focus on spatiotemporally encoded synchronized neural networks linking localized neuroanatomic centers where functional neuroactivity is occurring in the cerebral cortex while it is performing various mental tasks. This level of corticomorphic analysis actually represents the current high technology response to the age-long challenge to cognitive neuroscience of providing connections between human brain parenchymal morphology and the mind and to the dialog between cognitive neuroscience and mathematics in the study of the mental representation, or *matière à pensée* ([53]). In terms of the mathematics of geometrical quantization, the neurofunctional MRI modality depends on the direct projection on the singular observation plane $\nu = 0$ of focal points at infinity.

Despite its widespread use as a highly efficient medical imaging modality, clinical MRI is a remarkably recent technological development which appears to be in a constant state of flux and is therefore as far from maturation as it ever was. Few technologies have moved so rapidly, evolving from the first crude whole-body demonstration at 0.1 T by the seven-year construction of Raymond V. Damadian, Michael Goldsmith, and Larry Minkoff at Stanford and their implementation of the field-focused NMR (FONAR) technique in 1977 to the clinically powerful, sophisticated, high resolution imaging systems seen in most modern diagnostic institutions (Figure 14). The FONAR method in which an image is built up by moving the object through the resonance aperture of profiling coils is useful for acquiring chemical shifts of a localized area within an object but often does not lead to adequate spatial resolution. Therefore, FONAR has been widely replaced by the spin–warp version of Fourier MRI processing.

Spin–warp imaging is nowadays the most frequently applied MRI method. Developed by the Aberdeen University group and now mainly used commercially, this method is based on the Kepplerian spatiotemporal quadrature phase-sensitive strategy, allowing the synchronous and stroboscopic cross-sectional quadrature filtering of phase histories evolving in contiguous local frequency encoding subband multichannels of the semantic plane of incidence with respect to the rotating coordinate frame of quadrature reference:

- The basic objective of subband encoding is to decompose the image wavelet into uncorrelated frequency bands and then to encode each subband channel of the symplectic affine plane.

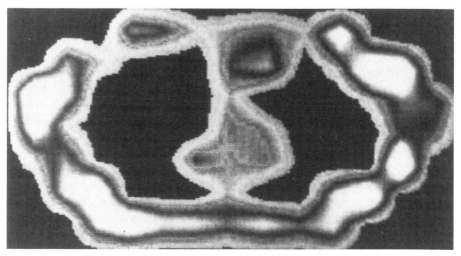

Figure 14. FONAR study of the thorax: Cross section at the level of the eighth corpus vertebrae thoracicae. The image shows the body wall, the pulmo dexter and sinister, the heart encroaching on the left lung field, the cardiac chambers, right atrium and a ventricle, and a section across the aorta descendens. The FONAR image is of great historical value.

- Multislice data acquisition in conjunction with the spin–warp Fourier MRI technique for decoding the symplectic affine plane in the confocal observation plane is used almost exclusively in current routine clinical MRI examinations.

Additional scanning techniques and the design of programmed pulse sequences acting as filter bank input are modified and updated on an almost daily basis. Although the feasibility of acquiring flow information by NMR had already been recognized during the 1950s, the technical prerequisites permitting selective pulse sequences suitable for the application of clinical MRI to blood flow imaging were not met until the past decade. Improved motion compensation has allowed magnetic resonance angiography to become a mainstream, if not a prerequisite, part of the evaluation of the cerebrovascular morphology and pathology.

The NMR spectroscopic imaging modality, often also referred to as chemical-shift imaging, is a subspeciality of NMR spectroscopy. In fact, NMR spectroscopic imaging is conceptionally an elegant combination of NMR spectroscopy and MRI with the goal of simultaneously characterizing chemical sites and constructing spatial maps. In NMR spectroscopic imaging, the local frequency encoding linear magnetic field gradient is replaced by additional phase encoding gradients, thereby preserving biochemical information on metabolites of interest. The NMR spectroscopic imaging uses the same equipment as clinical MRI to monitor the metabolic state of numerous regions but applies different pulse sequences to acquire the data sets from multiple ROIs in one or more tomographic slices within an MRI-defined FOV. The information either can be displayed as Larmor spectra from individual voxels, facilitating identification and quantitation of metabolites, or can be masked by conventional MRI, displaying the spatial distribution and intensity of individual metabolites throughout one or several slices. Since up to several thousand Larmor spectra can be simultaneously acquired from multislices, the image format is the most practical way to express the wealth of information on metabolic states obtained by NMR spectroscopic imaging.

The almost exclusively used reconstruction technique in NMR spectroscopic imaging is based on the two-dimensional Fourier transform method. Localizing pulse sequences such as STEAM (stimulated echo acquisition method), which now are commercially available for *in vivo* NMR spectroscopic imaging acquisitions, allow for routine evaluation of biochemical and functional damage to the CNS. Although the spatial resolution of proton spectroscopic images is below that of standard clinical MRI scans, the perspective in exciting metabolic maps masked by conventional MRI of the cerebral parenchyma for the diagnosis and biochemical assessment of brain disease holds great promise.

Routine clinical proton NMR spectroscopic imaging will become especially attractive as a complement to standard clinical MRI examinations, particularly for regionally heterogenous pathologies such as multifocal lesions, tissue perfusion, edema, and penumbra and for diseases affecting the cerebrum in a diffuse way. Although still in a experimental status, major clinical applications are expected for the assessment of intractable focal epilepsy, stroke, MS, neurodegenerative diseases such as morbus Alzheimer, human immunodeficiency virus (HIV) infection leading to dementia, and Parkinson's disease leading to movement disorders, coma, cerebral trauma, and finally brain death ([123], [282]).

In conclusion, MRI is surely one of the most exciting areas of clinical imaging, combining a dazzling, cutting edge technology with the challenges of the mathematical structure of the symplectic linear response theory of coherent tomography and the rewards of clinical practice. Although the progress in NMR coherent tomography and spectroscopy has taken place in less than 20 years, the pace shows little sign of slowing. If at any time a plateau of achievement appeared to have been reached, that notion was quickly dispelled by the next breakthrough. It is this virtual explosive development in technological equipment of the clinical MRI modality in conjunction with its unparalleled capability of contrast and spatial resolution, multiplanar imaging, extraordinary versatility, efficiency, and elegance which calls for a mathematical foundation of its syntax.

In an era of cost containment, the future of a high cost technology like clinical MRI does not solely depend on its extraordinary diagnostic performance. Independently, it has also an important socioeconomic aspect based on its cost efficacy. As the output of a billion-dollar industry, currently more than 4,000 clinical MRI scanners are available in the United States, where they are used as automated imaging systems for more than 16 million examinations per year. Presently there are about 700 clinical MRI scanners working in Germany to visualize the cross-sectional clinico-morphological anatomy of the human body. Unfortunately, it is unclear what the ideal number of MRI scanner systems should be. The greatest density of clinical MRI scanner systems is, in the United States and Japan, over 15 units per million inhabitants. In most West European countries, the density of MRI scanner systems averages between 3 and 7 units per million, although Switzerland averages 11 per million. The need for MRI examinations per million inhabitants is estimated at 50,000 per year. Assuming an annual throughput of 5,000 patients per year, this would necessitate 10 clinical MRI scanner systems per million.

The costs of per-patient examination play a critical role in the utilization of clinical MRI in response to the current situation of shrinking resources and retrenchments in health care. Magnetic resonance imaging technology is particularly visible and vulnerable to cost controllers because of the high purchase and maintenance price of instruments and the need for continuous system upgrades. Due to the extraordinary diagnostic power and the unsurpassed sensitivity of the highly involved MRI technique, most neurologists and orthopedists in the United States go straight to MRI exams, even in the era of shrinking clinical reimbursements. Several avenues have been explored to limit expenditures for clinical MRI. The most obvious way is to increase the utilization of existing resources by increasing the case load per MRI scanner. Since the introduction of clincal MRI, the average throughput has increased steadily. The progressive increase is a result of shorter examination times due to improved hardware and software. Nowadays, imaging times have been greatly reduced with new sequence types which increase patient throughput and reduce per-patient examination time. Nevertheless, the annual patient throughput for an MRI unit remains highly variable because it is determined to a large extent by the socioeconomic setting in which the clinical MRI scanner system is operating.

Another important cost factor is determined by the external magnetic flux density of the MRI scanner system. Because magnetic flux density is only one determinant of image quality, most manufacturers have made a dedicated effort in recent years to make available lower field MRI systems at highly competetive prices. The falling costs of purchase and housing as well as maintenance due to the tendency to lower external magnetic flux densities support the application of MRI as a clinical tool. The inherent economic advantages of MRI scanner systems at lower external magnetic flux densities are becoming increasingly relevant for the availability of clinical MRI as a tool of unprecedented and unparalleled radiodiagnostic accuracy for monitoring disorders and diseases affecting the human body. Even in a fast-changing medical environment and in the era of retrenchment, the future of clinical MRI research appears to be extremely bright.

Where the telescope ends, the microscope begins, which of the two has the grander view?

—Victor Hugo (1862)

People used to think that when a thing changes, it must be in a state of change and that when a thing moves, it is in a state of motion. This is now known to be a mistake.

—Bertrand Russell (1872–1970)

Johannes Kepler (1571–1630), *Astronom, Mathematiker und Musiker, der in den Bahnen der Planeten die "Weltharmonik" gehört und berechnet hat.*

—Joachim-Ernst Berendt (1992)

Reading the masters can mean entering a foreign paradigm, an unfamiliar mathematical world where alien values, language, definitions, tools, strategies, and assumptions frustrate our attempts to understand.

—Bruce Pourciau (1997)

It is not small physical size that defines the quantum level.

—Roger Penrose (1994)

Examination of the brain and spine with MRI *has many distinct advantages over* CT *imaging. . . . When a pathological process is encountered with* MRI, *it is usually detected by the presence of an abnormal signal and /or mass effect. If there is a focal space-occupying lesion, the multiplanar capability of* MRI *often helps to determine its position as intraaxial (within the brain parenchyma) or extraaxial (outside of the brain, distorting the brain's contour). This determination is the key to the formulation of a differential diagnosis.*

—Jim D. Cardoza and Robert J. Herfkens (1994)

Da wir aber auch allerhand vergessen haben, was wir nicht hätten vergessen sollen, ist unser Vorsprung nicht so riesenhaft, wie uns vorgeblasen wird.

—Erwin Chargaff (1992)

1.4 THE KEPPLERIAN PHASE-SENSITIVE QUADRATURE DETECTION STRATEGY

In the era of diminishing clinical importance of X-ray imaging in favor of noninvasive *in vivo* imaging and visualization, biomedical computing has rapidly emerged as a significant area of high technology research aimed at developing approaches for clinical radiodiagnostics and assessment of the cross-sectional parenchymal morphology of living organ systems and strategies for testing biomedical functional activities.

The ultimate goal of radiodiagnostic imaging procedures is to generate reliable images of the whole human body and its organ anatomy *in vivo* in a noninvasive way such that either tomographic morphology or biomedical functional activities can be accurately localized and quantified by the observer. As a consequence, X-ray imaging and specifically X-ray CT have to be made obsolete in diagnostic medicine.

If the semantically interpreting human observer is to recognize pathology on a clinical MRI scan, which is a two-dimensional gray scale representation, he or she must have an integrated three-dimensional concept of organ anatomy. However, there are two ways of learning anatomy, on a purely clinico-morphological basis and on a functional basis. The importance of including functional imaging aspects into anatomy and diagnosis is evident in the area of neuroimaging of CNS diseases because current estimates of false-positive rates for conventional diagnosis of cerebellar infarct (stroke) range up to 40%. This forms a challenge for clinical radiology which will be crucial for its survival as a clinical discipline ([72], [148]).

The final goal of diagnostic imaging procedures performed in patients with neurological symptoms is to identify the abnormal clinico-morphological and neurofunctional patterns of the human brain that correlate with the symptoms. In studying the correlation of human brain parenchymal morphology and cognition, by evaluating intra-axial and extra-axial cerebral parenchyma, and spine lesions and their mental influences, dynamical neuroimaging techniques for creating mental images during the performance of cognitive task are of paramount importance, for only the powerful techniques of neuroradiology can currently provide reliable topographic images of the active human brain *in vivo*, which is the least understood of human organ systems. Thus, the dynamical neuroimaging modality makes possible the determination of the principles underlying the formation and maintenance of topographic maps and the cerebral self-organization principles, which is one of the long-standing problems in neuroscience ([57]).

In clinical radiology, the point-by-point correspondence of morphological and functional images can be accomplished by NMR filter response techniques that are based on quantum holography. The benefit of the implementation of quantum holographic modalities is that the phase-sensitive quadrature detection of phase-coherent wavelets allows the representation of the physiological and biochemical processes displaying the underlying parenchymal morphology in a synergistic way.

An immediate advantage of this complementary approach is to assist the quantitative analysis of quantum holographic images, carried out by the definition of ROIs. As a direct consequence, the most critical factor in the resulting MRI protocols is the need for a highly accurate timing procedure to create an accurate reconstruction analysis–synthesis *filter bank*. The computer-controlled synchronization of its multichannels perform the subband coding of phase-coherent wavelet responses. A stable reference clock allows the image reconstruction. As indicated by the name, the magnetic resonance phenomenon in conjunction with stroboscopic sampling play a crucial role in clinical MRI.

It is the merit of the X-ray CT modality that it generated an awakening due to the potential of computer science in the field of radiodiagnostic imaging. The symbiosis of computer science with NMR coherent tomography, however, was assured with the realization that quantum holographic techniques could greatly improve the signal-to-noise ratio of the final image. Beyond coherent tomography, the phenomenon of resonance pervades the physical world. Phase-coherent wavelets allow for the generation of the following:

- constructive interference by stimulus-evoked parallel synchronization, and
- destructive interference by spoiled desynchronization.

Therefore, they are prominent candidates for the modeling of NMR at a mathematical level. To outline a cohesive history of the application of NMR coherent tomography to biomedical imaging problems and neuroimaging is an endeavor which merits a book of its own. It would show that the history of clinical MRI is one of the generation of ideas, their successful implementation, and their mathematical modeling ([223]). It is not necessarily the generator who actually implements or mathematically models.

Concerning quantum holography, it is important to notice that the basic idea of the acquisition of quantum holograms in differential phase–local frequency coordinate frames ([293]), as used for stroboscopic sampling purposes in SAR imaging, can be quite unexpectedly traced back to the dynamic physical astronomy of Johann Keppler. He was the first astronomer whose analysis reached laws of nature that were physical rather than mathematical or philosophical. The working hypothesis about the magnetic axis of solar planets and the ability of magnets to control direction in projective space was presented in his monumental Mars commentaries of 1609, entitled *Astronomia Nova* αιτιολογητος *seu Physica Coelestis, Tradita Commentariis de Motibus Stellæ Martis, ex observationibus Tychonis Brahe*. The *Astronomia Nova* has been prepared by the *Astronomiæ Pars Optica*. The important conceptual trick in MRI of referring spatial coordinates to a rotating frame had been already used by Keppler. It forces the conclusion that fictituously there is no external magnetic flux density, and the magnetization is stationary, albeit decaying, and does not precess with respect to the rotating coordinate frame of quadrature reference. *Learn from the masters!*

The attractive force of a magnet was known to Keppler from the famous book *De Magnete, Magneticisque Corporibus, et de Magno magnete tellure; Physiologia nova* (London, 1600) authored by Sir William Gilbert (1544–1603), Medicus Londinensis and physician to Queen Elizabeth I of England (Figure 15). Gilbert studied the flux lines of force, or "effluvia" as he termed them, around a small compass needle balanced on a pivot. In book six of *De Magnete* Sir William also demonstrated that the Earth itself was actually a giant magnet by noting that the ordinary magnetic needle maintains the north-south alignment because of the forces exerted by this giant magnet, and not because the spinning needle is "attracted by the stars."

> The Sun, chief inciter of action in nature, as he causes the planets to advance in their courses, so too doth bring about this revolution of the globe of the Earth, by sending forth the energies of his spheres.

The source of the magnetic forces remained a mystery until the last century, when Michael Faraday (1791–1867) discovered in 1831 that a voltage could be induced in a quiescent circuit subject to a changing magnetic field. Faraday's celebrated experiment concerning electromagnetic *induction* demonstrated that changing the amount of electric current flowing through one conductor could create an electromotive force, measured in volts, which could cause electric charge to move in a second conductor. The current was detected by its influence on a compass needle. During the change, caused by throwing open the switch, there was a momentary deflection of the spinning needle, proving that temporary current was flowing followed by a damped oscillation as the compass needle sought to regain its previous north-south alignment. Faraday's experimental set-up of electromagnetic induction demonstrated the prototype of a macroscopic *relaxation* phenomenon.

GVILIELMI GIL
BERTI COLCESTREN-
SIS, MEDICI LONDI-
NENSIS,

DE MAGNETE, MAGNETI-
CISQVE CORPORIBVS, ET DE MAG-
no magnete tellure; Phyſiologia noua,
plurimis & argumentis, & expe-
rimentis demonſtrata.

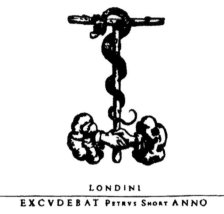

LONDINI
EXCVDEBAT Petrvs Short ANNO

Figure 15. Title page of Sir William Gilbert's famous book *DeMagnete* (1600), which influenced Keppler's physical astronomy.

At the nuclear spin level, Fourier duality leads to Bloch's nuclear induction decay-mode spectra and Purcell's nuclear magnetic resonance absorption-mode spectra. Indeed, Felix Bloch refers explicitly to the Faraday effect in a neighborhood of a *resonance* frequency in his fundamental 1946 paper on nuclear induction. Both the induction- and the absorption-mode spectra, acquired following phase-sensitive quadrature detection, are unaffected by any magnetic field gradient. The idea of linear gradient, however, is hidden in the epochal *Astronomia Nova* of 1609, which provides a detailed report of Keppler's "Martian struggle" to conquer the orbit of the planet Mars.

Keppler's conclusion from Sir William's experiments was that the attractive force of a magnet creates a sphere of attraction which attracts more strongly closer to the magnet. The virtue moving the planets, he continued, is propagated from the Sun into a sphere, and for the more remote parts of that sphere it is weaker. In terms of Gorter's magic word "oscillator" mentioned to Rabi, Keppler described in the *Astronomia Nova* the oscillator-driven dynamical system by an act of physical profanation 400 years before (translation from Latin):

Mein Ziel ist es, zu zeigen, daß die himmlische Maschinerie nicht von der Art eines göttlichen Lebewesens, sondern von der eines Uhrwerks ist, daß die ganze Mannigfaltigkeit ihrer Bewegungen von einer einfachsten magnetischen Kraft herrührt, so wie alle Bewegungen der Uhrwerkes allein von dem es treibenden Gewicht.

More than 400 years later, Sir Peter Mansfield, from the University of Nottingham, was knighted by Queen Elizabeth II for his contributions to diagnostic MRI. Sir Peter came up with the way for NMR to home in on particular tomographic slices of the sample by sequencing and pulsing affine linear magnetic field gradients. Basically this method is Keppler's stroboscopic stratification procedure of the orbit. Keppler used the perpendiculars from the apsidal line as the natural rotating frame of quadrature reference for the elliptical orbit forming an affine image of the circle, whereas Lauterbur achieved spatial localization by superposition of linear magnetic field gradients switched in the laboratory frame of reference.

This change of perspective actually leads from MRI to deeper insights into the Kepplerian dynamics of physical astronomy centered on the Sun. Keppler's stroboscopic timing strategy served as a unifying principle for his analysis, culminating in the development of his three fundamental laws of planetary motion. The helioeccentric frame of the Kepplerian dynamical system considerably extended the Copernican heliocentric static system ([302], [327]). It stimulated Galileo Galilei to give lectures on the sets of nested planetary spheres and the Platonic polyhedra outlined in the *Mysterium Cosmographicum* of 1596 without mentioning the true author.

By replacing the mean Sun of the Copernican astronomy by the physical center of the real Sun as the origin of the heliocentric frame (the "zeroth law" of planetary motion analysis, implicit already in Keppler's a priori astronomy and outlined in the *Mysterium Cosmographicum*), Keppler's procedure of phase history triangulation of eccentric circular orbits from a rotating coordinate frame of quadrature reference was based on the planet's periodic time and was derived without benefit of any optical instrument (Figure 16). As a matter of fact, Keppler's first two laws were stated in the same year that the telescope was invented. To quote the lucid description of the essence of the phase history triangulation method given by Albert Einstein in 1951, the profound as well as ingenious Kepplerian strategy of synchronous cross-sectional quadrature filtering of phase histories with respect to the rotating coordinate frame of quadrature reference proceeds as follows (communicated by Günter Doebel, 1983):

Das Leben Keplers war der Lösung eines doppelten Problems gewidmet. Sonne und Planeten ändern ihren scheinbaren Ort in bezug auf den Hintergrund der Fixsterne in einer komplizierten Weise, die sich unmittelbar der Beobachtung darbietet. Was man da mit großem Fleiß beobachtet und aufgezeichnet hatte, waren also nicht eigentlich die Bewegungen im Raume, sondern die zeitlichen Änderungen, die die Richtung Erde-Planet im Laufe der Zeit erfährt. Seit Kopernikus das Häuflein der Urteilsfähigen davon überzeugt hatte, daß die Sonne bei diesem Vorgang als ruhend, die Planeten aber—einschließlich der Erde—als um die Sonne bewegt aufzufassen seien, zeigte sich als erstes großes Problem: die Bestimmung der "wahren" Bewegungen der Planeten einschließlich der Erde, wie sie etwa auf dem nächsten Fixstern einem dort befindlichen Beobachter sichtbar wären.

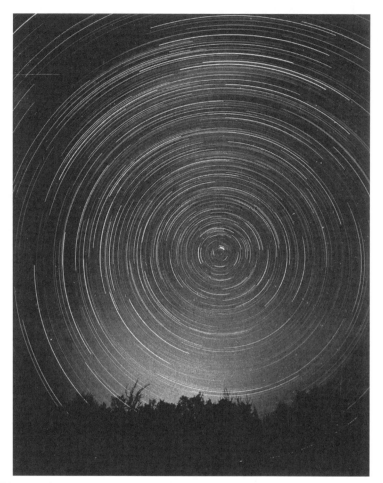

Figure 16. A rotating coordinate frame of reference. The coadjoint orbits $\mathcal{O}_\nu$ associated to the dual $\hat{G}$ of the Heisenberg nilpotent Lie group G provide in the natural way a rotating coordinate frame of reference ($\nu \neq 0$). The Kepplerian strategy to detect the differential phase coordinate of the planetary orbit is based on a rotating coordinate frame of reference.

Das zweite Problem lag in der Frage: Nach welchen mathematischen Gesetzen vollziehen sich diese Bewegungen? Es ist klar, daß die Lösung des zweiten Problems, wenn sie überhaupt dem menschlichen Geiste erreichbar wäre, die Lösung des ersten voraussetzte. Denn man muß einen Vorgang zuerst kennen, bevor man eine auf diesen Vorgang bezügliche Theorie prüfen kann.

Kepler erreichte die Lösung des ersten Problems durch einen wahrhaft genialen Einfall, der ihm die Bestimmung der "wahren" Gestalt der Erdbahn ermöglichte: Um die Erdbahn konstruieren zu können, braucht man neben der Sonne einen zweiten festen Punkt im planetarischen Raum. Hat man einen solchen Punkt, so kann man—indem man ihn und die Sonne als Fixpunkte von Winkelmessungen verwendet—die wahre Gestalt der

Erdbahn nach denselben Methoden der Triangulationsberechnungen (Dreiecksberechnung) bestimmen, die man allgemein bei der Herstellung von Landkarten zu verwenden pflegt.

Woher aber einen solchen zweiten Fixpunkt nehmen, wenn doch alle sichtbaren Objekte außer der Sonne (im einzelnen) unbekannte Bewegungen ausführen? Keplers Antwort: Man kennt mit großer Genauigkeit die scheinbare Bewegung des Planeten Mars und damit auch die Zeit seines Umlaufs um die Sonne ("Mars-Jahr"). Jedesmal, wenn ein Mars-Jahr vergangen ist, dürfte sich Mars an derselben Stelle des (planetaren) Raumes befinden. Beschränkt man sich zunächst auf die Benutzung solcher Zeitpunkte, so repräsentiert für diese der Planet Mars einen festen Punkt des planetaren Raumes, den man bei der Triangulation als Fixpunkt verwenden darf.

Dieses Prinzip benutzend bestimmte Kepler zunächst die wahre Bewegung der Erde im planetaren Raum. Da nun die Erde selbst zu jeder Zeit als Triangulationspunkt verwendet werden konnte, war er auch imstande, die wahren Bewegungen der übrigen Planeten aus den Beobachtungen zu bestimmen. Dadurch gewann Kepler die Grundlage für die Bestimmung der drei fundamentalen Gesetze, die mit seinem Namen für alle Zeiten verknüpft sind. Aus seinem wunderbaren Lebenswerke erkennen wir es besonders schön, daß aus bloßer Empirie allein die Erkenntnis nicht erblühen kann, sondern nur aus dem Vergleich von Erdachtem mit dem Beobachteten.

(English translation)

Kepler's life was devoted to solving a double problem. The sun and the planets alter their apparent position with respect to the background of the fixed stars in a complicated manner that is directly observable. What had been observed and recorded with great dilligence were not their actual motions in space, but rather the temporal changes that the direction pointing from the earth to the planet undergoes over the course of time. When that tiny group of those competent to judge were convinced by Copernicus that in this process it is the sun that is to be regarded as stationary and that the planets—including the earth—revolve about the sun, the first, major problem emerged: How to determine the "true" motions of the planets, including the earth, and how these motions would be perceived on the next fixed star to an observer located there.

The second problem lay in the question: According to which mathematical laws did these movements take place? It is obvious that the solution to the second question, if indeed it were fathomable to the human mind, presupposed the solution to the first question, for it would be necessary to know the process before it would be possible to test a theory relating to this process.

Kepler found the solution to the first problem through a truly ingeneous insight which made it possible for him to determine the "true" shape of the earth's orbit. In order to be able to construct the orbit of the earth one needs to have a second fixed point in planetary space in addition to the sun. If one has such a point, then using this point and the sun as fixed points for angular measurements, one can determine the true shape of the earth's orbit using the same methods of triangulation calculation (trigonometric calculations) that are generally used in the production of maps.

But where to find such a fixed point when all visible objects except for the sun (in particular) make unknown movements? Kepler's answer: The apparent motion of the planet Mars is known with great precision and thus also the period of time for its rotation around the sun (the "Mars year"). Every time that a Mars year passes, Mars is presumably at the same point in (planetary) space. If one initially restricts oneself to using such time points, then the planet Mars represents for these time points a firm point in planetary space that can be used as a fixed point in the triangulation calculations.

Using this principle, Kepler first determined the true motion of the earth in planetary space. Since now the earth itself could be used at any time as a triangulation point, he was then able to determine from his observations the true movements of the other planets as well. In this way Kepler derived the basis for the determination of the three fundamental laws with which his name has been linked for all time. From his wonderful life's work we can see especially clearly that knowledge cannot sprout from empirical data alone, but only from the comparison of what has been theorized with that which has been observed.

It is actually the synchronization effect of the determination of the baseline through the Sun, clearly described by Einstein, which makes Keppler's planetary dynamics only fictituously static. Even Hermann Weyl did not observe these dynamical aspects in his commentaries to the geometrical symmetries discovered in the *Mysterium Cosmographicum* ([369]). However, Keppler's dynamic physical astronomy, exposed in the form of a planetary clockwork in his greatest book, *Astronomia Nova*, is basically not a gravitational theory, but a spatiotemporal cross-correlational phase–frequency analysis of intralevel causal interaction control in quadrature format. In terms of coherent signal processing, the Keppler phase history triangulation procedure of eccentric circular orbits takes the form of intralevel in-plane encoding of resonant interactions. The stratigraphic time is clocked by the cycle times:

- The Kepplerian spatiotemporal strategy of the dynamics of physical astronomy forms a phase cycling scheme for the holographic reconstruction of planetary motions. It imposes a cyclic ordering structure by synchronous cross-sectional quadrature filtering of the phase histories of eccentric circular orbits in contiguous local frequency encoding subband multichannels with respect to the rotating coordinate frame of quadrature reference.

The Kepplerian spatiotemporal synchronization procedure allows for the bearings of the observer's location on the moving Earth to be taken from an immobilized orbiting platform by strobing the motion of the platform. This most ingenious *inversion* of the perspective via reflection of the baseline of an internal observer by an external observer and adopting a spatiotemporal cross-correlational point of view by freezing the motion of a phase quadrature reference to achieve an external observer residing on a stationary platform led Keppler, as a radical Copernican astronomer, to the stroboscopic and synchronous cross-sectional quadrature filtering of the phase histories of the Earth's orbit in the ecliptic plane of the helioeccentric frame. By an application of the numerical L^2 exhaustion technique of Archimedes and a treatment of the Earth as a planet like the others, he succeeded in triangulating the orbits of the other solar planets as well.

The Kepplerian quadrature conchoid trajectory construction, as presented in the *Astronomia Nova* ([305], [327]), determines the planetary orbits with respect to the helioeccentric frame by an a posteriori approach. As a response to the revolutionary geometrical language of the planetary spheres used in the *Mysterium Cosmographicum*, such an approach was called for by Tycho de Brahe, who disposed of a reliable phase-sensitive data base of planetary motion reconstruction. Tycho, however, as an ingenious observer, was not able to evaluate his data base in a congenial way so that it could provide deeper insight into the laws governing celestial dynamics.

Keppler interrupted his work on the Mars commentaries in order to complete his book *Paralipomena quibus Astronomiæ Pars Optica Traditur* (1604), which was geared toward the preparation of the tools from projective geometry and vision necessary to evaluate Tycho de Brahe's careful data base. It introduces the fundamental concept of *focus* and allows the practicing observational astronomer to understand Keppler's quadrature conchoid trajectory construction by an embedding of the focal plane at infinity into the set of leaves of the foliated superencoded projective space which is parametrized by the stratigraphic line of cycle times. Unfortunately, the projective ansatz of Keppler's physical astronomy and its impact have not been acknowledged by the interpreters of the *Astronomia Nova*.

The basic idea of testing the area law approximation is to cross-correlate the true orbit with respect to the helioeccentric frame with a rotating coordinate frame of quadrature reference. In terms of Keppler's vocabulary of planetary motion analysis, the procedure is accomplished by a straightening of the reference unit circle. The unrolling of the circumference gives rise to an associated pulse timing diagram of control along the stratigraphic time line $\mathbb{R}$. As a consequence, the setting underlying the quadrature conchoid trajectory method is a spatiotemporal Hilbert bundle. It may be conceived as a duality construction valid for the Heisenberg group $G \hookrightarrow \mathbf{Sp}(4, \mathbb{R})$. The historian Bruce Stephenson notes ([327], p. 109):

> Only now did he realize that those shortened distances, laid out along diameters of a circle which was not the orbit, were just about right to extend from the sun to the oval that *was* the orbit. The impact of this realization, as he wrote, was like awakening from sleep. Keppler did not remark here, although it must have been obvious to him from his earlier work, that the circular sectors with vertex at the sun *exactly* measured the sum of however many of these new distances were contained in them.

Apart from the Archimedes exhaustion, another root of Keppler's way of thinking lies in Greek philosophy, derived primarily from Aristotle. By adopting the point of view of Aristotelian physics, in which the elements of the spatiotemporal space are infinitesimal magnitudes but never zero, and so by envisaging time ($\chi\rho\acute{o}\nu o\varsigma$) not as a flowing instant as in the Newtonian dynamics but as a clocked sequence of *coexistences* on the stratigraphic time line $\mathbb{R}$, Keppler's reconstruction of the planetary motion required an accumulation of the time delays in paths ([3]) to generate the perfect reconstruction analysis–synthesis filter bank output by accumulating the phase histories evolving in subband channels. The time interval required to traverse an arc of the planet's orbit, the time delay, or *mora*, corresponds to the concept of phase, which is fundamental in quantum holography and clinical MRI. In mathematical terms, the Kepplerian quadrature conchoid trajectory construction performs a fibration over the bi-infinite stratigraphic time line $\mathbb{R}$ with respect to the rotating frame of quadrature reference and a synchronous cross-sectional quadrature filtering of phase histories of eccentric circular orbits. The noncommutative geometrical analysis approach suggests the introduction of a projectively completed, symplectic affine plane $\mathbf{P}(\mathbb{R} \times \mathcal{O}_\nu)$ ($\nu \neq 0$) of resonant intralevel interaction control in phase-sensitive quadrature format in order to encode the differential phases by stroboscopic and synchronous observations as well as the local frequencies of the planetary motion. These variables of the planar coordinatization are monotonically increasing along the apsidal line. In the helioeccentric context, the apsidal line is directed from the aphelion through the real Sun to the perihelion and presents the natural symmetry axis of the orbital plane:

- The phase-sensitive quadrature format is accomplished by an orthogonal projection of the phase-shifted distances onto the contiguous fibers formed by the implicit radii of reference within the orbital plane.
- The symmetry axis of the orbital plane provokes a decomposition $\mathcal{O}_+ \cup \mathcal{O}_-$ into disjoint open half-planes which implement linear gradients of opposite polarity.
- Keppler's quadrature conchoid trajectory construction performs the coadjoint orbit merging by cutting the orbital plane along the apsidal line through the real Sun.

Specifically, the Kepplerian spatiotemporal procedure amounts to the introduction of a stroboscopic and synchronous sampling lattice into the phase histories. The helioeccentric circle forms the reference for the bank of contiguous local frequency encoding subband multichannels separating stroboscopic and synchronous observations by *integral* revolutions:

- The quadrature conchoid trajectory construction implements the Kepplerian spatiotemporal strategy of stroboscopic and synchronous cross-sectional quadrature filtering of phase histories of helioeccentric orbits by means of the dual $\hat{G}$.
- The phase histories are evolving in contiguous local frequency encoding subband multichannels in quadrature format. With respect to the rotating coordinate frame of quadrature reference the channels form a filter bank of matched filter type in a projectively completed, symplectic affine plane of resonant intralevel control.

Thus the first law is a consequence of the second fundamental law of planetary motion, which was found chronologically earlier than the first law by Keppler's analysis. Conversely, the flatness of the planetary orbits implies the square integrability of the quadrature phase histories. As a consequence it follows that the Kepplerian spatiotemporal quadrature Hilbert bundle strategy admits a coherent signal processing interpretation which can be used for the perfect orbit reconstruction and consequently for navigational purposes. Keppler was the first astronomer whose heliocentric frame approach transformed the dynamics of physical astronomy into a theory which provided predictions of an error not exceeding the maximal error estimates of the measurements.

From a mathematical point of view, the quadrature conchoid trajectory construction suggests a pairing of the differential phase x and the local frequency y as real coordinates with respect to the rotating frame of quadrature reference. The swapped copy of this pairing leads to the real quadrature cell matrix

$$\begin{pmatrix} x & -y \\ y & x \end{pmatrix},$$

which represents a direct linear similitude of the plane $\mathbb{R} \oplus \mathbb{R}$. Considered as an element of the realification

$$\mathbb{C}(\mathbb{R} \oplus \mathbb{R})$$

of the field $\mathbb{C}$ of complex numbers, it represents the Kepplerian dynamics of the heliocentric frame in the symplectic affine plane $\mathbb{R} \oplus \mathbb{R}$ of intralevel causal interaction control in quadrature format. In the multiplicative group $\mathbf{GO}^{+}(2, \mathbb{R})$ of the commutative field $\mathbb{C}(\mathbb{R} \oplus \mathbb{R})$, the multiplication law of the quadrature cell matrices which are intrinsic to the quadrature conchoid trajectory construction reads

$$\begin{pmatrix} x & -y \\ y & x \end{pmatrix} \begin{pmatrix} x' & -y' \\ y' & x' \end{pmatrix} = \begin{pmatrix} xx' - yy' & -(yx' + xy') \\ yx' + xy' & xx' - yy' \end{pmatrix}.$$

The quadrature cell matrices admit the decomposition

$$\begin{pmatrix} x & -y \\ y & x \end{pmatrix} = \begin{pmatrix} x & 0 \\ 0 & x \end{pmatrix} + \begin{pmatrix} y & 0 \\ 0 & y \end{pmatrix} \begin{pmatrix} 0 & -1 \\ 1 & 0 \end{pmatrix}$$

corresponding to the decomposition of the real and imaginary part. Identification of the numbers $r \in \mathbb{R}$ with the diagonal matrices

$$r \begin{pmatrix} 1 & 0 \\ 0 & 1 \end{pmatrix} = \begin{pmatrix} r & 0 \\ 0 & r \end{pmatrix}$$

embeds the additive group $\mathbb{R}$ into the multiplicative group of homothetic transformations of the symplectic affine plane $\mathbb{R} \oplus \mathbb{R}$. The infinitesimal generator of the one-dimensional compact Lie group

$$\mathbf{SO}(2, \mathbb{R}) \hookrightarrow \mathbf{SL}(2, \mathbb{R})$$

of planar rotations which describes the circular dynamical symmetry of the quadrature reference by the compact orbit

$$\mathbb{T} \hookrightarrow \mathbb{R} \oplus \mathbb{R},$$

the Kepplerian reference circle group, is given by the alternating matrix

$$J = \begin{pmatrix} 0 & -1 \\ 1 & 0 \end{pmatrix}$$

of phase-sensitive quadrature detection. Due to the identity

$$J^4 = \mathrm{id}_{\mathbb{R} \oplus \mathbb{R}},$$

it admits period 4.

With respect to the orthonormal energetic frame of reference of the plane $\mathbb{R} \oplus \mathbb{R}$, the set of quadrature cell matrices represents the *Abelian* subgroup $\mathbf{GO}^+(2, \mathbb{R}) \hookrightarrow$ $\mathbf{GL}(2, \mathbb{R})$ of nonzero direct linear similitudes of the symplectic affine plane $\mathbb{R} \oplus \mathbb{R}$, which reflect the stroboscopic and synchronous quadrature format design of the eccentric Kepplerian clockwork dynamics. In clinical MRI, this clockwork is implemented by the traces of the tuned-in Heisenberg helices:

- The group $\mathbf{GO}(2, \mathbb{R})$ of all bijective linear similitudes of the symplectic affine plane $\mathbb{R} \oplus \mathbb{R}$ is the direct product of its normal subgroups consisting of the homothetic transformations of $\mathbb{R} \oplus \mathbb{R}$ of ratio > 0, isomorphic to the multiplicative group $\mathbb{R}^{\star}_+$ of strictly positive real numbers, and the orthogonal group $\mathbf{O}(2, \mathbb{R})$.
- The centralizer of the orthogonal group $\mathbf{O}(2, \mathbb{R})$ in $\mathbf{GL}(2, \mathbb{R})$ is the multiplicative group of homothetic transformations of $\mathbb{R} \oplus \mathbb{R}$.
- The group $\mathbf{GO}(2, \mathbb{R})$ is the normalizer in $\mathbf{GL}(2, \mathbb{R})$ of its subgroup $\mathbf{O}(2, \mathbb{R}) \hookrightarrow$ $\mathbf{GO}(2, \mathbb{R})$ of orthogonal transformations or linear isometries of $\mathbb{R} \oplus \mathbb{R}$.
- The commutative group $\mathbf{GO}^+(2, \mathbb{R})$ forms a normal subgroup of index 2 of the non-Abelian group $\mathbf{GO}(2, \mathbb{R}) \hookrightarrow \mathbf{GL}(2, \mathbb{R})$.

The commutative multiplication law of the quadrature cell matrices in $\mathbf{GO}^+(2, \mathbb{R})$ reads

$$\begin{pmatrix} x & -y \\ y & x \end{pmatrix} \begin{pmatrix} x' & -y' \\ y' & x' \end{pmatrix} = \begin{pmatrix} xx' - yy' & -(yx' + xy') \\ yx' + xy' & xx' - yy' \end{pmatrix}.$$

The conjugation identity

$$\begin{pmatrix} 1 & 0 \\ 0 & -1 \end{pmatrix} \begin{pmatrix} x & -y \\ y & x \end{pmatrix} \begin{pmatrix} 1 & 0 \\ 0 & -1 \end{pmatrix}^{-1} = \begin{pmatrix} x & y \\ -y & x \end{pmatrix}$$

yields the area law via the central angular momentum form

$$|w|^2 = \det w,$$

the invariance of the multiplicator

$$\mu \begin{pmatrix} x & -y \\ y & x \end{pmatrix} = x^2 + y^2,$$

as well as the moment map associated to the rotational *curvature* form

$$(w, w') \rightsquigarrow \mathfrak{I} w \bar{w}'$$

for $w, w' \in \mathbb{C}$. The mapping

$$\mu : \mathbf{GO}(2, \mathbb{R}) \longrightarrow \mathbb{R}_+^\star$$

defines a group homomorphism of $\mathbf{GO}(2, \mathbb{R})$ onto the multiplicative group $\mathbb{R}_+^\star$ so that the identity

$$\mathbf{O}(2, \mathbb{R}) = \ker(\mu)$$

holds. The mapping $\det / \mu$ defines a group homomorphism of $\mathbf{GO}(2, \mathbb{R})$ onto the multiplicative group $\mathbb{Z}/2\mathbb{Z} = \{1, -1\}$ so that

$$\mathbf{GO}^+(2, \mathbb{R}) = \ker\left(\frac{\det}{\mu}\right).$$

For the realification of $w \in \mathbb{C} - \{0\}$ in $\mathbf{GO}^+(2, \mathbb{R})$, the inverse of the associated quadrature cell matrix reads, in terms of the complex conjugate with reciprocal multiplicator,

$$\left(\mu\begin{pmatrix} x & -y \\ y & x \end{pmatrix}\right)^{-1} = \mu\left(\begin{pmatrix} x & -y \\ y & x \end{pmatrix}^{-1}\right),$$

as follows:

$$\begin{pmatrix} x & -y \\ y & x \end{pmatrix}^{-1} = \frac{1}{x^2 + y^2}\begin{pmatrix} x & y \\ -y & x \end{pmatrix}.$$

- The bijective similitudes w belonging to the subgroup $\mathbf{GO}^+(2, \mathbb{R}) \hookrightarrow \mathbf{GO}(2, \mathbb{R})$ represent exactly those endomorphisms of the symplectic affine plane $\mathbb{R} \oplus \mathbb{R}$ which commute with the direct linear similitude of the alternating matrix J of phase-sensitive quadrature detection.
- The group $\mathbf{GO}^+(2, \mathbb{R})$ of nonzero direct linear similitudes of the symplectic affine plane $\mathbb{R} \oplus \mathbb{R}$ is the centralizer in $\mathbf{GL}(2, \mathbb{R})$ of any direct linear similitude which is not a homothetic transformation of $\mathbb{R} \oplus \mathbb{R}$.
- The set $\mathbf{GO}^+(2, \mathbb{R}) \cup \{0\}$ of direct linear similitudes of the symplectic affine plane $\mathbb{R} \oplus \mathbb{R}$ is a commutative subfield $\mathbb{C}(\mathbb{R} \oplus \mathbb{R}) \cong \mathbb{C}$ of the real algebra of endomorphisms of $\mathbb{R} \oplus \mathbb{R}$ with the standard symplectic form $(w, w') \rightsquigarrow \Im w \bar{w}'$ as the rotational curvature form.
- The rotational curvature form is just the second fundamental form of the set of direct similitudes $\mathbb{C}(\mathbb{R} \oplus \mathbb{R})$.

The endomorphisms of the symplectic affine plane $\mathbb{R} \oplus \mathbb{R}$ which commute anti-symmetrically with the direct linear similitude represented by the alternating matrix J of quadrature phase detection show that the indirect linear similitudes of the plane $\mathbb{R} \oplus \mathbb{R}$ can be represented with respect to an orthogonal frame of reference of $\mathbb{R} \oplus \mathbb{R}$

as self-adjoint endomorphisms of quadrature cell matrices

$$\begin{pmatrix} x & y \\ y & -x \end{pmatrix} \in \mathbf{GO}(2, \mathbb{R})$$

with determinant form and multiplicator

$$-|w|^2 = -\det w.$$

In particular, the reflections

$$\begin{pmatrix} \cos \varphi & \sin \varphi \\ \sin \varphi & -\cos \varphi \end{pmatrix} \in \mathbf{GO}(2, \mathbb{R})$$

through the axes of angles $\frac{1}{2}\pi$ to $\mathbb{R} \times 0$ include the involutory flip matrix

$$\begin{pmatrix} 1 & 0 \\ 0 & -1 \end{pmatrix} \in \mathbf{GO}(2, \mathbb{R}).$$

Inspection of the spectrum shows that each indirect linear similitude of the plane $\mathbb{R} \oplus \mathbb{R}$ forms a reflection or symmetry about the homogeneous line spanned by the vector

$$(y, 1 - x).$$

For $x = 1, y = 1$, the indirect linear similitude

$$\begin{pmatrix} 1 & 1 \\ 1 & -1 \end{pmatrix} \in \mathbf{GO}(2, \mathbb{R})$$

of multiplicator -2 gives rise to the unique continuous involutory automorphism

$$w \rightsquigarrow \bar{w}$$

of the realification $\mathbb{C}(\mathbb{R} \oplus \mathbb{R})$ of the field $\mathbb{C}$.

The multiplicator homomorphism μ allows for a transition from the direct affine isometries of multiplicator $a = +1$ to the indirect affine isometries of multiplicator $a = -1$. It implies the rephasing or forcing to reconverge the process of the spin echo teleportation phenomenon by means of Hahn echoes. The spin echo pulse sequence was devised by Erwin Louis Hahn for nuclear magnetic resonance spectroscopy in 1950. It is the most commonly used pulse sequence in clinical MRI (Figure 17). Although faster spin echo techniques are available, such as FSE imaging, which use the idle time to measure phase-coherent wavelet responses from adjacent tomographic slices or different phase-encoding levels, the spin echo pulse sequence, as applied in the two-dimensional Fourier MRI reconstructive method, is still a workhorse of routine clinical MRI examinations. Most magnetic resonance images of body organs and the musculoskeletal system are presented using spin echo sequences which also are extensively used in nuclear magnetic resonance spectroscopy:

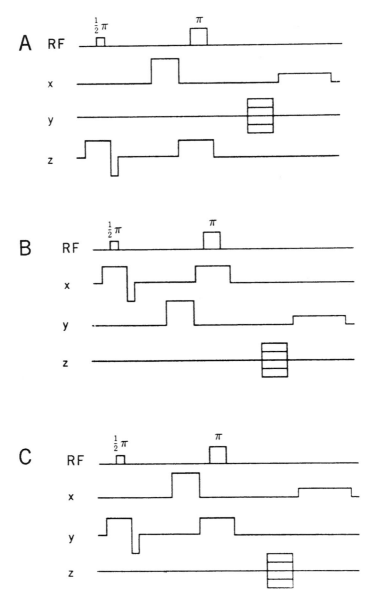

Figure 17. Timing diagrams of standard spin echo pulse sequences along the stratigraphic time line $\mathbb{R}$: Transverse (A), sagittal (B), and coronal MRI scans (C). RF means radiofrequency. The pulse sequences have to be synchronized with the switching protocol of the affine-linear magnetic field gradients.

- The refocusing procedure of conventional spin echo imaging by phase conjugation flip depends upon the fact that the connected normal subgroup $\mathbf{Is}^+(2, \mathbb{R})$ of direct affine isometries has index 2 in the non-Abelian, disconnected Lie group $\mathbf{Is}(2, \mathbb{R}) \hookrightarrow \mathbf{GA}(2, \mathbb{R})$ of all affine isometries of the symplectic affine plane $\mathbb{R} \oplus \mathbb{R}$.

- The quotient group $\mathbf{Is}(2, \mathbb{R})/\mathbf{Is}^+(2, \mathbb{R})$ is isomorphic to the group $\mathbb{Z}/2\mathbb{Z}$.

In gradient recalled echo imaging, the analogy to the refocusing procedure by spatial linear rewinder gradients should be observed. This procedure actually depends upon the fact that the group $\mathbf{SA}(\mathbb{R})$ of affine transvections has index 2 in the subgroup of $\mathbf{GA}(\mathbb{R})$ which is generated by the reflections or symmetries of the real line $\mathbb{R}$ about an arbitrary point. To increase the tissue differentiation and enhance the signal-to-noise ratio, a spoiled gradient recalled echo sequence can be used.

In conventional spin echo imaging, the spin echoes between water and fat come back into phase at the center of every echo, even though they differ in local frequency and are spatially misregistered. In gradient echo imaging, however, water and fat protons do not generally come into phase coherence at the center of the echo, since gradient recalled echo imaging lacks the refocusing pulse which accomplishes the rephasing task in conventional spin echo imaging. Therefore, fat and water fall out of phase in gradient recalled echo scans. The characteristic appeareance of this type of artifact is a sharply defined black rim around objects such as muscle fascicles on gradient recalled echo images. This artifact arises from boundary pixels that contain both fat and water protons and is manifest by an eerie black halo in all pixels along the entire fat-water interface.

For neurofunctional MRI of cerebral cortical activities it is important to observe that gradient recalled echoes do not refocus the dephasing effects of local inhomogeneities of magnetic flux density associated with the presence of deoxyhemoglobin. If spin echoes are used instead of gradient recalled echoes, then such dephasing effects will be refocused, provided that there is no significant diffusion of water molecules through the linear magnetic field gradients. However, if the water molecules diffuse through local magnetic field gradients during the echo time, then this will result in imperfect refocusing effects and hence to response loss in conventional spin echo pulse sequences:

- The direct linear similitude in $\mathbf{GO}^+(2, \mathbb{R})$ admitting the alternating matrix J of quadrature phase detection generates the subgroup $\mathbf{SO}(2, \mathbb{R}) \hookrightarrow \mathbf{O}(2, \mathbb{R})$ of planar rotations. It is isomorphic to the maximal compact, connected component $K \cong \mathbb{T}$ of the Iwasawa decomposition of $\mathbf{SL}(2, \mathbb{R})$.

- The torus group $K \hookrightarrow \mathbf{SL}(2, \mathbb{R})$ is driven by the center frequency $\nu \neq 0$ of the unitary character χ_ν associated with the planar coadjoint orbit $\mathbf{P}(\mathbb{R} \times \mathcal{O}_\nu) \hookrightarrow \mathbf{P}(\mathbb{R} \times \mathrm{Lie}(G)^\star)$ through the driving frequency $\nu \in \hat{C} - \{0\}$ of the rotating coordinate frame of quadrature reference of the projectively completed, tomographic slice $\mathbf{P}(\mathbb{R} \times \mathcal{O}_\nu)$, and frequency selected from the canonical foliation in projective space.

- At the Lie algebra level, any unitary linear representation of the group of dynamical symmetries $\mathbf{Mp}(2, \mathbb{R})$ is diagonalizable under the action of the generator $J \in \mathbf{GO}^+(2, \mathbb{R})$ of K with eigenvalues in the set $\frac{1}{2} i \mathbb{Z}$.

The area law suggests a relationship between the alternating matrix J of phase-sensitive quadrature detection and the special linear group $\mathbf{SL}(2, \mathbb{R})$. Let $\{e_+, e_-, h\}$ denote the standard basis of the three-dimensional non-Abelian simple Lie algebra Lie $(\mathbf{SL}(2, \mathbb{R}))$. Then the traceless matrices

$$e_+ = \begin{pmatrix} 0 & 1 \\ 0 & 0 \end{pmatrix}, \qquad e_- = \begin{pmatrix} 0 & 0 \\ 1 & 0 \end{pmatrix}, \qquad h = \begin{pmatrix} 1 & 0 \\ 0 & -1 \end{pmatrix}$$

are complex linear combinations of the famous Pauli spin matrices and satisfy the commutation relations

$$[h, e_+] = +2e_+, \qquad [h, e_-] = -2e_-, \qquad [e_+, e_-] = h.$$

These equations characterize Lie $(\mathbf{SL}(2, \mathbb{R}))$ completely. Notice that conjugation by J acts by transpositions on the set $\{e_+, e_-\}$ and reverses the sign of the element h as used by the nuclear spin echo method. More precisely, the adjoint representation $\mathrm{Ad}_{\mathbf{SL}(2,\mathbb{R})}$ of $\mathbf{SL}(2, \mathbb{R})$ acts on Lie $(\mathbf{SL}(2, \mathbb{R}))$ by conjugation as

$$\mathrm{Ad}_{\mathbf{SL}(2,\mathbb{R})} J(e_+) = -e_-, \qquad \mathrm{Ad}_{\mathbf{SL}(2,\mathbb{R})} J(e_-) = -e_+, \qquad \mathrm{Ad}_{\mathbf{SL}(2,\mathbb{R})} J(h) = -h.$$

Moreover, the element

$$(e_+ - e_-) \in \mathrm{Lie}\,(\mathbf{SL}(2, \mathbb{R}))$$

is the infinitesimal generator of the maximal compact subgroup $K \cong \mathbf{SO}(2, \mathbb{R})$ inside the Lie group $\mathbf{SL}(2, \mathbb{R})$. It generates the one-dimensional Lie algebra of $\mathbf{SO}(2, \mathbb{R})$ and provides the identity

$$J = \exp\left[\frac{1}{2} \pi (e_+ - e_-) \right] \in \mathbf{SL}(2, \mathbb{R}).$$

Identification of J with the imaginary unit i establishes that the Kepplerian quadrature conchoid trajectory construction in quadrature format is far from being obvious. Its fibration over the bi-infinite stratigraphic time line $\mathbb{R}$ with respect to the rotating frame of quadrature reference gives rise to a coordinatization of the symplectic affine plane of intralevel causal interaction control in terms of the complex variable

$$w = x + yi \in \mathbb{C}.$$

Thus the construction of the field $\mathbb{C}$ of complex numbers, based on the coordinatization process of the Kepplerian quadrature conchoid trajectory construction, is *dynamically* in character and therefore independent of the historically earlier, stationary, algebraic constructions due to Geronimo Cardano's *Ars Magna* of 1545 and Rafaele Bombelli's *Algebra* of 1572:

- The quadrature conchoid trajectory construction in the symplectic affine plane implements the quadrature format design of the stroboscopic and synchronous cycling system.
- The eccentric phase-frequency cycling scheme representing the conchoid trajectory is accomplished by transition from the polar coordinates of the Kepplerian unit circle to the symplectic coordinates of the unitary representation induced from a one-dimensional representation.

Transition to the reverse-phase history in the symplectic affine plane of intralevel causal interaction control in quadrature format is accomplished by the nonlinear mapping

$$w \rightsquigarrow \bar{w}.$$

The complex conjugate $\bar{w} \in \mathbb{C}$ which gives rise to the area law or central angular momentum identity

$$|w|^2 = \bar{w}w = \det w$$

is given by the conjugation action of the element $h = -\mathrm{Ad}_{\mathbf{SL}(2,\mathbb{R})}J(h) \in \mathrm{Lie}\,(\mathbf{SL}(2,\mathbb{R}))$ as

$$\begin{pmatrix} 1 & 0 \\ 0 & -1 \end{pmatrix} \begin{pmatrix} x & -y \\ y & x \end{pmatrix} \begin{pmatrix} 1 & 0 \\ 0 & -1 \end{pmatrix}^{-1} = \begin{pmatrix} x & y \\ -y & x \end{pmatrix}.$$

In particular, conjugation transfers the alternating matrix J of quadrature phase detection into its inverse

$$J^{-1} = -J.$$

More generally, for $w \neq 0$ the inverse of the associated quadrature cell matrix in terms of the complex conjugate reads

$$\begin{pmatrix} x & -y \\ y & x \end{pmatrix}^{-1} = \frac{1}{x^2 + y^2} \begin{pmatrix} x & y \\ -y & x \end{pmatrix}.$$

An application of the corner turn isomorphism which leaves as its pivot line the center line C of the Heisenberg nilpotent Lie group G pointwise fixed yields the real *isotropic* realization of G in block form as the group of unipotent upper triangular matrices

$$\left\{ \begin{pmatrix} 1 & -y & x & z \\ 0 & 1 & 0 & x \\ 0 & 0 & 1 & y \\ 0 & 0 & 0 & 1 \end{pmatrix} \,\middle|\, x, y, z \in \mathbb{R} \right\}.$$

The real isotropic realization implements the area law via the central angular momentum form

$$\det \begin{pmatrix} x_1 & y_1 \\ x_2 & y_2 \end{pmatrix}.$$

Indeed, the multiplication law of G reads

$$
\begin{pmatrix} 1 & -y_1 & x_1 & z_1 \\ 0 & 1 & 0 & x_1 \\ 0 & 0 & 1 & y_1 \\ 0 & 0 & 0 & 1 \end{pmatrix}
\begin{pmatrix} 1 & -y_2 & x_2 & z_2 \\ 0 & 1 & 0 & x_2 \\ 0 & 0 & 1 & y_2 \\ 0 & 0 & 0 & 1 \end{pmatrix}
$$

$$
= \begin{pmatrix} 1 & -(y_1 + y_2) & x_1 + x_2 & z_1 + z_2 + \det \begin{pmatrix} x_1 & y_1 \\ x_2 & y_2 \end{pmatrix} \\ 0 & 1 & 0 & x_1 + x_2 \\ 0 & 0 & 1 & y_1 + y_2 \\ 0 & 0 & 0 & 1 \end{pmatrix}.
$$

The inverse in G therefore is given by the matrix

$$
\begin{pmatrix} 1 & -y & x & z \\ 0 & 1 & 0 & x \\ 0 & 0 & 1 & y \\ 0 & 0 & 0 & 1 \end{pmatrix}^{-1}
= \begin{pmatrix} 1 & y & -x & -z \\ 0 & 1 & 0 & -x \\ 0 & 0 & 1 & -y \\ 0 & 0 & 0 & 1 \end{pmatrix}.
$$

In block form, the one-dimensional center of G is given by the subgroup of matrices

$$
C = \left\{ \begin{pmatrix} 1 & 0 & 0 & z \\ 0 & 1 & 0 & 0 \\ 0 & 0 & 1 & 0 \\ 0 & 0 & 0 & 1 \end{pmatrix} \;\middle|\; z \in \mathbb{R} \right\}
$$

and therefore is isomorphic to the real line $\mathbb{R}$:

- The three-dimensional Heisenberg group G is a closed subgroup of the symplectic group $\mathbf{Sp}(4, \mathbb{R})$.
- The Kepplerian spatiotemporal procedure of phase history triangulation of eccentric circular orbits leads to the real isotropic realization of G.

The differential operator associated to the natural left-invariant metric of the sub-Riemannian manifold G is the left-invariant sub-Laplacian $\mathcal{L}_G$ on G. Notice that the sub-Riemannian geometry is to the sub-Laplacian differential operator in the subelliptic realm what Riemannian geometry is to the Laplacian differential operator in the elliptic realm. In terms of the coordinates of the dual pairing presentation of G, the left-invariant sub-Laplacian differential operator $\mathcal{L}_G$ takes the form of a

Hörmander sum of squares

$$\mathcal{L}_G = -\frac{1}{2}\left[\left(\frac{\partial}{\partial x} - y\frac{\partial}{\partial z}\right)^2 + \left(\frac{\partial}{\partial y} + x\frac{\partial}{\partial z}\right)^2\right].$$

The analytic hypoellipticity of the left-invariant sub-Laplacian differential operator $\mathcal{L}_G$ implies Chow's condition of geometrical control theory in terms of Lie brackets. The solutions of the system of Hamilton-Jacobi equations associated with the principal symbol of $\mathcal{L}_G$ project onto the constant-velocity local length-minimizing curves with respect to the natural left-invariant sub-Riemannian metric of G:

- The natural left-invariant sub-Riemannian metric of G is the Legendre transform of the principal symbol of $\mathcal{L}_G$.
- The topology induced on G by the left-invariant sub-Riemannian metric is the original topology of G.
- The geodesics with respect to the natural left-invariant sub-Riemannian metric of G are either lines in the confocal plane or Heisenberg helices.
- Any two points of G can be joined by a minimizing geodesic.

The Heisenberg group G has two presentations that are particularly important in applications. It is standard that the radical of a bundled alternating bilinear form is the only invariant of the bundled form. Therefore, the dual pairing presentation of G is isomorphic to the *basic* presentation of the Heisenberg group G, which is given by the multiplication law of the unipotent matrices

$$\left\{\begin{pmatrix} 1 & \bar{w} & \frac{1}{2}|w|^2 + zi \\ 0 & 1 & w \\ 0 & 0 & 1 \end{pmatrix} \,\middle|\, w \in \mathbb{C}, z \in \mathbb{R}\right\}.$$

Computations are usually easiest in the basic presentation of G because the straight lines through the origin are the one-parameter subgroups. Therefore projective geometry provides an adequate point of view which is in accordance with Einstein's description of Keppler's strategy. Due to the planetary orbit stratification, the Kepplerian temporospatial phase detection strategy leads to the following basic presentation:

- There is a realization of the Heisenberg group G by a faithful matrix representation $G \longrightarrow \mathbf{Sp}(4, \mathbb{R})$ defining the image group as an extension via matrix multiplication.

In terms of the left-invariant vector fields

$$W = \frac{\partial}{\partial w} - \bar{w}\frac{\partial}{\partial z}, \qquad \bar{W} = \frac{\partial}{\partial \bar{w}} + w\frac{\partial}{\partial z},$$

the left-invariant sub-Laplacian differential operator $\mathcal{L}_G$ takes the form

$$\mathcal{L}_G = -\tfrac{1}{2}(W\bar{W} + \bar{W}W).$$

The spectrum of the subelliptic differential operator $\mathcal{L}_G$ is absolutely continuous with uniform multiplicity on the longitudinal center frequency axis $\mathbb{R}$, transverse to the symplectic affine plane $\mathbb{R} \oplus \mathbb{R}$. The density of the spectrum on the longitudinal center frequency axis $\mathbb{R}$ is given by the Pfaffian P_G of G:

- The symmetries of the left-invariant subelliptic differential operator $\mathcal{L}_G$ are reflected in the time reversal, which is implicit in the spin echo methods and the gradient echo imaging methods.

The preceding coordinatization is in accordance with the conventions of stereotaxy. Stereotaxy is a technique of neurosurgery developed for accessing regions in the brain on a predetermined trajectory for the purpose of advanced image-guided diagnosis and therapy. In three-dimensional MRI, the same coordinatization procedure is used by the stereotactic frames of MR-compatible localizer systems attached to a patient's head in a normal supine position ([1]). The stereotactic x axis is directed to the patient's left- to right-hand side, the y axis to the front posterior to anterior, and the z axis to the top of the head inferior to superior. Relying on reference markers, modern stereotactic localizer systems allow access of neuroanatomical target points with an image-guided precision of less than 1 mm in space.

For $w \in \mathbb{C}$, the complex isotropic realization of G reads as the group of matrices

$$
\begin{pmatrix}
1 & \bar{w} & \frac{1}{2}\,|w|^2 + zi \\
0 & 1 & w \\
0 & 0 & 1
\end{pmatrix}.
$$

- The scaling factor $\frac{1}{2}$ in front of the area $|w|^2 = \det w$ adjusts the central angular momentum form of the area law to the Kepplerian phase history triangulation procedure of eccentric circular orbits.

- The complex isotropic realization of G in block form has the advantage that it displays the complex conjugation as a manifestation of the time structure. With respect to the rotating coordinate frame of quadrature reference associated with the spatiotemporal quantization procedure of quantum holography, it is at the basis of the nuclear spin echo teleportation phenomenon.

The multiplication law of the complex isotropic realization is given as

$$
\begin{pmatrix}
1 & \overline{w_1} & \frac{1}{2}\,|w_1|^2 + z_1 i \\
0 & 1 & w_1 \\
0 & 0 & 1
\end{pmatrix}
\begin{pmatrix}
1 & \overline{w_2} & \frac{1}{2}\,|w_2|^2 + z_2 i \\
0 & 1 & w_2 \\
0 & 0 & 1
\end{pmatrix}
$$
$$
= \begin{pmatrix}
1 & \overline{w_1 + w_2} & \frac{1}{2}\,|w_1 + w_2|^2 + \left(\Im(\overline{w_1} w_2) + z_1 + z_2\right)i \\
0 & 1 & w_1 + w_2 \\
0 & 0 & 1
\end{pmatrix},
$$

so that the center consists of the matrices

$$\left\{ \begin{pmatrix} 1 & 0 & zi \\ 0 & 1 & 0 \\ 0 & 0 & 1 \end{pmatrix} \middle| z \in \mathbb{R} \right\}.$$

Therefore the pivot line C is isomorphic to the purely imaginary line

$$C \cong \mathbb{R}i.$$

The inverse of an element in G reads

$$\begin{pmatrix} 1 & \bar{w} & \frac{1}{2}|w|^2 + zi \\ 0 & 1 & w \\ 0 & 0 & 1 \end{pmatrix}^{-1} = \begin{pmatrix} 1 & -\bar{w} & \frac{1}{2}|w|^2 - zi \\ 0 & 1 & -w \\ 0 & 0 & 1 \end{pmatrix},$$

so that the commutator of two elements in G is given as

$$\left[\begin{pmatrix} 1 & \overline{w_1} & \frac{1}{2}|w_1|^2 + z_1 i \\ 0 & 1 & w_1 \\ 0 & 0 & 1 \end{pmatrix}, \begin{pmatrix} 1 & \overline{w_2} & \frac{1}{2}|w_2|^2 + z_2 i \\ 0 & 1 & w_2 \\ 0 & 0 & 1 \end{pmatrix} \right]$$

$$= \begin{pmatrix} 1 & 0 & \left(\Im\left(\det \begin{pmatrix} \overline{w_1} & w_1 \\ \overline{w_2} & w_2 \end{pmatrix} \right) \right) i \\ 0 & 1 & 0 \\ 0 & 0 & 1 \end{pmatrix}.$$

The commutator $[\cdot,\cdot]$ measures the extent to which noncommutativity governs the group law of G. Obviously, the commutator subgroup $[G,G]$ coincides with C.

    The Kepplerian quadrature conchoid trajectory construction is based on equal increments of time rather than of distance in accumulating the phase histories of eccentric circular orbits in contiguous channels. By an application of the libration theory to the problem of planetary motion reconstruction, transvections (*Zeilenscherungen* in German) of the symplectic affine plane of resonant intralevel interaction control in quadrature format are used to reconstruct the orbital positions of the planets from the multichannel filter bank. Transvections, defining ramps with respect to the apsidal line, allow the construction of the distances of the planetary orbit on the contiguous fibers where the phase histories of an eccentric circular orbit are evolving (the modern usage of the notion of distance is unlike Keppler's concept of *distantia*, which is a stand-in for an interval on a line). Scaling the altitude proportions of the elliptical orbit with respect to the rotating coordinate frame of quadrature reference is performed in accordance with the area law. An application of a phase shift of the rotating coordinate frame of quadrature reference from the aphelion and quadrant at eccentric anomalies, $\{0, \frac{1}{2}\pi\}$, to the octants at eccentric anomalies, $\{\frac{1}{4}\pi, \frac{3}{4}\pi\}$, of the conchoid trajectory construction within the symplectic affine plane accomplished the detection of the famous eccentric anomaly of as much as 8 min discrepancy to the reference frequency cycle. This procedure finally established the first fundamental law for the Martian orbit (*revocare ellipses*, in Keppler's terms) as a consequence of the area law ([371]). This process realized, without benefit of any optical instrument, an improvement of nearly two orders of magnitude in the reconstruction of planetary orbital positions.

The quadrature conchoid trajectory construction is an outcome of the "Martian struggle" to conquer the Mars. The conquest of Mars portrays Keppler's dauntlessness, resolve, and determination to reconstruct the orbit, providing spectacularly improved results for the "indomitable" planet. Remarkably, the rotational curvature form, which is visualized by the moment map, seems to have almost escaped notice in the literature. Although the quadrature format admits a broad range of applications from the modern point of view, such as quadrature mixers, single-sideband generation, and coherent lock-in detection in microcircuitry electronics ([106], [107], [158]), the secondary literature does not reflect the importance of this powerful Kepplerian method of determining the planetary motion. Even one of the most devoted commentators of Keppler's work, the editor of his *Collected Papers*, Max Caspar, did not recognize the quadrature conchoid trajectory construction as a duality formulation of the area law but suggested that it only formed a sort of enjoyable play ([Johannes Kepler: Gesammelte Werke, Vol. 3], p. 470):

> Die Überlegungen bekunden die Eindringlichkeit, mit der Kepler seine geometrisch anschauliche Methode anwendet; er braucht diese Überlegungen im folgenden nicht mehr, hat aber seine Freude an ihnen.

(English translation)

> These ideas demonstrate the vigor with which Kepler applied his dynamic geometric method; he no longer needed these ideas in the following but he derived his pleasure from them.

Specifically, Caspar did not recognize the projective character of Keppler's approach so that it is no surprise that Keppler is not recognized as one of the founders of projective geometry, which gave rise to the line

$$\text{Keppler} \Longrightarrow \text{Desargues} \Longrightarrow \text{Poncelet.}$$

Reference to transvections in the determination of planetary orbital positions by use of the libration theory presents an anticipation of the target-induced local Doppler frequency shift in SAR high resolution imagery and the Lauterbur linear gradient switching for the subband encoding of spin-warp Fourier MRI processing. It basically corresponds to the angularly selective property of photonic holograms recorded in thick materials of systems with holographic mass memory. Mathematically, two in-plane encoding transvections, combined with a third transvection encoding a direction C transversal to the symplectic affine plane of resonant intralevel interaction control, generate the noncommutative geometry of the three-dimensional Heisenberg nilpotent Lie group G with one-dimensional center $C \hookrightarrow G$:

- Conversely, the symplectic affine plane of intralevel causal interaction control in which the Kepplerian strategy takes place is obtained by factoring out the center C of the structure group G. The plane G/C is endowed with the structure of the symplectic polarized cross section of G mod C.

- The symplectic affine plane G/C allows the stroboscopic and synchronous cross-sectional quadrature filtering of phase histories with respect to the rotating coordinate frame.

- The rotating coordinate frame of quadrature reference of the coadjoint orbit $\mathcal{O}_\nu$ ($\nu \neq 0$) defined by the symplectic polarized cross section G/C implements analysis of the second Kepplerian fundamental law of planetary motion, the area law, by the spatiotemporal quantization procedure of quantum holography.

The dilations of transversal line C implemented by G accomplish the selection of the tomographic slices. Computer control performs resonance with the hierarchical fibration of contiguously excited, adjacently decoupled, energetic strata $\mathbf{P}\left(\mathbb{R} \times \mathcal{O}_\nu\right)$ of center frequency ν. The canonical symplectic form

$$\omega_\nu = \nu \, d\kappa \qquad (\nu \neq 0)$$

with respect to the frame coordinates is defined by the parallel baselines of the transvections of the planar coadjoint orbits $\mathbf{P}\left(\mathbb{R} \times \mathcal{O}_\nu\right) \hookrightarrow \mathbf{P}\left(\mathbb{R} \times \mathrm{Lie}(G)^\star\right)$:

- The dual $\hat{G}$ of the Heisenberg group G organizes the parameters of the Kepplerian spatiotemporal quadrature Hilbert bundle strategy in terms of the spatiotemporal quantization procedure of quantum holography in a way consistent with transvections.

- Transition from the Heisenberg group to the compact Heisenberg nilmanifold is accomplished by performing the cross section of G modulo the stroboscopic and synchronous principal lattice subgroup.

If the rotating coordinate frame of quadrature reference admits the center frequency $\nu \neq 0$, the realification

$$\begin{pmatrix} x & -y \\ y & x \end{pmatrix}$$

of $w \in \mathbb{C}$ suggests an application *in stages* of the bundle-theoretic inducing construction to the unitary characters of the corresponding closed normal Abelian subgroups (N, M) of G. Both are isomorphic to $\mathbb{R} \oplus \mathbb{R}$, and there are injections

$$C \hookrightarrow N \hookrightarrow G, \qquad C \hookrightarrow M \hookrightarrow G,$$

respectively. Then the associated homogeneous manifolds $(G/N, G/M)$ are fibrations of G sitting over the semidirect factors (T, S), which both are isomorphic to the additive group $\mathbb{R}$. In the usual diagram notation for fiber bundles sitting over their base manifold

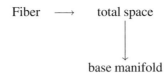

the situation can be displayed as follows:

$$\mathbf{P}\,(\mathbb{R} \times \mathcal{O}_\nu) \quad \longrightarrow \quad G/N \qquad \mathbf{P}\,(\mathbb{R} \times \mathcal{O}_\nu) \quad \longrightarrow \quad G/M$$

$$\downarrow \qquad\qquad\qquad\qquad\qquad \downarrow$$

$$T \qquad\qquad\qquad\qquad\qquad\quad S$$

The standard inducing construction of unitary linear representations of Lie groups from closed normal subgroups is patterned on the embedding of unitarily induced representations as locally square integrable, irreducible, linear subrepresentations in the quasi-regular representations on homogeneous base manifolds. In the case of the Kepplerian quadrature conchoid trajectory construction, the geometrical interpretation of the L^2-inducing construction yields a pair of induced Hilbert bundles sitting over the additive group $\mathbb{R}$ as baselines and a quadrature pair (U^ν, V^ν) $(\nu \neq 0)$ of isomorphic irreducible unitary linear representations of G. They are associated with the projectively completed, symplectic affine plane $\mathbf{P}\,(\mathbb{R} \times \mathcal{O}_\nu)$ of central character

$$\chi_\nu = U^\nu \mid C = V^\nu \mid C,$$

which displays the driving frequency $\nu \neq 0$. The quadrature pair (U^ν, V^ν) satisfies the Weyl commutation relations

$$U^\nu \circ V^\nu = e^{4\pi i \nu xy}\, V^\nu \circ U^\nu.$$

Let χ_ν^N denote any extension of χ_ν from C to N, and similarly, let χ_ν^M be any extension of χ_ν from C to M. The unitarily induced representations

$$U^\nu \cong L^2 - \mathop{\mathrm{Ind}}_{\underset{N}{\uparrow}}^G \chi_\nu^N, \qquad V^\nu \cong L^2 - \mathop{\mathrm{Ind}}_{\underset{M}{\uparrow}}^G \chi_\nu^M$$

of G are acting in the natural way as matched bank filters on the cross sections. The Fourier-transformed pair of tempered distributions $(1_\nu, \varepsilon_0)$ of soft and hard pulse types, respectively, attached to the rotating coordinate frame of quadrature reference of the projectively completed coadjoint orbit $\mathbf{P}\,(\mathbb{R} \times \mathcal{O}_\nu)\,(\nu \neq 0)$, gives rise to a pair of quadrature phase histories

$$\left(x_0,\, e^{2\pi i \nu [z + (x - x_0)y]} \cdot 1_\nu \right) \qquad (x_0 \in T),$$

and

$$\left(y_0,\, e^{2\pi i \nu [z - x(y - y_0)]} \varepsilon_{(-y)} \right) \qquad (y_0 \in S),$$

which are defined on the pair (T, S) of affine Lagrangian lines immersed into the projectively completed symplectic affine plane $\mathbf{P}(\mathbb{R} \times \mathcal{O}_\nu)$. The punch line of the transvectional encoding is that the induced Hilbert bundles are G-homogeneous complex vector space bundles. The G-homogeneity allows the adjustment of the stroboscopic phase cycling of the orbit by a shift of the initial phase x_0. Similarly, the adjustment of the local frequencies by a choice of the intermediate frequency y_0 is performed by a linear magnetic field gradient switched in the laboratory frame of reference. The phase shifter as well as the intermediate frequency of the clockwork dynamics via the transition

$$\text{Fourier transform} \Longrightarrow \text{Mellin transform}$$

is an ingredient of the method of lock-in detection via the localization pair

$$\text{Fourier transform} \perp \text{Mellin transform}.$$

Then the gradient echo is associated to the reflection

$$\begin{pmatrix} -1 & 0 \\ 0 & 1 \end{pmatrix} \in \mathbf{O}(2, \mathbb{R}) - \mathbf{SO}(2, \mathbb{R})$$

with respect to the basis defined by the pair (T, S) of affine Lagrangian lines spanning the projectively completed, symplectic affine plane $\mathbf{P}\left(\mathbb{R} \times \mathrm{Lie}(G)^\star\right)$:

- The Hilbert bundle over the bi-infinite stratigraphic time line implements, in quadrature format, the intralevel causal interaction control which is governed by the second fundamental law of planetary motion, the law of conservation of the central angular momentum form.
- The action of its structure group, the Heisenberg nilpotent Lie group G, moves the fibers around by unitary linear transformations; these act as cross-sectional matched bank filters on the phase histories.
- The phase histories evolve in contiguous local frequency encoding subband multichannels with respect to the rotating coordinate frame of quadrature reference. The adjustment of the local frequency is performed by the Mellin transform along an affine Lagrangian line.

Performing averages along the cross sections, the pair of isomorphic irreducible unitary linear representations (U^ν, V^ν) of G defines the holographic transform $\mathcal{H}_\nu$. As the coefficient function of U^ν mod C, or what amounts to the same coefficient function of V^ν mod C, $\mathcal{H}_\nu$ implements the stroboscopic and synchronous cross-sectional bank filters of phase histories in quadrature format. They lead to the implementation of filter banks of matched filter type in the projectively completed, symplectic affine planes $\{\mathbf{P}(\mathbb{R} \times \mathcal{O}_\nu) \mid \nu \neq 0\}$ of resonant intralevel interaction control in quadrature format, which are accessible to subtle *lock-in* techniques (Figure 18). Thus the cross-sectional procedure *modulo center* of spatiotemporal quantization by means of the rotating coordinate frame of quadrature reference, replete with the illusion of a

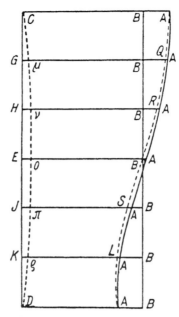

Figure 18. Keppler's phase sensitive quadrature detection strategy for the localization of the planet's position on its orbit. Original drawing from the *Astronomia Nova* (1609) which contains the first and the second Kepplerian laws on the planetary orbits. The point E located "in quadrature position" provides a phase difference of $\frac{\pi}{2}$.

stationary motion, is of the utmost importance in the mathematical modeling of the Kepplerian spatiotemporal strategy and in its application to matched bank filters.

In antiquity, a tradition had developed of distinguishing between mathematical and physical theories. Astronomy was concerned with uniform motion in epicycles and deferents. The coordinatization of planetary motion in terms of continuously changing variables was an entirely new problem, for the solution of which Keppler developed his own technique of filtering observations in projective space. Because his matched filter technique had to detect small deviations of the planetary orbit from the circular shape in order to validate the helioeccentric model, its accuracy exceeded by far all the results previously available. The depth of originality and strong impact of the basic ideas of Kepplerian planetary motion analysis in projective space upon the whole dynamics of physical astronomy centered on the Sun cannot be overemphasized (Figure 19).

The Kepplerian strategy involved neither a particular insight into the causes of planetary motion nor the consideration of the order they imposed on the nonuniform motion in a noncircular orbit. Due to the equivalence of the area law and the law of conservation of the orbital angular momentum form, the Kepplerian strategy is applicable to *planar* orbit configurations without reference to the law of gravitation describing the intralevel causal interaction control. The only specific assumption Keppler had to make about the planet Mars was its sidereal period of 687 days.

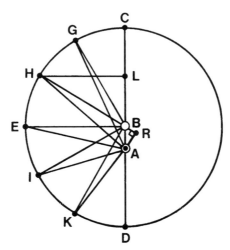

Figure 19. Explanation to Keppler's conchoid construction as displayed in Figure 18: The line segment $\overline{AR}$ is perpendicular to the segment $\overline{RH}$ prolongating the radius $\overline{BH}$. A = real sun; B = center of the Kepplerian reference circle, the punctum equans; $\overline{CD}$ = apsidal line, connecting the apsides, which are the aphelion C and the perihelion D. The Kepplerian reference circle is parametrized by the mean anomaly. Mathematically, mean anomaly is equivalent to time, with the normalization that the planet's periodic time equals 2π. Note the area of the enclosed rectangular triangle ABR at the mean anomaly CBH.

Therefore this strategy reveals an extraordinary flexibility covering periodic motion beyond the traditional planetary motion realm of the area law.

In contrast to some philosophers of science ([124], [271]), the completely different approach to a planetary theory created by Isaac Newton (1643–1727) cannot refute the Kepplerian strategy. In other words, due to the difference in their methodologies, Newton's gravitational planetary theory cannot logically falsify Keppler's holographic filtering analysis of planetary motion caused by magnetic forces which control the local frequencies. Because the planetary orbit is a conic section in projective space, Keppler's second law is compatible with Newtonian dynamics:

- The Kepplerian dynamics of physical astronomy centered on the Sun, and the magnetic hypothesis include the assumption that the magnetic axis of the solar planet maintains a constant direction with respect to the orbital plane through the Sun, perpendicular to the apsidal line, to provide geometrical symmetry through the ability of the magnet to control direction in projective space.

In view of the magnetic hypothesis, logic falsification is an inappropriate method for the evaluation of Keppler's results or for pointing out the difference between the scientific achievements of Keppler and Newton in the dynamics of physical astronomy. Due to the magnetic hypothesis and the development of the MRI modality, appreciation of the revolutionary Kepplerian planetary clockwork approach to dynamic physical astronomy requires a complete revision (Figure 20).

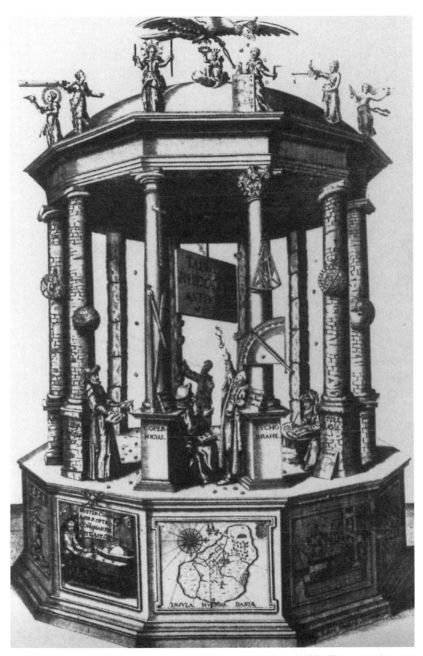

Figure 20. Title page of Johannes Keppler's book *TabulæRudolphinæ* (1627). The copperplate engraves by small etchings the main strategies of planetary orbit localization: The adjustment of the apsidal line through the eccentric sun, and the transition from the circular to the elliptic orbit performed by affine-linear mapping.

Although the matched bank filter idea for the planetary orbit reconstruction is profoundly original and fundamental for the development of modern science, Keppler's pioneering work unfortunately always remained in the shadow of Newton's gravitational inverse square law. Keppler's contributions as an observer are little-recognized, as well. His place in science has been abated by Isaac Newton, who remarked, *wrongly*, that Keppler knew the orbit to be noncircular and guessed it to be elliptical.

The misguided interpretation of Keppler's new astronomy has actually its origin in Newton's nine-page tract entitled *De Motu Corporum in Gyrum* of 1684 where he states as a scholium ([The Mathematical Papers of Isaac Newton, Vol. VI], p. 49): "The major planets orbit, therefore, in ellipses having a focus at the centre of the Sun, exactly as Keppler supposed."

In 1685 Newton gave to the qualitative description of the planetary intralevel causal interaction due to Giovanni Alfonso Borelli (1608–1679) its quantitative form and had even earlier derived it from the Kepplerian third fundamental law of planetary motion. Keppler's adherence to the Aristotelian hypothesis of a force tangential to the planet's orbit, his adoption of the viewpoint of projective geometry, his "failure" to use an inverse square law for his central solar force, the "awkward magnetic arrangement" of his libration theory, and the absence of the formalism of the integral calculus have prevented many from understanding his strategy for quadrature filtering the phase histories of eccentric circular orbits in contiguous local frequency encoding subband multichannels with respect to the rotating coordinate frame of quadrature reference.

Moreover, thinking in terms of the coordinatization by the variables of phases and local frequencies and, ultimately, in terms of the bundle-theoretic inducing construction of Lie group representations is less intuitive. Therefore the unbelievable depth of Keppler's approach obscured his mathematical achievements, not only as an ingenious geometrical and numerical approximator, but also as a scientist who included the holographic aspects of the reconstruction of planetary motion into his reasoning.

The emergence of Newton's monumental work *Philosophiae Naturalis Principia Mathematica* in 1687 would be historically unimaginable without the profound analysis of planetary motion that Keppler brought about, his introduction of orbits traversed under the action of magnetic forces, and his bold and innovative advances in the field called mathematical physics. However, Newtonian gravitational planetary theory blinded scientists of later generations to Keppler's underlying cross-correlational theory of intralevel causal interaction control in quadrature format. The mistake has been to envisage Keppler's dynamics of physical astronomy merely as a precursor of Newton's *Principia Mathematica* and the first and second laws only as empirical premises for Newton's argument.

Newton suggested that Keppler's discovery of the first law is an empirical one. Although the philosopher Georg Wilhelm Friedrich Hegel (1770–1831) could not foresee that Keppler's approach to the underlying mathematical structure of the causal connection between micro- and macrolevels was fully confirmed by clinical MRI, he criticized the transition of the fame from Keppler to Newton in his *Enzyklopädie der philosophischen Wissenschaften* §270 (1817–1830) (G.W.F. Hegel, *Werke in Zwanzig Bänden*, Vol. 9, p. 86):

Die Gesetze der absolut-freien Bewegung sind bekanntlich von Kepler entdeckt worden; eine Entdeckung von unsterblichem Ruhme. Bewiesen hat Kepler dieselbe in dem Sinne, daß er für die empirischen Daten ihren allgemeinen Ausdruck gefunden hat.... Es ist seitdem zu einer allgemeinen Redensart geworden, daß Newton erst die Beweise jener Gesetze gefunden habe. Nicht leicht ist der Ruhm ungerechter von einem ersten Entdecker auf einen anderen übergegangen.

(English translation)

The laws of absolute free movement were, as is well-known, discoverd by Keppler—a discovery conferring immortal fame. Keppler proved these laws in the sense that he found general expression for the empirical data.... It has since become a commonplace that only with Newton was the proof of those laws found. T'would not be easy for fame to have passed more unjustly from the original discoverer to another.

Newton neglects Keppler's appreciation of planetary motion to be understood in terms of time delays. Actually, Keppler was not satisfied with a geometrical theory of planetary orbits, even though his stratification approach and quadrature detection were profoundly original. In fact a dynamical physics of attracting forces was necessary to discover his laws of planetary motion as a physical process by exploiting the precision of Tycho's observations during the Martian struggle and replacing the Ptolemaic epicycle construction of uniformly rotating circles as well as the Copernican models, instead of merely supplementing these approaches. Newton's statement impeded any fair analysis of Keppler's innovative mathematical techniques. Therefore many of Keppler's ingenious applications, such as the quadrature conchoid trajectory construction in the ecliptic affine symplectic plane, which he deduced by the L^2 exhaustion technique of Archimedes in order to verify the area law, received no notice in the elapsed centuries. Ingenious as they are, the Kepplerian geometrical and numerical approximation techniques, based on a fibration with respect to the rotating frame of quadrature reference sitting over the bi-infinite stratigraphic time line $\mathbb{R}$ of cycle times, have never been translated into the vocabulary of the mathematical discipline of noncommutative geometrical analysis, nor have his methods been taken as a *cue* to the conceptions of modern technology such as those of signal analysis, quantum holography, SAR, and MRI.

The development of Bloch's dynamics in a clinical MRI modality in terms of the foliated superencoded projective space represents the most remarkable renaissance of Keppler's dynamical ideas. It finally established that Kepplerian physics in terms of time delays or local frequencies is at least as profound and as fruitful as the Newtonian physics of acceleration. Indeed, the Kepplerian dynamics of time delays is directly applicable to MRI, whereas the Newtonian dynamics of acceleration is not. Specific results of an approach are one aspect; the range of a different scientific theory and its associated methodology are the other one.

Although the magnetic hypothesis of his Mars commentaries includes the assumption that the magnetic axis of the planet maintains a constant direction in projective space, orthogonal to the orbital plane through the Sun, in order to provide geometrical symmetry through the magnet's directive power, Keppler has never been recognized as an early pioneer of NMR and clinical MRI ([223]). The cleft beween the macrolevel of physical astronomy and the microlevel of nuclear spin isochromats stimulated by the filter bank input seems to be too wide to reverse the lack of his unbelievably deep spatiotemporal insights. Who would expect that elliptical orbits are excited by the stepped phase-encoding linear gradients in the pulse timing diagram of control along the stratigraphic time line $\mathbb{R}$ for two-dimensional gradient echo and fast spin echo MRI? Who would expect that the "awkward magnetic arrangement" of Keppler's libration theory would at long last lead to a powerful high technology application of nuclear spin isochromats? Everybody, however, who understands Keppler's spatiotemporal strategy to encode the planetary motions along the event line of cycle times will understand the basic principles of the MRI encoding process. *Learn from the masters*!

Keppler's fame rests primarily on the tortuous path to the discovery of the laws of planetary motion during the struggle to conquer Mars. The three fundamental laws represent one of the greatest scientific accomplishments. However, the true picture of their discovery is still not well known. There was incomprehension of Keppler's research work by his contemporaries as well as misunderstanding of early commentators which has continued to the present day, so that major unclarities and misinterpretations continue to be disseminated in the literature ([3]). Newton's remark in the *De Motu Corporum* treatise is a particularly prominent misinterpretation in a long series of misunderstandings. When a change of paradigms actually occurred in the development of science, it was landmarked by the Mars commentaries of Johann Keppler. However, even science historians of no less stature as Thomas S. Kuhn (1922–1996) have been inclined to Newton's point of view to a degree which has impeded any profound mathematical analysis of the Kepplerian dynamics of physical astronomy. The inner logic of Keppler's account of his prolonged struggle with the Martian motion, his holographic approach to the dynamical symmetries governing planetary motions and the global geometrical shape of the orbits of the solar planets, and the quantum physical aspects of his stroboscopic and synchronous approach did not find the recognition they actually deserve.

As Einstein observed, Johann Keppler would never have been able to complete his research work without his background of order philosophy. Keppler believed that the natural world, because it has been created, was organized according to basic principles more fundamental than those of mere physics. His astronomical work, however, was directed at finding the order that was objectively within nature. In view of these principles he was lonely in his research work. The chief importance of his work in science does *not* lie merely in the numerical precision of the careful evaluation and the diligent condensation of vast amounts of astronomical observational data, as emphasized by Richard Philips Feynman (1967) as well as by the textbook literature ([115]) which emphasizes a trial-and-error interpretation. The importance of his work is based on the revolutionary novelty of the resonance application of the area law by *reversing* the directions in projective space along which Tycho de Brahe had observed Mars from Earth. This strategy required a virtuous numerical efficacy in the application of the L^2 exhaustion technique of Archimedes in order to derive the first fundamental law of planetary motion by summation of the effects of the pulses pushing the planet along infinitesimal orbital elements. It is this novelty which led to the line

$$\text{Keppler} \Longrightarrow \text{Newton} \Longrightarrow \text{Einstein}$$

and pointed beyond the invariant differential submanifold solution of the two-body problem defined by the law of spin conservation for motions in a central field of gravitation to the holographic *path integral* approach to the Green propagator of the central field and even anticipated the global approach by Feynman (Nobel Prize winner in 1965) to the Bohr-Sommerfeld quantization rules. In view of the fact that the most original of Keppler's thoughts were four centuries ahead of his time and actually led to the bundle-theoretic inducing construction of unitary linear group representations from the unitary characters of closed normal Abelian subgroups, the Newtonian gravitation theory should be replaced by the Fourier system theory ([87]) in the preceding falsification line. Then Fourier analysis, when considered as a symplectic linear response theory, and quantum mechanics in its transactional interpretation ([56]) give rise to another line:

$$\text{Keppler} \Longrightarrow \text{Fourier} \Longrightarrow \text{Feynman}.$$

Unfortunately, the roots of symplectic linear response theory has never been traced back to Keppler's libration theory. Similarly, the modern treatises of the Feynman path integral or L^2 summation over the phase histories neither mention the considerable ancestry of this global functional integral line of ideas nor indicate its application to SAR or practical clinical MRI.

To conclude these historical remarks, it should be mentioned that in 1952 Otto E. Neugebauer discovered that the Babylonian astronomers had already used a primitive kind of Fourier series for the prediction of celestial events. The Fourier transform, however, grew from the desire to understand black body radiation in the context of the cooling characteristics of military cannons. The application of the operational calculus of Fourier integral operators underlying the Kepplerian spatiotemporal strategy of the dynamics of physical astronomy to the visualization of clinical MRI scans is of considerably higher benefit to humankind.

The phase-coherent wavelets received from the spin isochromats of the sample present very weak signals which have to be detected by the clinical MRI scanner. One of the implications of this weakness is that clinical MRI presents a noninvasive imaging modality. Therefore clinical MRI is superior to X-ray CT. A fascinating aspect of the art of electronic engineering is to find that the symmetries inherent in the Kepplerian spatiotemporal strategy reappear in the integrated circuit technology in order to implement high sensitivity detection devices.

The RF hardware of the clinical MRI scanner includes the pulse programmer, the transmitter with its single-sideband modulator, the set of radiofrequency receiver coils including the standard surface coils placed parallel to the magnetic axis as well as the quadrature phased array multicoils, and the receiver, which includes a spectrum analyzer. The pulse programmer controls the entire automated imaging organization, the transmitted pulse sequences create the excitation of the nuclear spins during the transmission mode, and the receiver coils collect the NMR phase-coherent wavelet responses during the detection process. Advances and refinements in the design of pulse sequences and surface coils have enhanced the ability of MRI diagnosticians to identify a wide variety of soft tissue structures. These advances have affected all subspecialties of clinical radiodiagnostics including proton NMR spectroscopic imaging:

- For low magnetic flux density MRI systems of 0.12 T to high magnetic flux density systems of 4.0 T, sequences of RF excitation pulses of central frequencies ν from 5 MHz through about 180 MHz are required.

The most efficient way of generating pulse sequences of clinical MRI protocol is to leave the program stored in the first-in/first-out (FIFO) memories and switch control of the operation to a second set of FIFO queue buffers. In the architecture of the pulse programmer, an FIFO buffer operates like a shift register in that data entered at the input appear at the response output in the same order. The important difference between the two, however, is that with a shift register the data get pushed along as additional data are entered and clocked, but with an FIFO buffer the data fall through to the output queue with only a small delay of about 1 to 25 μs. Input and response output are controlled by separate clocks, and the FIFO memory keeps track of what data have been entered and what data have been removed. The program in the set of secondary FIFO queue buffers is cycled in accordance with the protocol, and the control is returned to the principal FIFO architecture.

In the Kepplerian spatiotemporal strategy of stroboscopic and synchronous filtering of phase histories evolving in multichannels in the plane, time is not envisaged as a flowing instant but as an event line of coexistences in which the libratory motions take place. In the synchronous discipline of large scale integrated system design, sequence and time are connected through the use of a systemwide clock signal. The purposes of the clock signal are twofold. The clock serves as a sequence reference and also as a time reference. As a sequence reference, its transitions serve the logical purpose of defining successive increments of time at which system state changes may occur. As a stratigraphic time reference, the duration between transitions serves the physical purpose of accounting for delays in paths from the output to the input of clocked elements:

- In MRI scanner architectures, phase coherence of the wavelets is performed by deriving the timing procedure from a single master oscillator for the pulse programmer, the pulse synchronizer, the RF reference for the transmitter, and the RF reference for the phase-sensitive detector.

For the utmost stability, a quartz crystal oscillator is mounted in a constant-temperature oven. A typical high performance modular oscillator can deliver 10 MHz at a frequency stability of one part in 10^{11} per day and makes it a natural basis of the frequency synthesizers used in clinical MRI scanners.

The transmitter as well as the receiver need reference RFs to be strictly controlled. Due to the Kepplerian spatiotemporal strategy, the phase-sensitive detection is of crucial importance in MRI processing. The procedure of a rotating coordinate frame of quadrature reference makes for the *reduction* of the Larmor frequency to a manageable level from a computational point of view. Reduction is not at the source of the external magnetic flux density but is obtained by subtraction of an intermediate frequency y_0 from the reference RF which enables both the observer and the computer equipment of the clinical MRI scanner to view the projectively completed, symplectic affine plane $\mathbf{P}\,(\mathbb{R} \times \mathcal{O}_\nu)$ of the rotating coordinate frame of quadrature reference, with the hologram encoded in magnetization phase and local frequency coordinates.

The accurate control of phase coordinates is a hardware problem when a variety of frequencies are required, for most electronic circuits generate a phase shift that is frequency dependent. A delay line forms a typical example for this dependence. Thus the phase should be controlled at a single frequency. This can be accomplished by heterodyning a fixed intermediate frequency y_0 with the variable local frequency to produce the Larmor frequency y in the transmitter chain of the clinical MRI scanner.

Another practical aspect of the hardware is that despite shielding efforts some RF leakage may enter the receiver chain in the clinical MRI scanner and produce artifacts of fluctuating intensity sweeping across the entire scan in the phase encoding direction ([133]). For this reason, baseband detection is not to be recommended, unless the echo signal is so strong that little amplification is called for, a situation only encountered in high magnetic flux density proton imaging. Thus the Larmor frequency itself is never generated in the scanner's electronics during the wavelet reception process. The signal issuing from a low noise preamplifier has its frequency changed to an intermediate frequency y_0 by means of a phase-sensitive detector. The intermediate frequency, which should be chosen higher than the highest Larmor frequency to be encountered, and the Larmor frequency should be up converted to avoid spurious signals in the receiver. Then low pass filtering allows for restriction to single-sideband processing.

The architecture of quadrature phase-sensitive detection avoids the loss in narrow frequency subbands by correspondingly splitting the reference of the rotating coordinate frame into two quadrature references and performing detection in two circuit branches. The pairs of phase-coherent wavelet responses (ψ, φ) in the complex modulation space $L_\mathbb{C}^2(\mathbb{R})$ of mod C square integrable cross-sectional and swapped cross-sectional phase history channels, respectively, are transvectionally encoded in quadrature format via the unitary forms of the cross sections

$$\left(x_0,\ e^{2\pi i\nu[z+(x-x_0)y]}\psi(x) \right) \qquad (x_0 \in T)$$

and

$$\left(y_0,\ e^{2\pi i\nu[z-x(y-y_0)]}\varphi(-y) \right) \qquad (y_0 \in S).$$

Due to the phase conjugation associated with the reflection of the spin echo teleportation phenomenon

$$\begin{pmatrix} 1 & 0 \\ 0 & -1 \end{pmatrix} \in \mathbf{O}(2, \mathbb{R}) - \mathbf{SO}(2, \mathbb{R}),$$

the frequency-encoded subband channels are accessible to the lock-in and read-out by the trace filter sweep of quantum holography

$$1_\nu \oplus 1_\nu,$$

provided the phase coordinates of the channels with respect to the rotating frame of quadrature reference are accurately detected:

- In quadrature phase-sensitive detection, the reference for the second detector represents a swapped copy of the first reference. The phase shift through the angle of $\frac{1}{2}\pi$ is performed by data routing.

A broadband ring modulator, the circular symmetry of which serves as provision for *holographically* changing the phase of both quadrature reference inputs while maintaining their $\frac{1}{2}\pi$ phase difference, realizes electronically the infinitesimal generator

$$J = \begin{pmatrix} 0 & -1 \\ 1 & 0 \end{pmatrix}$$

of the compact Lie group $\mathbf{SO}(2, \mathbb{R})$ describing the circular symmetry of the quadrature reference. The circuit diagram of the phase-sensitive detector is implemented by four diodes connecting the four alternately grounded nodes of a matched Schottky quad or balanced mixer ([158]). Then the output is filtered to remove the ultrahigh frequency components of the RF spectra and is amplified. The phase-coherent wavelets of the remaining frequencies form a phase hologram which is ready for viewing down the center C of G, and storage in the computer provided each point corresponds with a spatial location in the laboratory coordinate frame by the solvable affine Lauterbur encoding technique of spin–warp Fourier MRI processing.

In the lock-in technique, the output of the quadrature phase-sensitive detector controls the frequency by a subsequent integrated circuit, the phase-locked loop ([158]). This building block causes the frequency source rapidly to lock to the reference frequency:

- Phase-locked loops perform excitation pulse synchronization by pulling in to resonance.

Moreover, they ensure long-term stability of the magnetic field under the switching of linear magnetic field gradients. The ensuing Lauterbur encoded quantum hologram can be displayed by a raster scan on an oscilloscope screen. As the electron beam in the cathode ray tube sweeps across the screen, there is a correspondence between beam position and spatial position within the selected tomographic slice of center frequency $\nu \neq 0$. The $\mathbb{R}$-linear isomorphism

$$(x, y) \rightsquigarrow \begin{pmatrix} x & -y \\ y & x \end{pmatrix}$$

of the projectively completed, generic coadjoint orbit $\mathbf{P}\left(\mathbb{R} \times \mathcal{O}_1\right)$ onto the realification $\mathbb{C}(\mathbb{R} \oplus \mathbb{R})$ of the field $\mathbb{C}$ of complex numbers suggests an extension to the skew field $\mathbb{H}$ of quaternions. The $\mathbb{R}$-linear mapping

$$(w, w') \rightsquigarrow \begin{pmatrix} w & w' \\ -\bar{w}' & \bar{w} \end{pmatrix}$$

provides an isomorphism from the image $\mathbb{H}(\mathbb{C} \oplus \mathbb{C})$ of $\mathbb{C} \times \mathbb{C}$ onto the skew field $\mathbb{H}$. In terms of the matrices of the type $\mathbb{H}(\mathbb{C} \oplus \mathbb{C})$, the multiplication in $\mathbb{H}$ reads

$$\begin{pmatrix} w_1 & w_1{}' \\ -\bar{w}'_1 & \bar{w}_1 \end{pmatrix} \begin{pmatrix} w_2 & w_2{}' \\ -\bar{w}'_2 & \bar{w}_2 \end{pmatrix} = \begin{pmatrix} w_1 w_2 - w_1{}'\bar{w}'_2 & w_1 w_2{}' + w_1{}'\bar{w}_2 \\ -\left(\bar{w}_1\bar{w}'_2 + \bar{w}'_1 w_2\right) & \bar{w}_1\bar{w}_2 - \bar{w}'_1 w_2{}' \end{pmatrix}.$$

The capability to obtain scans in a variety of planes has been heralded as a fundamental advantage of clinical MRI. In a single multislice sequence, each tomographic slice angle of obliquity and interslice interval can be selected independently. Oblique imaging has been applied to numerous areas of diagnosis, including the spine, knee, heart, and orbits:

- The group $\mathbb{S}_3$ is the nontrivial covering $\mathrm{Spin}(3, \mathbb{R})$ of the rotation group $\mathbf{SO}(3, \mathbb{R})$. The compact group $\mathbf{SO}(3, \mathbb{R})$ contains two normal subgroups, both isomorphic to $\mathbb{S}_3$, which give rise to the Clifford translations acting transitively on the real projective space $\mathbf{P}\left(\mathbb{R} \times \mathrm{Lie}(G)^\star\right)$.
- Identification of the group $\mathbb{S}_3 \hookrightarrow \mathbb{R}^4$ with the unit sphere of the skew field $\mathbb{H}$ provides the multiplanar imaging capability of the MRI modality via the Abelian groups $\mathbf{SO}(2, \mathbb{R})$ of Clifford translations of tomographic slices in the elliptic non-Euclidean space $\mathbf{P}\left(\mathbb{R} \times \mathrm{Lie}(G)^\star\right)$.
- Identification of the unit sphere $\mathbb{S}_3 \hookrightarrow \mathbb{R}^4$ with the compact group $\mathbf{SU}(2, \mathbb{C})$, or the compact homogeneous manifolds $(\mathbf{SU}(2, \mathbb{C}) \times \mathbf{SU}(2, \mathbb{C})) / \mathbf{SU}(2, \mathbb{C})$, or $\mathbf{SO}(4, \mathbb{R}) / \mathbf{SO}(3, \mathbb{R})$ provides the design of pairs of surface coils of the MRI scanner bore via zonal spherical harmonics.

Because the multiangle, variable-interval, oblique imaging technique supposes a spherically homogeneous magnetic field, the $\mathbf{SU}(2, \mathbb{C})$ approach to the design of surface coils is at the basis of the multislice imaging technique. The symplectic structure associated with the phase-sensitive quadrature detection implies the rotational symmetry of the traces of the Heisenberg helices on the transversal plane. The rotational symmetry of the trace filter sweep of quantum holography

$$1_\nu \oplus 1_\nu \qquad (\nu \neq 0)$$

gives rise to the zonal spherical harmonics which allow for an implementation of spherically homogeneous magnetic fields inside the MRI scanner bore.

2

THE STRUCTURE–FUNCTION PROBLEM IN CLINICAL MRI

Everyone knows what a curve is, until he has studied enough mathematics to become confused through the countless number of possible exceptions.

—Felix Klein (1849–1925)

Theorien kommen zustande durch ein vom empirischen Material inspiriertes Verstehen, welches am besten im Anschluß an Plato als Zur–Deckung–Kommen von inneren Bildern mit äußeren Objekten und ihrem Verhalten zu deuten ist. Die Möglichkeit des Verstehens zeigt aufs Neue das Vorhandensein regulierender typischer Anordnungen, denen sowohl das Innen wie das Außen des Menschen unterworfen sind.

—Wolfgang Pauli (1961)

The Heisenberg group is remarkably little known considering its ubiquity. What I call "the Heisenberg group" is not in fact one object, but a collection of similar objects, rather like a functor, or a scheme in algebraic geometry, or even a combination of several overlapping functors.

—Roger Howe (1980)

2.1 THE PLANAR COADJOINT ORBIT STRATIFICATION OF THE HEISENBERG DUAL

Shortly after Werner Heisenberg introduced the canonical commutation relations in quantum physics, which underlie his uncertainty principle of 1925, Hermann Weyl showed they could be interpreted as the structure relations for the Heisenberg Lie algebra $\text{Lie}(G)$. In the context of application to clinical MRI, the interference of phase-coherent wavelets ([291], [297], [310], [350]) with real synchronization parameters of macroscopic quantum field theory is based on the simply connected Heisenberg

122

nilpotent Lie group G. A coordinatization of the nonsplit central group extension

$$\mathbb{R} \lhd G \longrightarrow \mathbb{R} \oplus \mathbb{R}$$

of the transversal plane $\mathbb{R} \oplus \mathbb{R}$ by the central line $\mathbb{R}$ with respect to the laboratory frame is constructed by a flag (L, H) of the real vector space E of dimension $n = \dim_{\mathbb{R}} E = 3$. By definition ([291]), the pair (L_1, H_1) consists of a homogeneous line L_1 and a plane H_1 in E containing L_1. Thus

$$L_1 \hookrightarrow H_1 \hookrightarrow E.$$

In clinical MRI, H_1 denotes an oblique tomographic slice. The subgroup of the linear group GL(E) globally preserving L_1 and H_1 can be identified with the standard Borel subgroup of upper triangular matrices

$$\begin{pmatrix} x_{11} & x_{12} & x_{13} \\ 0 & x_{22} & x_{23} \\ 0 & 0 & x_{33} \end{pmatrix}$$

with real entries such that

$$\det \begin{pmatrix} x_{11} & x_{12} & x_{13} \\ 0 & x_{22} & x_{23} \\ 0 & 0 & x_{33} \end{pmatrix} = x_{11} x_{22} x_{33} \neq 0.$$

The subgroup of the standard Borel subgroup consisting of the matrices of the type above, leaving all the points of the line L pointwise fixed, and acting on H_1 like the group $\Theta(H_1, L_1)$ of transvections of H_1 associated to the line L_1, is the group G with diagonal elements

$$x_{11} = x_{22} = x_{33} = 1.$$

Then G admits the symplectic polarized realization which reads, in terms of unipotent upper triangular matrices,

$$G = \left\{ \begin{pmatrix} 1 & x & z \\ 0 & 1 & y \\ 0 & 0 & 1 \end{pmatrix} \,\middle|\, x, y, z \in \mathbb{R} \right\}.$$

Under its natural left-invariant sub-Riemannian metric, the isometry of G corresponding to the rotation of the symplectic affine plane $\mathbb{R} \oplus \mathbb{R}$ of matrix

$$\begin{pmatrix} \cos \vartheta & -\sin \vartheta \\ \sin \vartheta & \cos \vartheta \end{pmatrix} \in \mathbf{SO}(2, \mathbb{R})$$

and infinitesimal generator J is given by the assignment

$$\begin{pmatrix} 1 & x & z \\ 0 & 1 & y \\ 0 & 0 & 1 \end{pmatrix} \rightsquigarrow \begin{pmatrix} 1 & x\cos\vartheta - y\sin\vartheta & z - xy\sin^2\vartheta + \frac{1}{2}(x^2 - y^2)\sin\vartheta\cos\vartheta \\ 0 & 1 & x\sin\vartheta + y\cos\vartheta \\ 0 & 0 & 1 \end{pmatrix}.$$

The circular cylinder of radius $\sqrt{x^2 + y^2}$ is left invariant. The isometry of G corresponding to the reflection of the circular ray traces

$$\begin{pmatrix} 1 & 0 \\ 0 & -1 \end{pmatrix} \in \mathbf{O}(2, \mathbb{R}) - \mathbf{SO}(2, \mathbb{R})$$

in the transversal symplectic affine plane $\mathbb{R} \oplus \mathbb{R}$ admits the block matrix

$$\begin{pmatrix} \boxed{\begin{matrix} 1 & 0 \\ 0 & -1 \end{matrix}} & \begin{matrix} 0 \\ 0 \end{matrix} \\ \begin{matrix} 0 & 0 \end{matrix} & -1 \end{pmatrix}.$$

The block $\square$ denotes the tracial reflection in the transversal symplectic affine plane $\mathbb{R} \oplus \mathbb{R}$. Explicitly it is given by

$$\begin{pmatrix} 1 & x & z \\ 0 & 1 & y \\ 0 & 0 & 1 \end{pmatrix} \rightsquigarrow \begin{pmatrix} 1 & x & -z \\ 0 & 1 & -y \\ 0 & 0 & 1 \end{pmatrix}.$$

In addition, the group of homothetic transformations of ratio $r > 0$ is given by the assignments

$$\begin{pmatrix} 1 & x & z \\ 0 & 1 & y \\ 0 & 0 & 1 \end{pmatrix} \rightsquigarrow \begin{pmatrix} 1 & rx & r^2z \\ 0 & 1 & ry \\ 0 & 0 & 1 \end{pmatrix}.$$

Note that the entry of the longitudinal center C of G is *quadratic* in the ratio r whereas the transverse coordinates are *linear* in r.

It follows that the group $\mathbf{GO}(2, \mathbb{R})$ of bijective linear similitudes of the symplectic affine plane $\mathbb{R} \oplus \mathbb{R}$ can be implemented by the group of isometries of the sub-Riemannian manifold G with respect to its natural left-invariant metric. Due to the group invariance, all points of G play the same role. Therefore, every point of the stratified Lie group G is the center of one-parameter subgroups of rotations and homothetic transformations. On the *spectral* side, the subgroup of homothetic transformations of G is at the origin of the *localization* procedure by linear magnetic field gradients which are temporally switched in the laboratory frame of reference.

The geodesics of G are the fiber projections of *bicharacterics* within the cotangent bundle $T^\star(G)$. Using the classical terminology due to Courant–Hilbert, the geodesics form the "characteristic rays," or locally minimizing curves of constant velocity. The problem of computing the geodesics amounts to the classical *isoperimetric* problem in the Euclidean plane $\mathbb{R} \oplus \mathbb{R}$ ([119]). The projection of the solution of the system of Hamilton–Jacobi equations associated with the principal symbol of the left-invariant sub-Laplacian differential operator $\mathcal{L}_G$, starting at the origin and parametrized by the symplectic affine coordinates of the foliation leaves

$$\left(t, \frac{1}{2\pi\nu} \begin{pmatrix} x & -y \\ y & x \end{pmatrix}, 2\pi\nu \right)$$

at the driving oscillator frequency $\nu \neq 0$, are either the homogeneous lines of the transverse symplectic affine plane $\mathbb{R} \oplus \mathbb{R}$ or the Heisenberg helix of longitudinal axis through the point of affine coordinates

$$\left(-\frac{x}{2\pi\nu}, -\frac{y}{2\pi\nu}, 0\right)$$

in the transverse plane. The punchline is that the homogeneous lines of the symplectic affine plane $\mathbb{R} \oplus \mathbb{R}$ are *resonant* lines. Specifically, the affine Lagrangian lines which span the plane $\mathbb{R} \oplus \mathbb{R}$ are revealed to be resonant lines:

- The directions of the affine Lagrangian lines in the projectively completed, symplectic affine plane $\mathbf{P}(\mathbb{R} \times \mathcal{O}_\nu)$ $(\nu \neq 0)$ are capable of controlling the ray traces of the nonresonant Heisenberg helices.

It is this feature which provides the fundamentals for the localization technique by linear magnetic field gradients temporally switched in the laboratory frame of reference. In fact, the nonsingular coadjoint orbits $\mathcal{O}_\pm$ of the affine Lie group $\mathbf{GA}(\mathbb{R})$ merge to the coadjoint orbits $\mathbf{P}(\mathbb{R} \times \mathcal{O}_\nu)$ $(\nu \neq 0)$ of G so that the linear gradient localization technique fits the transvectional encoding procedure. In this way, the merging of the coadjoint orbits gives rise to the trace filter encoding.

The Heisenberg helix adopts the explicit form

$$\begin{pmatrix} 1 & \dfrac{-x(1-\cos 2\pi\nu t) - y\sin 2\pi\nu t}{2\pi\nu} & \dfrac{r^2(2\pi\nu t - \sin 2\pi\nu t)}{2(2\pi\nu)^2} \\ 0 & 1 & \dfrac{x\sin 2\pi\nu t - y(1-\cos 2\pi\nu t)}{2\pi\nu} \\ 0 & 0 & 1 \end{pmatrix} \quad (t \in \mathbb{R})$$

in the symplectic polarized realization of G. Notice the central Coriolis component. In the real isotropic realization of G, however, the Heisenberg helix reads as follows:

$$\begin{pmatrix} 1 & -\dfrac{y\sin 2\pi\nu t}{2\pi\nu} & -\dfrac{x(1-\cos 2\pi\nu t)}{2\pi\nu} & \dfrac{r^2(2\pi\nu t - \sin 2\pi\nu t)}{2(2\pi\nu)^2} \\ 0 & 1 & 0 & \dfrac{x\sin 2\pi\nu t}{2\pi\nu} \\ 0 & 0 & 1 & -\dfrac{y(1-\cos 2\pi\nu t)}{2\pi\nu} \\ 0 & 0 & 0 & 1 \end{pmatrix} \quad (t \in \mathbb{R})$$

The energy cylinder carrying the Heisenberg helix has the radius $r \geq 0$ where

$$r^2 = \frac{1}{(2\pi\nu)^2}(x^2 + y^2).$$

- The center tube or bore of the superconducting magnet in the clinical MRI scanner hosts the energy cylinders of the Heisenberg helices.

The circular ray trace of the Heisenberg helix in the transverse plane $\mathbb{R} \oplus \mathbb{R}$ implements, in NMR spectroscopy, Gorter's fundamental idea of a driving oscillator of frequency $\nu \neq 0$:

- The circularity of the ray traces of the Heisenberg helices combined with the oddness of their time dependence in the longitudinal direction allows for spin echo refocusing and gradient echo rewinding.
- The circularity of the tracial grating array defines a phase-locked synchronized neural network by sandwich symmetry.

The ray trace is accessible to the phase-sensitive quadrature detection. Consequently the transition from the cotangent bundle $T^\star(G)$ to the unitary dual $\hat{G}$ will allow the read-out of the encoded differential phase and local frequency information by the trace filter sweep of quantum holography

$$1_\nu \oplus 1_\nu \,.$$

- Up to scaling and translation, the phase and local frequency encoding circular ray traces of the Heisenberg helices are given by the product of cell matrices:

$$\frac{1}{2\pi\nu} \begin{pmatrix} \cos\vartheta & -\sin\vartheta \\ \sin\vartheta & \cos\vartheta \end{pmatrix} \begin{pmatrix} x & -y \\ y & x \end{pmatrix},$$

where

$$\vartheta = 2\pi\nu t \qquad (t \in \mathbb{R})$$

denotes the azimuth angle and

$$1_\nu \oplus 1_\nu$$

denotes the trace filter sweep of quantum holography associated with the tomographic slice $\mathbf{P}(\mathbb{R} \times O_\nu)$ of Larmor precession frequency $\nu \neq 0$.

The multiplicator $r \geq 0$ of the foliation leaf coordinates

$$\left(t, \frac{1}{2\pi\nu} \begin{pmatrix} x & -y \\ y & x \end{pmatrix}, 2\pi\nu \right)$$

is given by

$$r^2 = \frac{1}{(2\pi\nu)} \mu \begin{pmatrix} x & -y \\ y & x \end{pmatrix} = \frac{1}{(2\pi\nu)} (x^2 + y^2) \geq 0\,.$$

For $r = 1$ the ray traces of the Heisenberg helices admit the angular frequency $2\pi\nu$ of the circular grating array, and they are minimizing over the interval $[-\pi, +\pi]$ if the local frequency satisfies the condition

$$|y| \leq 2\pi\,.$$

The time evolution matrix associated with the flip angle $\theta \in [-\pi, \pi]$ and the (T_1, T_2) spin–relaxation decomposition of the contact one-form κ as a section in the dual vector bundle $T^\star \left(T^\star(G) \right)$ reads

$$
\left(
\begin{array}{|cc|cc}
\hline
e^{-|t|/T_2} \sin \theta \cos 2\pi\nu t & -e^{-|t|/T_2} \sin \theta \sin 2\pi\nu t & & 0 \\
e^{-|t|/T_2} \sin \theta \sin 2\pi\nu t & e^{-|t|/T_2} \sin \theta \cos 2\pi\nu t & & 0 \\
\hline
0 & 0 & & 1 - e^{-|t|/T_1}(1 - \cos \theta)
\end{array}
\right) (t \in \mathbb{R}).
$$

Fiber multiplication of the relaxation weights provides the contrast encoding relaxation-weighted Heisenberg helices equipped with the tracial control parameters $(x, y) \in \mathbb{R} \oplus \mathbb{R}$ of the foliation leaf coordinates.

In the application to clinical MRI, the three-dimensional real Lie group G represents the noncommutative structure group to analyze and synthesize the convolutional structure of the phase-coherent wavelets in terms of the unitary dual $\hat{G}$ of G from the Fourier transform side of view, and in a similar way to analyze the frequency window of the affine wavelets which are originating from temporal switching of linear gradients in terms of the affine linear group $\mathbf{GA}(\mathbb{R})$. The relation

$$
\dim_\mathbb{R} G = \dim_\mathbb{R} E = 3
$$

indicates that MRI is an essentially three-dimensional imaging modality, and the dual aspect suggests using row vectors of upper triangular matrices instead of using column vectors of lower triangular matrices for the coordinatization of the nonsplit central group extension $\mathbb{R} \lhd G \longrightarrow \mathbb{R} \oplus \mathbb{R}$. Indeed, the isomorphism of the underlying three-dimensional real vector space onto its dual is not canonical, and the row vectors of a matrix indicate the coordinates with respect to a basis of the dual of the underlying vector space whose coordinates represent the column vectors of the transposed matrix with respect to the dual basis.

In view of the fact that clinical MRI exhausts the full group theoretical properties of the holographic transform $\mathcal{H}_\nu$ and the affine wavelet transform, a treatment of the noncommutative projective geometry and harmonic analysis of the nonsplit central group extension G of $\mathbb{R} \oplus \mathbb{R}$ by $\mathbb{R}$ will be needed.

It follows from the multiplication law

$$
\begin{pmatrix} 1 & x_1 & z_1 \\ 0 & 1 & y_1 \\ 0 & 0 & 1 \end{pmatrix}
\begin{pmatrix} 1 & x_2 & z_2 \\ 0 & 1 & y_2 \\ 0 & 0 & 1 \end{pmatrix}
=
\begin{pmatrix} 1 & x_1 + x_2 & z_1 + z_2 + x_1 y_2 \\ 0 & 1 & y_1 + y_2 \\ 0 & 0 & 1 \end{pmatrix}
$$

that the three-dimensional Heisenberg nilpotent real Lie group $G \hookrightarrow \mathbf{GL}_3(\mathbb{R})$ is noncommutative. The inverses of its elements are given by

$$
\begin{pmatrix} 1 & x & z \\ 0 & 1 & y \\ 0 & 0 & 1 \end{pmatrix}^{-1}
=
\begin{pmatrix} 1 & -x & -z + xy \\ 0 & 1 & -y \\ 0 & 0 & 1 \end{pmatrix}.
$$

The commutator of two elements of G is given by

$$\left[\begin{pmatrix} 1 & x_1 & z_1 \\ 0 & 1 & y_1 \\ 0 & 0 & 1 \end{pmatrix}, \begin{pmatrix} 1 & x_2 & z_2 \\ 0 & 1 & y_2 \\ 0 & 0 & 1 \end{pmatrix}\right] = \begin{pmatrix} 1 & 0 & \det\begin{pmatrix} x_1 & y_1 \\ x_2 & y_2 \end{pmatrix} \\ 0 & 1 & 0 \\ 0 & 0 & 1 \end{pmatrix}$$

so that commutation holds if and only if the area of the parallelogram spanned by the row vectors (x_1, y_1) and (x_2, y_2) vanishes.

Because G admits the one-dimensional center C of elementary matrices

$$C = \left\{ \begin{pmatrix} 1 & 0 & z \\ 0 & 1 & 0 \\ 0 & 0 & 1 \end{pmatrix} \;\middle|\; z \in \mathbb{R} \right\},$$

for the derived group it follows that

$$[G, G] = C.$$

An application of the concepts of the geometry of classical groups to the nonsplit central group extension $\mathbb{R} \lhd G \longrightarrow \mathbb{R} \oplus \mathbb{R}$ shows that the elementary matrices forming C are the coordinates with respect to the laboratory frame of automorphisms of the three-dimensional real vector space G which represent nontrivial transvections associated with the transversal homogeneous plane $\mathbb{R} \oplus \mathbb{R}$ of fixed points as the eigenspace in G associated to the unique eigenvalue 1. The homogeneous longitudinal center line C of G of coordinate $z \in \mathbb{R}^\times$ is transversal to the plane G/C:

- A homogeneous line L of G is mapped into itself under the transvection associated with the center line C if and only if it is contained in the plane $\mathbb{R} \oplus \mathbb{R}$ left pointwise fixed in which it forms a Lagrangian line; a homogenous plane of G is mapped into itself by the transvection if it coincides either with the plane left pointwise fixed or it contains the transversal center line C.

The subgroup of $\mathbf{GL}(G/C; L)$ of $\mathbf{GL}(G/C)$ consisting of all collineations of G/C letting an arbitrary line L in G/C be globally invariant is identified with the group of real matrices

$$\begin{pmatrix} \alpha & \beta \\ 0 & \gamma \end{pmatrix}$$

of determinant $\alpha\gamma \neq 0$ and $\Theta(G/C; L)$ with the subgroup

$$\left\{ \begin{pmatrix} 1 & \beta \\ 0 & 1 \end{pmatrix} \;\middle|\; \beta \in \mathbb{R} \right\}$$

isomorphic to $\mathbb{R}$. Therefore, the Heisenberg Lie group G intrinsically gives rise to the disconnected affine Lie group

$$\mathbf{GA}(\mathbb{R}) = \left\{ \begin{pmatrix} \alpha & \beta \\ 0 & 1 \end{pmatrix} \;\middle|\; \alpha \neq 0, \beta \in \mathbb{R} \right\}$$

of the real line $\mathbb{R}$:

- For any homogeneous line L in G/C, the real Lie group $\mathbf{GA}(\mathbb{R})$ forms a subgroup of the centralizer of $\Theta'(G; L)$ in $\mathbf{GL}(G)$ and its elements are implemented in the MRI scanner by linear gradients of slope $\alpha \neq 0$ of spatial local magnetic flux densities.

The Lie group $\mathbf{GA}(\mathbb{R})$ forms the RF modulation group acting on the modulation space $L_{\mathbb{C}}^2(\mathbb{R})$ of the solvable affine Lauterbur encoding procedure ([197]). Therefore the elements

$$\begin{pmatrix} \alpha & \beta \\ 0 & 1 \end{pmatrix} \in \mathbf{GA}(\mathbb{R})$$

are called *gradient matrices*.

In contrast to $\mathbf{GA}(\mathbb{R})$ the Lie group G is unimodular. Indeed, the Lebesgue measure

$$\mathrm{d}x \wedge \mathrm{d}y \wedge \mathrm{d}z = \mathrm{d}\left(\begin{pmatrix} x \\ y \end{pmatrix}, z \right)$$

defines a choice of left and right Haar measures of G. Note, however, that the natural sub-Riemannian metric of G, the Legendre transform of the principal symbol on $\mathrm{T}^\star(G)$ of the left-invariant sub-Laplacian differential operator $\mathcal{L}_G$, is only left-invariant and not bi-invariant.

Considered as a group extension, G sits in the exact sequence

$$0 \longrightarrow C \longrightarrow G \longrightarrow G/C \longrightarrow 0.$$

Clearly G is contractible, with a contraction being given by the parametrization

$$\mathbb{R} \times G \ni \left(t, \begin{pmatrix} 1 & x & z \\ 0 & 1 & y \\ 0 & 0 & 1 \end{pmatrix} \right) \rightsquigarrow \begin{pmatrix} 1 & tx & tz \\ 0 & 1 & ty \\ 0 & 0 & 1 \end{pmatrix} \in G.$$

Consequently $\pi_1(G) = 0$, and G is the universal covering group of the central extension

$$\mathbb{T} \lhd G_0 \longrightarrow \mathbb{R} \oplus \mathbb{R}.$$

The multiplication law of the Lie group G_0 underlying G reads

$$(x_1, y_1, \zeta_1)(x_2, y_2, \zeta_2) = (x_1 + x_2, y_1 + y_2, \zeta_1\zeta_2 e^{2\pi i x_1 y_2}).$$

Both G and G_0 admit the same Lie algebra of upper triangular matrices

$$\mathrm{Lie}(G) = \mathrm{Lie}(G_0) = \left\{ \begin{pmatrix} 0 & a & c \\ 0 & 0 & b \\ 0 & 0 & 0 \end{pmatrix} \middle| a, b, c \in \mathbb{R} \right\}$$

due to the identity for the one-parameter subgroups of G,

$$\exp_G\left(t \begin{pmatrix} 0 & a & c \\ 0 & 0 & b \\ 0 & 0 & 0 \end{pmatrix} \right) = \begin{pmatrix} 1 & ta & tc + \frac{1}{2}t^2 ab \\ 0 & 1 & tb \\ 0 & 0 & 1 \end{pmatrix},$$

which holds for all parameter values $t \in \mathbb{R}$ and all infinitesimal generators

$$\begin{pmatrix} 0 & a & c \\ 0 & 0 & b \\ 0 & 0 & 0 \end{pmatrix} \in \mathrm{Lie}(G).$$

In particular, the mapping $\exp_G : \mathrm{Lie}(G) \longrightarrow G$ is surjective,

$$\exp_G\big(\mathrm{Lie}(G)\big) = G,$$

hence a diffeomorphism. The canonical basis of $\mathrm{Lie}(G)$ consisting of the matrices

$$P = \begin{pmatrix} 0 & 1 & 0 \\ 0 & 0 & 0 \\ 0 & 0 & 0 \end{pmatrix}, \quad Q = \begin{pmatrix} 0 & 0 & 0 \\ 0 & 0 & 1 \\ 0 & 0 & 0 \end{pmatrix}, \quad I = \begin{pmatrix} 0 & 0 & 1 \\ 0 & 0 & 0 \\ 0 & 0 & 0 \end{pmatrix}$$

gives rise to the automorphisms associated to the elementary matrices

$$\exp_G P = \begin{pmatrix} 1 & 1 & 0 \\ 0 & 1 & 0 \\ 0 & 0 & 1 \end{pmatrix}, \quad \exp_G Q = \begin{pmatrix} 1 & 0 & 0 \\ 0 & 1 & 1 \\ 0 & 0 & 1 \end{pmatrix}, \quad \exp_G I = \begin{pmatrix} 1 & 0 & 1 \\ 0 & 1 & 0 \\ 0 & 0 & 1 \end{pmatrix}$$

of the three-dimensional real vector space G having the scalar 1 as their only eigenvalue. These automorphisms are nontrivial transvections with associated homogeneous lines and transversal homogeneous fixed-point planes as eigenspaces of the single-point spectrum $\{1\}$ in G. In the terminology of clinical MRI, the fixed-point planes are called the directions of tomographic sagittal planes, tomographic coronal planes, and tomographic transaxial planes, respectively. The Lie bracket $[\,\cdot\,,\cdot\,]$ of $\mathrm{Lie}(G)$ is defined by the linear commutator

$$\left[\begin{pmatrix} 0 & a & c \\ 0 & 0 & b \\ 0 & 0 & 0 \end{pmatrix}, \begin{pmatrix} 0 & a' & c' \\ 0 & 0 & b' \\ 0 & 0 & 0 \end{pmatrix} \right] = \begin{pmatrix} 0 & 0 & \det \begin{pmatrix} a & b \\ a' & b' \end{pmatrix} \\ 0 & 0 & 0 \\ 0 & 0 & 0 \end{pmatrix}.$$

In terms of the canonical basis $\{P, Q, I\}$ of $\mathrm{Lie}(G)$ the canonical commutation relations read

$$[P, Q] = I, \quad [P, I] = 0, \quad [Q, I] = 0.$$

The preceding equations characterize the Heisenberg Lie algebra $\mathrm{Lie}(G)$ completely. Quantum mechanics is steeped in symplecticism, owing to the anti-symmetry of the Lie bracket occurring in the canonical commutation relations.

The direction of the longitudinal center line C of G is defined by $\exp_G I$:

- In terms of transvections of the three-dimensional real vector space G, the commutation of P and I is equivalent to the fact that the direction of the longitudinal center line C is contained in the homogeneous tomographic sagittal plane, and the direction of the real line spanned by P is contained in the homogeneous tomographic transaxial plane.

In a similar way, the following geometrical result can be established:

- In terms of transvections of the three-dimensional real vector space G, the commutation of Q and I is equivalent to the fact that the direction of the longitudinal center line C is contained in the homogeneous tomographic coronal plane, and the direction of the real line spanned by Q is contained in the homogeneous tomographic transaxial plane.

Thus the direction of the longitudinal center line C is given by the intersection of the homogeneous tomographic coronal plane and the homogeneous tomographic sagittal plane.

It follows for the derivation associated with the Lie bracket $[\,\cdot\,,\cdot\,]$ of Lie(G) that

$$\mathrm{ad}_{\mathrm{Lie}(G)} \begin{pmatrix} 0 & a & c \\ 0 & 0 & b \\ 0 & 0 & 0 \end{pmatrix} = \begin{pmatrix} 0 & 0 & 0 \\ 0 & 0 & 0 \\ -b & a & 0 \end{pmatrix}.$$

The adjoint representation Ad_G of G acts by conjugation on Lie(G) as

$$\begin{pmatrix} 1 & x & z \\ 0 & 1 & y \\ 0 & 0 & 1 \end{pmatrix} \begin{pmatrix} 0 & a & c \\ 0 & 0 & b \\ 0 & 0 & 0 \end{pmatrix} \begin{pmatrix} 1 & x & z \\ 0 & 1 & y \\ 0 & 0 & 1 \end{pmatrix}^{-1} = \begin{pmatrix} 0 & a & c - \det\begin{pmatrix} a & x \\ b & y \end{pmatrix} \\ 0 & 0 & b \\ 0 & 0 & 0 \end{pmatrix}$$

so that again

$$\mathrm{Ad}_G \circ \exp_G = \exp_G \circ \, \mathrm{ad}_{\mathrm{Lie}(G)}$$

and explicitly,

$$\mathrm{Ad}_G \begin{pmatrix} 1 & x & z \\ 0 & 1 & y \\ 0 & 0 & 1 \end{pmatrix} = \begin{pmatrix} 1 & 0 & 0 \\ 0 & 1 & 0 \\ -y & x & 1 \end{pmatrix}.$$

In terms of the dual basis $\{P^\star, Q^\star, I^\star\}$ of Lie$(G)^\star$, the action of the coadjoint representation CoAd_G of G on Lie$(G)^\star$ reads

$$\begin{pmatrix} 1 & x & z \\ 0 & 1 & y \\ 0 & 0 & 1 \end{pmatrix}^{-1} (\alpha P^\star + \beta Q^\star + \nu I^\star) = (\alpha - \nu y)P^\star + (\beta + \nu x)Q^\star + \nu I^\star$$

so that

$$\mathrm{CoAd}_G \begin{pmatrix} 1 & x & z \\ 0 & 1 & y \\ 0 & 0 & 1 \end{pmatrix} = \begin{pmatrix} 1 & 0 & -y \\ 0 & 1 & x \\ 0 & 0 & 1 \end{pmatrix}.$$

This implies the flatness of CoAd_G for $\nu \neq 0$ so that its projective completion exists (Figure 21):

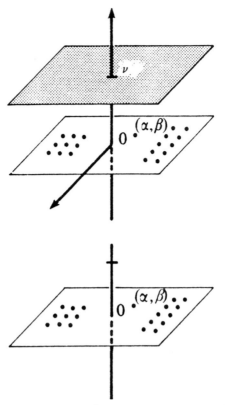

Figure 21. Coadjoint orbit picture of the dual $\hat{G}$ of the Heisenberg nilpotent Lie group G in the vector space dual Lie$(G)^\star$ of the Heisenberg Lie algebra Lie (G). The center frequencey $\nu \neq 0$ determines the whole tomographic slice of the foliation via resonance with the global frequency ν. The singular plane is determined by the condition $\nu = 0$. The projective completion of Lie$(G)^\star$ by the stratigraphic time line $\mathbb{R}$ provides the basic mathematical model of clinical MRI. The lower picture visualizes the quotient manifold Lie$(G)^\star/\mathrm{CoAd}_G(G)$.

- The nontrivial coadjoint orbit of G,

$$\mathcal{O}_\nu = \mathrm{CoAd}_G(G)(\nu I^\star) \qquad (\nu \neq 0),$$

  is the symplectic affine plane in the real vector space dual Lie$(G)^\star$ given by the set

$$\mathcal{O}_\nu = \mathbb{R}P^\star + \mathbb{R}Q^\star + \nu I^\star.$$

  The symplectic structure of $\mathcal{O}_\nu$ is given by the rotational curvature form ω_ν. The projective completion $\mathbf{P}(\mathbb{R} \times \mathcal{O}_\nu)$ by the stratigraphic time line $\mathbb{R}$ forms the tomographic slice of central frequency $\nu \neq 0$.

As opposed to the connected component

$$\mathbf{GA}^+(\mathbb{R}) = \left\{ \begin{pmatrix} \alpha & \beta \\ 0 & 1 \end{pmatrix} \,\middle|\, \alpha > 0, \beta \in \mathbb{R} \right\}$$

of the affine Lie group $\mathbf{GA}(\mathbb{R})$ of the real line $\mathbb{R}$ which, up to isomorphism, is the only connected non-Abelian Lie group of dimension 2 and admits only two nontrivial phase conjugate coadjoint orbits $\mathcal{O}_{\pm}$, the nontrivial coadjoint orbits of the Heisenberg nilpotent real Lie group G are parametrized by the *punctured* central line $C - \{0\}$. The functional self-organization by resonance is performed by the process of coadjoint orbit merging. This proves the central role played by the coadjoint orbit model of the associated unitary duals to clinical MRI.

For the applications to noninvasive clinical imaging and microvascular dynamical topographic neuroimaging, it is of paramount importance that the simply connected Heisenberg Lie group G admits infinitely many nontrivial, noninteractive, coadjoint orbits $\mathbf{P}(\mathbb{R} \times \mathcal{O}_\nu) \hookrightarrow \mathbf{P}(\mathbb{R} \times \mathrm{Lie}(G)^\star)$ $(\nu \neq 0)$ providing a stratified structure of the projectively immersed quotient $\mathrm{Lie}(G)^\star / \mathrm{CoAd}_G(G)$. The coadjoint orbits are transversal to the longitudinal center line C and synchronously revolving planar tomographic slices, uniquely determined by the central unitary character χ_ν of G ([243]),

$$\mathbf{P}(\mathbb{R} \times \mathcal{O}_\nu) \rightsquigarrow \chi_\nu \qquad (\nu \neq 0),$$

and uniquely determining the frequency of resonance ν of the whole tomographic slice.

In clinical MRI, for a given external magnetic flux density, it is in the planar coadjoint orbits $\mathbf{P}(\mathbb{R} \times \mathcal{O}_\nu)$ of G that the quantum coherent phenomenon of the dephasing of the free induction decay takes place after the spin relaxation time T_2. The transverse or spin–spin relaxation process is opposed to the longitudinal or spin–lattice relaxation process by which the magnetization of the coherently excited spin isochromats of the planar coadjoint orbits $\mathbf{P}(\mathbb{R} \times \mathcal{O}_\nu)$ return to the longitudinal direction of the center line C after the time T_1. Thus the free induction decay is the combined T_1 and T_2 weighted spin–relaxation response to a magnetization excitation of the dissipative spin system within the select planar coadjoint orbit $\mathbf{P}(\mathbb{R} \times \mathcal{O}_\nu) \hookrightarrow \mathbf{P}(\mathbb{R} \times \mathrm{Lie}(G)^\star)$ performed by resonance with a pulse of central frequency $\nu \neq 0$ (Figure 22 and Figure 23). The tissue specific spin–relaxation times satisfy

$$T_2 \leq T_1.$$

On a clinical MRI scan of the cerebral parenchymal morphology, for instance, the white matter appears white, the gray matter appears gray, and the CSF appears dark using acquisitions of T_1 spin–relaxation weight. The result is the opposite on T_2-weighted scans. A cerebral subdural hematoma or intraparenchymal bleed appears isodense on T_1-weighted MRI acquisitions and dark on T_2-weighted MRI scans during the first three days, gaining a high NMR filter response intensity later as the red blood cells break down and release their paramagnetic methemoglobin ([188], [287]):

- Because there are two tissue relaxation times, T_1 and T_2, available together with two waiting times, T_R and T_E, there are four basic MRI scan types. For T_1 weighting, the echo time T_E should be short to reduce differences in T_2-dependent NMR response loss.Likewise, for T_2 weighting, T_R must be as long

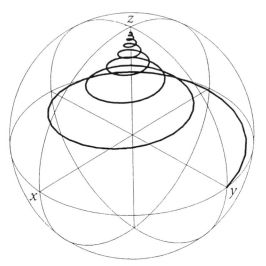

Figure 22. Relaxation weighted spherical trace of a Heisenberg helix. Note that the Heisenberg helices carried by the energy cylinders form the geodesics with respect to the sub-Riemannian geometry of the manifold G. The planar coadjoint orbit of the Heisenberg nilpotent Lie group G is a cross section of the cotangent bundle $T^\star S_2$ of the sphere $S_2 \hookrightarrow \mathbb{R}^3$ and therefore provides the multiplanar imaging capability of clinical MRI. To control the Heisenberg helices, the resonance in the planar coadjoint orbit can be accomplished by the application of spin echo or gradient echo techniques.

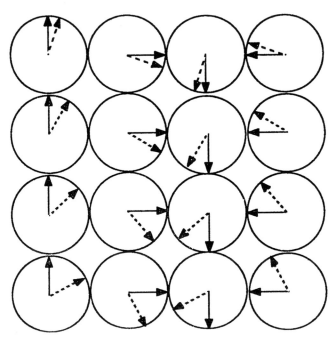

Figure 23. Planar traces of Heisenberg helices forming a Kepplerian clockwork. The global frequency is given by the Larmor frequency $\nu \neq 0$. The rows of the matrix visualization vary the differential phases, whereas the columns vary the local frequencies of the Kepplerian clockwork. The insuing filter bank structure is implemented by the interal symplectic affine structure associated to the planar coadjoint orbits of the Heisenberg Lie group G.

as possible to reduce T_1 weighting by allowing the spins to fully recover. For proton density weighting, both T_1 and T_2 relaxation effects are reduced by choosing T_E short and T_R long.

As an example, in the MRI-assisted diagnosis of white matter disorders, the demonstration of MS lesions can be performed by using moderately T_2 weighted spin echo sequences, a relatively long echo time T_E of 40 to 60 ms, and a relatively short repetition period T_R of 2,000 to 2,500 ms. The resulting images have good T_2 contrast, while CSF still has low NMR filter response (Figure 24). On such MRI scans, MS lesions have a higher intensity than anything else except subcutaneous fat, while fluidlike abnormalities, such as dilated perivascular spaces, have lower signal ([27], [152], [175], [289], [343], [345], [347]). The corpus callosum and subcallosalependymal surfaces are abnormal in most MS patients. The MS lesions vary from focal abnormalities to long confluent demyelinating plaques and radiate from the inferior surface of the corpus callosum.

It is this diversity of spin–relaxation rates

$$\frac{1}{T_k} \ (k \in \{1, 2\})$$

in different tissues that produces the superior soft-tissue image contrast of the Fourier MRI modality. However, the combination of long T_E and short T_R should not be used for the tracial encoding of image contrast.

Radiological tissue differentiation in accordance with the (T_1, T_2) spin–relaxation decomposition of κ does not seem to be of great value for realistic clinical MRI applications to the human body. The empirically established correlations between spin–relaxation rates of neoplastic tissues and histopathology shows that the *in vivo* values of the synchronized timing parameters T_k $(k \in \{1, 2\})$ actually are so wide ranged that their overlap between benign and malignant lesions makes it impossible to characterize human tumor tissue types simply by measurements of these values or a combination of these. Reasons for this insufficient distinction include biological causes since benign and malignant tissues have possibly similar biochemical composition:

- Spin isochromats form dissipative nuclear spin systems naturally associated with the (T_1, T_2) relaxation decomposition of κ. In spin isochromats the proton ensembles are precessing in synchrony.
- Spin isochromat manipulation by resonance with RF excitation pulses of central frequency $\nu = (1/2\pi)\dot{\vartheta}$ and filtering measurements of the signals responding to the induced magnetization perturbations are transversally performed by the vertical projection of the free induction decays along the lift of the longitudinal center line C of G to $\mathrm{Lie}(G)^\star$ to the planar coadjoint orbit $\mathbf{P}(\mathbb{R} \times \mathcal{O}_\nu)$ immersed into the stratified structure of the projectively completed, symplectic affine space $\mathbf{P}(\mathbb{R} \times \mathrm{Lie}(G)^\star)$ $(\nu \neq 0)$.

The central unitary character χ_ν allows for planar spin slice selection by computer-controlled linear gradients of spatial local magnetic flux densities along the longi-

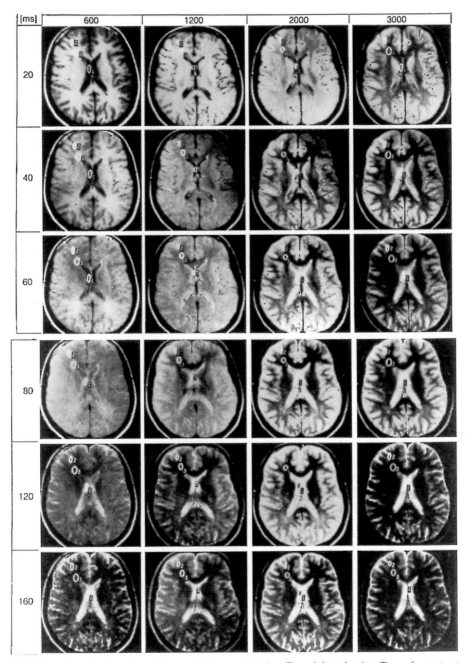

Figure 24. Visualization of the influence of the repetition time T_R and the echo time T_E on the contrast of CNS, grey, and white matter. The series of transverse cerebral MRI scans has been acquired by a conventional spin echo pulse sequence. Scan parameters $\Rightarrow T_R$ in ms, $\Downarrow T_E$ in ms.

tudinal center line C and resonance with a RF excitation pulse of central frequency $\nu = \dot{\vartheta}/2\pi$. Thus the in-plane linear gradient coordinate frames of spatial local magnetic flux densities within selectively excited planar tomographic slices create a linkage between spatial position and frequency ν of the central unitary character in such a way that the two are essentially synonymous. This linkage (in Greek, $\tau o \zeta \epsilon \nu \gamma \mu \alpha$) between the spatial scale along the logitudinal center line C and the parallel affine linear scale of nuclear Larmor reference frequencies forms the origin of Paul C. Lauterbur's term "zeugmatography" for MRI. It is one of the purposes of this text to make the fundamental Lauterbur $\tau o \zeta \epsilon \nu \gamma \mu \alpha$ link mathematically precise by establishing that the Heisenberg nilpotent real Lie group G forms the structure group of the spin isochromats which are the dissipative nuclear spin systems naturally associated with the (T_1, T_2) relaxation decomposition of κ:

- The image contrast of T_k-weighted MRI scans ($k \in \{1, 2\}$) is based on the (T_1, T_2) relaxation decomposition of κ.

From the electrical engineering point of view, the wavelets give rise to the wide-band and narrow-band ambiguity functions, respectively. The wide-band width capabilities of photonic fiber channel networks are attractive features of photonic telecommunication systems, whereas narrow-band width frequencies are used in spatially localized MRI for selective planar spin slice excitation purposes. It is this variety of approaches and the perspectives of neurofunctional MRI to cognitive neuroscience which make wavelet theory such an exciting area of multidisciplinary research.

Similar to the affine Lie group approach to affine wavelet sets, there exist trivial orbits in $\mathbf{P}(\mathbb{R} \times \mathrm{Lie}(G)^\star)$ apart from the planar coadjoint orbits $\mathbf{P}(\mathbb{R} \times \mathcal{O}_\nu), (\nu \neq 0)$. The trivial coadjoint orbits of G are single points of spatial coordinates

$$(\alpha, \beta) \in \mathbb{R} \oplus \mathbb{R}$$

with respect to $\{P^\star, Q^\star\}$ located in the homogeneous singular plane $\nu = 0$ of $\mathrm{Lie}(G)^\star$. As a spatial Fourier filter, the homogeneous singular plane $\mathbf{P}(\mathbb{R} \times \mathcal{O}_\infty)$ within the stratified structure of the projectively completed dual $\mathbf{P}(\mathbb{R} \times \mathrm{Lie}(G)^\star)$ admits an important application to optical microscopy. Indeed, in confocal scanning microscopy, the singular plane $\nu = 0$ is called the confocal plane of $\mathrm{Lie}(G)^\star$. The one-dimensional representations of G which are generated by the two-dimensional distributional Fourier transforms $\mathcal{F}_{\mathbb{R} \oplus \mathbb{R}} \, \varepsilon_{(\alpha, \beta)}$ of the Dirac measures

$$\{\varepsilon_{(\alpha, \beta)} | (\alpha, \beta) \in \mathbb{R} \oplus \mathbb{R}\}$$

located as von Neumann bottlenecks within the confocal plane are implemented by a spinning disc containing a raster pattern of pinhole apertures through which light is sent and collected and an objective lens to speed the scanning process of plane inside the specimen. In a confocal scanning microscope, the lens optically acts as a massively parallel, two-dimensional Fourier transform processor. The disc revolves to ensure that every spot $\varepsilon_{(\alpha, \beta)}$ in the homogeneous singular plane which forms the array of bottlenecks will be visited and to speed the scanning process ([234],

[302]). The result has given microscopists the ability to see into objects and to create three-dimensional high resolution images from confocal planar scannings:

- The most important property of confocal scanning microscopy is its ability to form a three-dimensional image of an object possessing appreciable depth. The three-dimensional imaging capability results from the strong optical tomographic property of confocal scanning microscopy.

In biological microscopy, for example, this allows the investigation of the structure inside a cell. In material science or semiconductor device technology it allows the measurement of surface topography. This ability to form a three-dimensional image is extremely powerful, especially when coupled with the improved resolution and contrast of confocal microscopy.

The three-dimensional imaging capability due to the tomographic property is of a completely different nature from the restricted depth of field in conventional microscopy, the difference being that in a conventional microscope out-of-focus information is merely blurred, while in the confocal scanning microscope it is actually detected much less strongly: Light scattered at some place axially separated from the focal plane is defocused at the detector plane and hence fails to pass efficiently through a raster placed there.

It is a remarkable fact that according to the classification of the coadjoint orbits of G there exist no finite-dimensional irreducible unitary linear representations of dimension greater than 1. A consequence is the double-slit experiment of photonics, which is the archetypal example of the wave–particle duality ([303]). Quantum holography rigorously proves that the interference pattern is destroyed by a localization of the path of each photon. Thus the observer has no right to maintain that any given photon actually follows a definite path.

Unser Bildner hat den Seinen den Geist gefügt, nicht bloß damit sich der Mensch seinen Lebensunterhalt erwerbe, sondern auch dazu, daß wir vom Sein der Dinge, die wir mit den Augen betrachten, zu den Ursachen ihres Seins und Werdens vordringen, auch wenn weiter kein Nutzen damit verbunden ist.

—Johann Keppler (1571–1630)

How, to have a × *b not equal b* × *a is something that does not fit in very well with geometrical ideas.*

—Paul A. M. Dirac (1902–1984)

Years of hard work will surely be necessary to put an end to the clichés, there being no task more difficult than that of modifying accepted ideas.

—Jean A. Dieudonné (1906–1995)

The great Johannes Kepler . . .

—Roger Penrose (1989)

Timing is everything.

—The MRI Manual, 1998

The full information needed to reconstruct the state of an object can be divided into two parts, quantum and classical.

—Tony Sudbery (1997)

2.2 QUANTUM COMPUTATIONAL ASPECTS

Quantum theory was developed originally as a theory to explain the behavior of ensembles of microscopic objects. Recently considerable interest has developed in the application of quantum theory to individual systems and its extension to macroscopic system hierarchies. In part, this interest has been stimulated by the progress in experimental physics and computer-intensive system engineering. The quantum theoretic approach to macroscopic system engineering has its mathematical foundation in the discipline of noncommutative geometrical analysis, which provides the appropriate orbital calculi.

An example of an important application of noncommutative geometrical analysis to Lie group actions which is beyond the frontier of pure mathematics is that of *quantum holography*. As an initially purely academic idea, the spatiotemporal quantization strategy of quantum holography leads to the nuclear resonance absorption-mode spectra and the reconstructive tomographic procedure of computerized pulsed Fourier MRI. The quantized calculi associated with the geometrical analysis of quantum holography form the climax in elegance of the subject matter.

The advantage of studying the interaction of resonances and the dynamical symmetries of mode-locked dissipative spin systems via a connected Lie group action is that it is easier to identify periodic, quasi-periodic, and chaotic motions by iterating a one-parameter circle map than by an application of a cumbersome integration procedure to the underlying Bloch–Riccati differential equation. Furthermore, for the *cognoscente* of Lie group and group $C^\star$–algebra theory, another advantage is that the coadjoint orbit visualization, also known by the more fashionable term *geometrical quantization*, conveys much more of group representations than would otherwise be possible by assigning to each classical dynamical system for a connected Lie group action a corresponding quantum dynamical system. In this way, classical dynamical systems seem to be inextricably linked to the class of *square integrable* representations of connected Lie groups whenever their actions occur. A coadjoint orbit forms an affine *linear variety* in the dual of the Lie algebra if and only if the corresponding equivalent irreducible unitary linear representations are square integrable modulo kernel. The geometrical characterization of square integrability by *flat* coadjoint orbits allows for an extension of the classical Weyl theory from compact to nilpotent Lie group representations. In particular, it allows for an explicit *direct* integral decomposition of *tensor product* square integrable representations performing holographic *encryption* by mixing deterministic propagators of quantum theory.

Important applications of the spatiotemporal quantization strategy for the benefit of humankind as well as impressive visualizations of the canonical foliation of planar coadjoint orbit leaves associated with the unitary dual $\hat{G}$ of the Heisenberg group G seemed to be out of reach of noncommutative geometrical analysis. The canonical foliation carries the holographic *decryption* performed by mixing deterministic propagators of Fourier MRI.

The objective of computerized pulsed Fourier MRI is to evaluate, via the *symplectic* linear response theory of *coherent* tomography, the planar interference patterns, or quantum holograms, selected and coherently excited by the MRI scanner system. The reconstructive read-out procedure from the canonically foliated three-dimensional superencoded projective space $\mathbf{P}(\mathbb{R} \times \mathrm{Lie}(G)^{\star})$ is performed by an application of the quantized calculus in terms of the symplectically formatted Fourier transform. Since its introduction in the early 1980s, the reconstructive tomographic procedure of computerized pulsed Fourier MRI has become the method of choice in a continuously increasing area of noninvasive radiodiagnostic tests, leaving virtually no internal organ system untouched. Frequently, clinical MRI is the definitive examination procedure, providing invaluable information to help the surgeon not only understand the underlying pathology but also make the critical decision regarding surgical intervention. Patients the world over enjoy a higher quality of life, and many lives have been saved, thanks to clinical MRI, which forms the most sensitive and reliable diagnostic imaging modality in computer-assisted clinical medicine presently available. As a consequence, an extension of its traditional geographical distribution in North America, Western Europe, and Japan to other parts of the world seems necessary.

Although the main topic of Fourier analysis is the study of spectra, most mathematicians are unaware of the practical application of spectral transform techniques to the site identification by NMR scanning signals, the correlations between sites, and the more sophisticated methods of spectral localization analysis, applied in computerized pulsed Fourier MRI of clinically relevant human anatomy and pathophysiology. The key point is that spin isochromats allow to perform *implicitly* the Fourier transform. The spectral transform for the left-invariant sub-Laplacian differential operator $\mathcal{L}_G$ of the sub-Riemannian manifold G establishes that quantum computation can perform the Weyl symbol and quantum information can be represented in planar tomographic slices carrying a rotational curvature form.

Outside the realm of physical chemistry it is not well known how to consider modern spin choreography as a prelude to NMR quantum computation and computerized pulsed Fourier MRI, and even MRologists do not realize that the symplectically formatted Fourier transform represents the reconstructive procedure of NMR tomography.

Physical chemists are used to applying the Bargmann–Fock model for the eventual realization of the real Heisenberg Lie algebra $\text{Lie}(G)$ in terms of shift operators, otherwise known as *creation* and *annihilation* or raising and lowering operators. As adjoints, this pair of operators actually represent complex conjugates with respect to the complexification of the transverse symplectic affine plane $\text{Lie}(G)/\text{center}$. Instead of using a projective geometrical analysis approach to Fourier NMR spectroscopy, physical chemists consider the Fourier transform as a black box and therefore do not touch the metaplectic group $\mathbf{Mp}(2, \mathbb{R})$ acting on the Heisenberg Lie group

$$G = \exp_G \text{Lie}(G), \qquad \exp_G \mid \text{center} = \text{id}_{\mathbb{R}}$$

to embed, via the covariance identity of $\mathbf{Mp}(2, \mathbb{R})$, the quadrature phase duality of the Bloch nuclear induction decay-mode spectrum and the Purcell nuclear resonance absorption-mode spectrum. The quadrature phase-sensitive detection of phase-coherent response wavelets revolutionized NMR spectroscopy and finally chemical analysis as well as noninvasive clinical radiodiagnostics for the benefit of patients.

The contact geometry of G can be obtained from the contact one-form

$$\kappa = \mathrm{d}z + \tfrac{1}{2}\left(x \,\mathrm{d}y - y \,\mathrm{d}x\right)$$

where

$$\mathrm{d}\kappa = \mathrm{d}x \wedge \mathrm{d}y$$

is the rotational curvature form

$$\omega_1 = P_G(1)\,\mathrm{d}\kappa$$

with respect to the laboratory coordinate frame of reference. The scaled rotational curvature form

$$\omega_\nu = \nu\,\omega_1 = P_G(\nu)\,\mathrm{d}\kappa \quad (\nu \neq 0)$$

then allows to holographically record the circular grating arrays formed by the traces of the Heisenberg helices.

The holographic reconstruction is performed from the rotating coordinate frame of reference attached to the coadjoint orbit $\mathbf{P}\left(\mathbb{R} \times \mathcal{O}_\nu\right) (\nu \neq 0)$ of G at the Larmor precession frequency ν of the driving oscillator. *Both* of the coordinate frames of references represent cross sections of the one-dimensional center in G so that the *transition* from one coordinate frame to the other can be performed by phase-sensitive detection. The dynamical transition by an application of quadrature and stroboscopic phase-sensitive detection strategies has its roots in Keppler's change of perspective for the localization of planetary orbits. It is basic not only for his physical astronomy but also for a spatiotemporal analysis of nuclear spin and antiecho responses and related quantum teleportation phenomena.

The transfer from one coordinate frame to the other one within the selected coadjoint orbit is performed by the linear isomorphism $\log_{\mathrm{Lie}(G)} \mid (G/\text{center})$. The reconstructive read-out procedure performed by fast Fourier transform (FFT) processors from the coadjoint orbit unveils the intellectual beauty and efficacy of this unique interdisciplinary achievement and provides a perspective for the realization of a quantum computer based on NMR spectroscopic techniques.

The computerized pulsed Fourier MRI modality requires a creative combination of spatiotemporal quantization strategies. Its coherent excitation–acquisition procedures offer a new view to the elliptic non-Euclidean *line bundle* geometry by the transvectional action of G on the canonical foliation of the three-dimensional superencoded projective space $\mathbf{P}\left(\mathbb{R} \times \mathrm{Lie}(G)^{\star}\right)$ which is parametrized by the bi-infinite stratigraphic *time* line $\mathbb{R}$ of the MRI protocol.

The fundamental idea of associating a Lie algebra to a given connected Lie group is akin to associating the derivative ψ' and, via duality, the differential one-form $\psi'(t)\,dt$ on a given continuously differentiable function $\psi : \mathbb{R} \longrightarrow \mathbb{C}$ of density $\psi(t)\,dt$ with respect to Lebesgue measure dt of the one-parameter laboratory frame of calculus. Specifically the Heisenberg Lie algebra $\mathrm{Lie}(G)$ implements:

1. the location operator $\psi \rightsquigarrow 2\pi i \nu t \psi(t)\,dt \quad (\nu \neq 0)$, and
2. the momentum operator $\psi \rightsquigarrow \psi'(t)\,dt$.

It is a remarkable fact that quantum holography allows for a new interpretation of the coadjoint orbit picture of the Heisenberg group G. The group G, which can be defined as the only connected, simply connected, three-dimensional, nilpotent, *non-Abelian* Lie group, admits a realization by a faithful matrix representation $G \longrightarrow \mathbf{Sp}(4, \mathbb{R})$. It provides the coadjoint action on the projective completion $\mathbf{P}\left(\mathbb{R} \times \mathrm{Lie}(G)^{\star}\right)$ of the dual vector space $\mathrm{Lie}(G)^{\star}$ by the bi-infinite stratigraphic time line $\mathbb{R}$. The planar coadjoint orbits $\mathbf{P}\left(\mathbb{R} \times \mathcal{O}_{\nu}\right) \hookrightarrow \mathbf{P}\left(\mathbb{R} \times \mathrm{Lie}(G)^{\star}\right)$ $(\nu \neq 0)$ of G form a *decomposition* by the canonical foliation of contiguously excited, adjacently decoupled, energetic strata which are parametrized by the bi-infinite stratigraphic time line $\mathbb{R}$.

A specific application of quantum holography, namely computerized pulsed Fourier MRI, is based as an efficient noninvasive radiodiagnostic imaging modality on an originally purely academic idea. The nuclear spin and gradient echo responses allow for a surprising interpretation of the planar coadjoint orbit leaves $\mathbf{P}\left(\mathbb{R} \times \mathcal{O}_{\nu}\right) \hookrightarrow \mathbf{P}\left(\mathbb{R} \times \mathrm{Lie}(G)^{\star}\right)$ $(\nu \neq 0)$. They represent a hierarchy of tomographic slices forming the canonical foliation of energetic strata which are selected and then phase sensitively encoded by the coherent excitation–acquisition cycles along the bi-infinite stratigraphic time line $\mathbb{R}$.

The coadjoint orbit and group $C^\star$–algebra realizations of the unitary dual

$$\hat{G} \cong \mathrm{Lie}(G)^\star / \mathrm{CoAd}_G(G) \cong C^\star(G)\hat{\ }$$

establish geometrically the phase-coherent wavelet collapse phenomenon of the infinite dimensional irreducible unitary linear representations of G, which are square integrable modulo center, *down* to the non–square integrable, one-dimensional representations, which are unitary characters of G. Since the Plancherel measure of $\hat{G}$ is concentrated on the square integrable representations of G, the coherent wavelet collapse phenomenon affords a Plancherel-negligible subset of $\hat{G}$.

It is one of the advantages of the coadjoint orbit visualization of the unitary dual $\hat{G}$ that it includes the energetic edge consisting of the single-point coadjoint orbits of G. For a quantum computer operating in parallel on all of its inputs, the *singular* observation plane forms the bottleneck for the amount of information that can be extracted from quantum computations performed in parallel.

The Hilbert space for a system of distinguishable particles must be taken as the tensor product of the Hilbert spaces of the individual particles, to model the correlations among them. The phenomenon of phase-coherent wavelet collapse suggests a geometrical analysis of tensor product representations of G by use of the conjugation symmetry which restores phase coherence in the *planar* affine coadjoint orbit leaves of the canonically foliated projective space $\mathbf{P}(\mathbb{R} \times \mathrm{Lie}(G)^\star)$. The energetic edge separates the coadjoint orbit $\mathbf{P}(\mathbb{R} \times \mathcal{O}_\nu)$ from the coadjoint antiorbit or echo orbit $\mathbf{P}(\mathbb{R} \times \mathcal{O}_{-\nu})$, by sandwich symmetry which derives from the reflection

$$\begin{pmatrix} \begin{array}{cc|c} 1 & 0 & 0 \\ 0 & -1 & 0 \\ \hline 0 & 0 & -1 \end{array} \end{pmatrix}$$

used to describe the standard spin echo experiment. The sandwich symmetry is determined by the singular observation plane $\mathbf{P}(\mathbb{R} \times \mathcal{O}_\infty)$ consisting of the Plancherel-negligible set of *single*-point coadjoint orbits of G. Crossing the energetic gap creates the collapse of the *generic* coadjoint orbit dimension

$$\dim_{\mathbb{R}} \mathbf{P}(\mathbb{R} \times \mathcal{O}_\nu) = 2 \qquad (\nu \neq 0)$$

down to dimension zero. It establishes that the nuclear spin echo and gradient echo phenomena of NMR spectroscopy and clinical MRI form a genuine quantum self-interference effect which generates quantum teleportation states by time reversal.

What has given preference to the geometrical construction of the canonically foliated three-dimensional super-encoding projective space $\mathbf{P}(\mathbb{R} \times \mathrm{Lie}(G)^\star)$ over the standard bra–ket procedures of quantum mechanics? One fundamental answer is that the space $\mathbf{P}(\mathbb{R} \times \mathrm{Lie}(G)^\star)$ contains the singular observation plane $\mathbf{P}(\mathbb{R} \times \mathcal{O}_\infty)$ in which the coherent wavelet collapse phenomenon occurs. Thus the projective space $\mathbf{P}(\mathbb{R} \times \mathrm{Lie}(G)^\star)$ includes the bottleneck for the amount of information that can be extracted from quantum computing by NMR spectroscopy.

The analogies between NMR spectroscopy and optical spectroscopy are often unhappily neglected. Following Bloembergen's procedure, an extension from NMR spectroscopy to photonics should be possible. Such an extension can be achieved by the Frobenius concept of *weak* containment and *central* integral decomposition of unitary Lie group representations.

For any connected, simply connected nilpotent Lie group, the tensor product $U_1 \hat{\otimes} U_2$ is square integrable modulo its kernel provided the irreducible unitary linear representations U_1 and U_2 are square integrable modulo their kernels. Note that the mixed representation $U_1 \hat{\otimes} U_2$ admits as its coadjoint orbit the composite of the coadjoint orbits $\mathcal{O}_{U_1}$ and $\mathcal{O}_{U_2}$, given by the closed hull $\overline{\mathcal{O}_{U_1} + \mathcal{O}_{U_2}}$. Its central integral decomposition establishes that the weak containment, and specifically the containment for *perfect* reconstruction, of the one-dimensional *identity* representation 1 implies the unitary isomorphy

$$U_2 \cong \check{U}_1$$

of U_2 with the *contragredient* representation $\check{U}_1$ instead of U_1.

- The one-dimensional identity representation 1 has the single-point coadjoint orbit $\{0\} \in \mathcal{O}_\infty$.

It follows from the weak containment of 1 in the tensor product representation $U \hat{\otimes} \check{U}$ that the composite coadjoint orbit associated with the mixing procedure $\hat{\otimes}$ takes the sandwich symmetric form $\overline{\mathcal{O}_U - \mathcal{O}_U}$. The *entangling* equivalence of the square integrable representations U_2 and U_1 of the Heisenberg Lie group G is valid across the energetic gap of the associated quantum states. The energetic edge is determined by the phase-coherent wavelet collapse phenomenon associated with the Plancherel-negligible set of *single-point* coadjoint orbits inside $\mathcal{O}_\infty$.

An important point of concern is the distinction of positive and rewinding negative frequencies, because resonance takes place only at the Larmor precession frequency ν and *not* at the opposite frequency. The reflection

$$P_G \rightsquigarrow -P_G$$

of the Pfaffian polynomial function indicates the conjugation transition

$$U \rightsquigarrow \bar{U}$$

of *entangled*, non-isomorphic representations in $\hat{G}$. Realized by rewinding gradients, the reflection allows to emulate the sandwich symmetric bilinear rotations. These include the implementation of the π pulses which are used to perform the spin echo teleportation effect by time reversal, as well as the photonic teleportation phenomenon.

The transition

$$\bar{U} \rightsquigarrow \check{U}$$

leads from the *conjugate* representation $\bar{U}$ of U to the contragredient representation $\check{U}$ of U, via the canonical anti-isomorphism of the representation Hilbert space onto its dual. Notice that the contragredient representation is created by the reflection ˅ through the neutral element of G. In contrast to $\bar{U}$, which acts on the antidual, the representation $\check{U}$ acts on the dual of the representation Hilbert space ([308], [309]). Due to the *trace formula* for square integrable representations modulo center, the contragredient representation $\check{U}$ of G is of central importance for the reconstructive read-out procedure of quantum holography.

The associated orbital calculus establishes that the mode mixing of a phase-coherent wavelet ψ evolving under a propagator with a probing mode allows for a *nonlocal* holographic read-out, or collapse detection inside the observation plane $\mathbf{P}(\mathbb{R} \times \mathcal{O}_\infty)$, solely of the original wavelet ψ or its phase conjugate mode $\bar{\psi}$:

- The quantum states associated with spin isochromats can be quantum computationally realized by a coherent superposition of phase-locked, synchronized neural network organizations.

- The spin density reconstruction can be performed by a coherent superposition of phase-locked, synchronized neural networks with three sandwich symmetric layers, followed by an amplification to the macroscopic system level via classical parallelism.

Within the decoherence time scale, the reconstructed phase-coherent wavelets reflect *quantum dynamics* at the *macroscopic* level of the receiver coil. This quantum computational observation is fundamental in the areas of NMR spectroscopy and clinical MRI.

Due to the Bargmann–Fock model of the Heisenberg Lie algebra Lie(G), the link between quantum holography and synchronized parallel neural networks explains the redundancy of quantum holograms and the quantum parallelism at the molecular level. In this way, geometrical analysis on the canonically foliated, three-dimensional projective space $\mathbf{P}(\mathbb{R} \times \mathrm{Lie}(G)^\star)$ exhibits the quantum physical nonlocality character of quantum holography. As emphasized by the work in NMR spectroscopy done by Bloch and Hahn and validated by experiments in quantum teleportation, quantum holography goes beyond the realm of phase-coherent wavelet analysis.

The conjugation and reversion anti-involutions that arise naturally in geometrical quantization theory prove the extraordinary power of the coadjoint orbit visualization in terms of the symmetries of the canonically foliated projective space $\mathbf{P}(\mathbb{R} \times \mathrm{Lie}(G)^\star)$. The standard bra–ket manipulations of quantum mechanics, however, do not provide a clear rule as to when the wavelet collapse should be invoked, in place of the deterministic propagators:

- The weak containment of the one-dimensional identity representation 1 in the square integrable tensor product representation $U \otimes \check{U}$ implies that the observation states are the weak limits of nontrivial linear combinations of quantum states coherently superposed by ensemble quantum computers.

- The cross-correlation of the observation states is independent of the distance of the locations where the measurements have been made.
- The amplification of the observation states to the macroscopic system level via classical parallelism can be performed by means of a symplectic Fourier transform along the projective fiber connections.
- It is impossible to completely reconstruct the quantum states from a finite number of observation states on identically prepared copies of the spin quantum system.

Restriction to the one-dimensional identity representation 1 proceeds in opposite direction to the induction procedure. Induction of 1 from the uniform *lattice* introduced by quadrature phase-sensitive detection leads to the natural unitary linear representation of G by translations modulo stroboscopic lattice. It contains square integrable representations modulo center of integral multiplicity $|P_G|$, and their intertwining operators implement the Kepplerian stroboscopic localization procedure for planetary orbits.

Specifically for computerized pulsed Fourier MRI, the key importance of the canonically foliated three-dimensional super-encoded projective space $\mathbf{P}(\mathbb{R} \times \mathrm{Lie}(G)^\star)$ derives from the fact that it is capable of offering three closely related, mutually compatible G-actions for the implementation of Fourier MRI which are required to go beyond NMR spectroscopy:

1. the coadjoint G-action,
2. the transvectional G-action, and
3. the frequency modulation G-action.

The first among these G-actions establishes the canonical foliation of the projective completion $\mathbf{P}(\mathbb{R} \times \mathrm{Lie}(G)^\star)$ of the dual vector space $\mathrm{Lie}(G)^\star$ by the bi-infinite stratigraphic time line $\mathbb{R}$. The transvections, implemented on a modular basis by the energetic stratification of G, factor into dilations. The transvections together with the dilations preserve the square integrability modulo center and form the classical group of projective homologies. Their actions on the real projective space $\mathbf{P}(\mathbb{R} \times \mathrm{Lie}(G)^\star)$, canonically foliated by the coadjoint G-action, map projective lines onto projective lines and leave the projective plane at infinity, $\mathbf{P}(\mathbb{R} \times \mathcal{O}_\infty)$, pointwise fixed. An important point of concern is that the projective plane at infinity carries the de Rham evaluation current $\varepsilon_{(\alpha,\beta)} \, d\alpha \otimes d\beta$. Of course, the de Rham evaluation current ω_∞ is expressed in terms of the stationary frame of reference. In addition, the dilations with longitudinal axis preserve the canonical foliation of contiguously excited, adjacently decoupled, energetic strata $\mathbf{P}(\mathbb{R} \times \mathcal{O}_\nu) \hookrightarrow \mathbf{P}(\mathbb{R} \times \mathrm{Lie}(G)^\star)$ $(\nu \neq 0)$.

The identification of the unitary dual $\hat{G}$ with the orbit space $\mathrm{Lie}(G)^\star/\mathrm{CoAd}(G)$ allows to adopt the dual point of view: The interpretation of the energy transitions which are performed by the homologies as modulations of the Larmor precession frequencies provides the spectral localization. It is this crucial procedure of spectral localization analysis in energetic coordinates, the least understood of the basic

MRI concepts, which justifies the noncommutative geometrical analysis approach to clinical MRI.

The symplectic Fourier transform reconstructive procedure of quantum holograms is another crucial topic of clinical MRI which justifies the Heisenberg group approach. This procedure is based on the read-out of the frequency encoding subband multi-channels of spectral localization analysis which decomposes the planar coadjoint orbit leaves $\mathcal{O}_\nu \hookrightarrow \mathbf{P}(\mathbb{R} \times \mathrm{Lie}(G)^\star)$ ($\nu \neq 0$). The leaves of the canonical foliation, different from the projective plane at infinity $\mathbf{P}(\mathbb{R} \times \mathcal{O}_\infty)$, are planar symplectic manifolds due to the fact that the cotangent bundle $\mathsf{T}^\star(G/\mathrm{center})$ has a natural symplectic structure while the tangent bundle $\mathsf{T}(G/\mathrm{center})$ does not.

The read-out is then performed by an application of the symplectic Fourier transform. In fact, this procedure generates a phase-adjusted average of the de Rham evaluation currents along the planar coadjoint orbit leaves, lifted up along the projective fiber connections from the dispersion-free set of foci in the projective plane at infinity, $\mathbf{P}(\mathbb{R} \times \mathcal{O}_\infty)$. The homeomorphism of $\mathbf{P}(\mathbb{R} \times \mathrm{Lie}(G)^\star)$ to the compact unit sphere $\mathbb{S}_3 \hookrightarrow \mathbb{R}^4$, with antipodes identified via the action of the group $\{\mathrm{id}, -\mathrm{id}\}$, provides the direct multiplanar imaging capability of the clinical MRI modality. The immersion of the leaves into the real projective space $\mathbf{P}(\mathbb{R} \times \mathrm{Lie}(G)^\star)$ basically establishes the three-dimensional rendering character of MRI.

Although radiologists are skilled at semantically interpreting original cross-sectional scans, more advanced clinical applications of computerized pulsed Fourier MRI, such as retroperitoneal MRI or magnetic resonance angiography, reveal that the three-dimensional rendering is of utmost importance. Despite formidable challenges, technical advances have already made it possible to develop multiple surface and volume algorithms which generate clinically useful three-dimensional renderings from MRI data sets. Because such an imaging strategy provides excellent-quality reconstructions that are viewed interactively on a satellite console, clinical MRI is tending toward three-dimensional imaging with continuous acquisition of the examination volume.

The revolutionary advances in clinical MRI, such as dynamic MRI, have expanded options for image-guided interventional radiology and operative endoscopic approaches utilized in surgery. Surgeons try to reduce the operative trauma by exposing and isolating the smallest segment of human anatomy possible while still allowing safe access to the target volume with minimal injury. Small incisions or craniotomies are a characteristic of good surgeons. Such reduced-access field for less traumatizing procedures requires the precise spatial localization facilitated by imaging modalities. Because computerized pulsed Fourier MRI provides the best tissue characterization and image control of any existing imaging modality, clinical MRI scans can be used to serve as exact noninvasive road maps to improve visualization during surgical or interventional procedures in the operating room and reduce complications associated with the access to high risk areas of the human body.

Traditionally, stereotactic methods, with and without the use of reference frames, have been utilized only for image-guided interventions in neurosurgery, but now the tendency is to utilize the same principles of image guidance for accurately localizing biopsy specimens and performing resections of lesions throughout the whole body. The more recent emergence of minimally invasive surgical procedures was initially accomplished with relatively low technology. However, target definition, spatial localization for biopsy and chemotherapy of tumors, preoperative trajectory planning, minimally invasive interventions, and telesurgery require improved image-guided facilities. The most versatile clinical imaging device, the MRI modality, is exemplary for precise image guidance in interventional radiology and teleradiology.

MRI-guided nonferromagnetic fine needle aspiration is an example of a minimally invasive procedure to obtain cytologic specimens of suspicious lesions in the breast. Because contrast-enhanced MRI of the breast is able to reveal suspicious lesions that are not palpable and are not depicted with X-ray mammography or ultrasonic imaging, they must be spatially localized under MRI guidance and then either aspirated, biopsied, or excised. Presently, MRI-guided nonferromagnetic needle localizations are going to assume a role as the initial procedure in the evaluation and management of breast disorders. Moreover, recent studies have demonstrated that MRI-guided nonferromagnetic fine needle aspiration biopsy has accuracy exceeding that of adrenal biopsy for distinguishing adenomas from metastases. In this sense, clinical MRI is being used to screen adrenal masses.

The vision of MRI-guided, minimally invasive surgery is a relatively new concept for the integration of noninvasive imagery with therapy devices. The integration of real-time monitoring MRI into therapy systems will revolutionize the field of therapy and dominate the operating room of the next century. The vision of intraoperative image-guided facilities will take surgery into the twenty-first century, when tomographic microtherapy may eventually be conducted by radiological surgeons, or surgical radiologists. For the rapidly progressing treatment of cancer using gene therapy, for example, augmenting the immune system with genes such as interferon will help the tumor become more antigenic and enable the patient to reject the tumor. Here clinical MRI will serve to visualize the injected gene therapy material within the tumor.

Imaging means visualization, *not* to make visible and reconstruct what is already visible. The clinical applications of MRI were first emphasized by the capability to detect and visualize MS plaques of demyelination in the cerebral white matter and the spinal cord. Since that time, computerized pulsed Fourier MRI has been the imaging procedure of choice for the assessment of MS and for monitoring its short-term and long-term evolutions as well as the therapeutic efficacy of doses of beta-interferon or copolymer 1.

At the time of writing, over 6,000 whole-body MRI scanner systems are available for clinical imaging purposes with hardware and software specifically designed to meet the unique needs of neuroimaging, imaging of the human body, and pediatric imaging. Today no top neurosurgeon or orthopedic surgeon in North America, Western Europe, and Japan will operate without having planned his intervention on the basis of selected clinical MRI scans which identify the target and reconstruct its spatial extent. One of the best examples of presurgical planning is provided by the neurosurgical removal of lesions that are close to the primary sensory or motor cortex and the resection of difficult lesions such as skull base tumors or intraspinal neoplasms. It can often be difficult to predict the exact location of these primary cortical areas, due to normal biological variation and the distorting effects of the lesion itself. Fusion of two data sets generated by MRI and magnetic resonance angiography is necessary to visualize both the parenchymal and vascular structures in order to improve or complement the surgeon's ability by reliable preoperative assessment and to decrease the operation risk.

Since about the mid-1980s the identification of the projective split $\mathbf{P}(\mathbb{R} \times \mathbb{R}^3)$ with the orientable projective space $\mathbf{P}(\mathbb{H})$ of the real quaternion skew field $\mathbb{H}$ is standard in computer vision and robotics. Antipode identification with the compact unit sphere $\mathbb{S}_3 \hookrightarrow \mathbb{R}^4$ gives rise to the real Clifford algebra $C\ell_{(3,0)}(\mathbb{R})$ spanned over $\mathbb{R}$ by the three Pauli spin matrices. The conjugation and reversion anti-involutions of $C\ell_{(3,0)}(\mathbb{R})$ reflect its basic symmetries. The language of projective geometry, applied to the volume-rendering capability of the clinical MRI modality, fits the elliptic realm of noncommutative geometrical analysis.

Image processing tools are fundamental to computerized pulsed Fourier MRI, from the design of data acquisition strategies through filter bank design. For the noncommutative Fourier analysis approach to the design of matched bank filters via Keppler's spatiotemporal quadrature phase-sensitive detection strategy, familiarity with the inducing construction of unitary linear representations of Lie groups from closed normal subgroups would be a helpful background. However, the understanding of the bundle-theoretic approach to the concept of unitarily induced representation has been made easier by recalling many well-known facts from noncommutative projective geometry and the coadjoint orbit technique of Lie group representation theory. In addition to the mathematical prerequisites, a basic knowledge of optical and digital signal processing, familiarity with quantum physics of NMR spectroscopy phenomena, and interest in the principles of clinical radiodiagnostics and neuroradiological applications to cognitive neuroscience and the development of modern science from its historical origins would be helpful.

A large number of texts and videotapes are presently available which describe, along with an array of interactive reference tools on CD-ROMs, the affine wavelet algorithms of digital signal processing, the basic NMR spectroscopy phenomena, and the clinical MRI strategies in terms of a bewildering array of acronymic appellations. Because many radiologists are reluctant to get into computerized pulsed Fourier MRI, in some of the introductory texts of the MRI modality the physical background of the NMR spectroscopy phenomenon and its instrumentation technology is presented in a simplistic style which sacrifices the fundamental concepts behind clinical MRI.

An even more severe shortcoming is the neglect of the geometrical quantization strategy of assigning to a classical dynamical system for a connected Lie group action a corresponding quantum dynamical system. In computerized pulsed Fourier MRI, the consistency of classical and quantum dynamical system descriptions is based on the fact that the separation of the spectroscopic energy levels is much greater than the mean thermal energy. Although the associated transition to square integrable Lie group representations might be confusing at times, it is unavoidable for the final justification of the frequently used characteristic mixture of quantum physical and classical treatments in terms of the quantized calculus. The interactive software, however, can serve as a diagnostically useful companion. The extensive list of references, although it is not at all comprehensive, should be beneficial to acquire an overview and to delve into the highly promising and fascinating multidisciplinary MRI research and its applications to efficient noninvasive radiodiagnostic imaging procedures and the emerging fields of cognitive neuroscience and image-guided, minimally invasive therapy. It should lead to the advanced applications of clinical MRI that have gained maturity over the last few years and to those modalities which are just now coming into the mainstream.

Formalism often is viewed as standing on its own, without regard for the applications insight that breathes life into it.

—Carver A. Mead (1989)

The new aspect is that the signal content *is carried by the temporal response structure, whereas it is the signal* importance *that is represented by the spike trains.*

—Jürgen Krüger (1991)

Zu viele Symptome sind des Diagnostikers Verderben. Er muß eine Auswahl getroffen haben, und dann muß es die richtige gewesen sein.

—Erwin Chargaff (1992)

Dans la mathématique moderne, l'étude des symétries d'une structure mathématique donnée a toujours fourni les résultats les plus puissants. Les symétries sont les applications qui conservent certaines propriétés. Dans notre cas ce seront des applications conservant la "direction."

—Emil Artin (1962)

Es gibt nur Linien.

—Gilles Deleuze und Félix Guattari (1992)

2.3 PROJECTIVE HOMOLOGIES: AFFINE DILATIONS AND TRANSVECTIONS

Reflections have become indispensable to all who are interested in the theory of semisimple Lie groups. Recall that a reflection in a real Euclidean vector space is an endomorphism which sends some nonzero vector to its negative while fixing pointwise the homogeneous hyperplane orthogonal to the vector under consideration. There is a more general concept called *transvection* which has found less attention in the mathematical literature. The present section is concerned with the factorization of transvections into a product of dilations in a more general setting than is actually needed for the Hamiltonian action within the Heisenberg group approach to clinical MRI. The punchline on the *spectral* side is this: The factorization of a transvection acting on a symplectic affine plane into a product of dilations allows to merge the nonsingular coadjoint orbits of the affine linear group $\mathbf{GA}(\mathbb{R})$ to the projectively completed, symplectic affine coadjoint orbits $\mathbf{P}\big(\mathbb{R} \times \mathcal{O}_\nu\big)$ ($\nu \neq 0$) of the Heisenberg group G. Because the three-dimensional two-step nilpotent Lie group G is, up to isomorphy, the *only* connected, simply connected *stratified* real Lie group with affine linear Pfaffian $\nu \rightsquigarrow P_G(\nu)$, the localization technique of temporally switching affine linear gradients fits the transvectional encoding procedure and gives rise to the trace filter encoding:

- The merging procedure for the nonsingular coadjoint orbits of $\mathbf{GA}(\mathbb{R})$ and G gives rise to the Mellin transformation along Lagrangian lines of $\mathbf{P}\big(\mathbb{R} \times \mathcal{O}_\nu\big)$ ($\nu \neq 0$).
- The merging procedure transforms the transvectional encoding into the trace filter encoding.

- The merging process generates a multiresolution analysis by temporally switching linear magnetic field gradients in the laboratory coordinate frame of reference.

Conversely, the compatibility of the spectra of the dilations with the symplectic
structure justifies the phase-sensitive quadrature detection by the trace filter sweep of
quantum holography $1_\nu \oplus 1_\nu$.

As observed earlier, clinical MRI scanners are basically devices to perform measurements of planar spin excitation profiles or quantum holograms. The quantum
holograms form circular grating arrays of traces of Heisenberg helices within the
tomographic slices according to the symplectic linear response theory of coherent
tomography. Measurements of the rotational curvature form of the trivial line bundle
of the selected tomographic slice require a coordinate frame of reference inside the
three-dimensional superencoding projective space $\mathbf{P}(\mathbb{R} \times \mathrm{Lie}(G)^\star)$, specifically a
direction line of the tomographic slices which are considered to be canonically im-
mersed as linear symplectic affine varieties. Following Keppler's *Paralipomena*, the
viewpoint of projective geometry is particularly useful for a deeper understanding of
his ingenious quadrature conchoid trajectory construction of the rotational curvature
form. Starting with the baseline in projective space which he had determined via the
stroboscopic effect, he succeeded in filtering out the elliptical orbit of the planet Mars
from the traditional epicyclic model of planetary motion ([327]).

In view of the immersion into the superencoded projective space $\mathbf{P}(\mathbb{R} \times \mathrm{Lie}(G)^\star)$,
the coordinate frame of reference has to be adapted to the underlying geometry of
the nonsplit central group extension $\mathbb{R} \lhd G \longrightarrow \mathbb{R} \oplus \mathbb{R}$ and, by duality, the basic
symmetries in its projective completion $\mathbf{P}(\mathbb{R} \times \mathrm{Lie}(G)^\star)$. Due to the aforementioned
linearity of the Pfaffian P_G, the transvectional G-action on $\mathbf{P}(\mathbb{R} \times \mathrm{Lie}(G)^\star)$ implies
the consideration of the projective dimension

$$n = 3$$

for the interlevel selection of tomographic slices from the foliation of contiguously
excited, adjacently decoupled, energetic strata $\mathcal{O}_\nu$ ($\nu \neq 0$) in the complement of the
plane at infinity, $\mathbf{P}(\mathbb{R} \times \mathcal{O}_\infty) \hookrightarrow \mathbf{P}(\mathbb{R} \times \mathrm{Lie}(G)^\star)$, and the projective dimension

$$n = 2$$

for the quantum holographic in-plane encoding of intralevel causal interactions.
Because there is a natural action of the Heisenberg group G on the three-dimensional
real projective space $\mathbf{P}(\mathbb{R} \times \mathrm{Lie}(G)^\star)$ which admits a coordinatization in terms of
transvections, the intrinsic transvectional geometry can be considered as part of the
quantum geometry which gives rise to the quantized calculus suitable to treat Fourier
MRI in the superencoded projective space $\mathbf{P}(\mathbb{R} \times \mathrm{Lie}(G)^\star)$:

- Motivated by the read-out process of photonic holograms, the coadjoint orbits
  $\mathcal{O}_\nu \hookrightarrow \mathrm{Lie}(G)^\star$ ($\nu \neq 0$) of G under their structure of symplectic affine planes
  are considered to be immersed as linear symplectic affine varieties into the

complement of the projective plane at infinity $\mathbf{P}(\mathbb{R} \times \mathcal{O}_\infty)$ of the superencoded projective space $\mathbf{P}(\mathbb{R} \times \mathrm{Lie}(G)^\star)$.

- *Scholium:* Considered as a linear symplectic affine variety in the real projective space $\mathbf{P}(\mathbb{R} \times \mathrm{Lie}(G)^\star)$ canonically associated with the dual vector space $\mathrm{Lie}(G)^\star$, the flatness of the coadjoint orbit $\mathcal{O}_\nu \hookrightarrow \mathbf{P}(\mathbb{R} \times \mathrm{Lie}(G)^\star)$ ($\nu \neq 0$) of G plays a pivotal role in the encoding procedure of resonant intralevel interactions in the modulation space $L^2_{\mathbb{C}}(\mathbb{R})$ effected by the discrete series trace formula on the transverse plane G/C for the holographic transform of the RF modulation G-action.

For the sake of a unified treatment, it is convenient to leave the projective dimension $n \geq 2$ unspecified. Because the solvable affine Lauterbur encoding procedure of clinical MRI is based on imposing linear magnetic field gradients in sequence instead of simultaneously, the noncommutative geometry of dilations and transvections in projective spaces of dimension $n \in \{2, 3\}$ has to be developed. Each transvection is the product of dilations of the same fixed hyperplane, the ratio of one being described arbitrarily.

The transvectional action from the Heisenberg group G, apart from the RF modulation action, gives a geometrical reason for the tremendous importance of G in a quantized calculus approach to clinical MRI. In terms of projective spaces, the interpretation of transvections as translations, which leaves the projective plane at infinity $\mathbf{P}(\mathbb{R} \times \mathcal{O}_\infty)$ pointwise fixed, seems to be more intuitively accessible. Due to the fact that in the Lauterbur encoding process affine dilations control the transvections implemented by G, these affine linear bijections are included into the classification of those automorphisms belonging to the linear group $\mathrm{H}(\mathbb{R}) = \mathbf{GA}(\mathbb{R})$ of homologies of the projective real line $\mathbf{P}_1(\mathbb{R}) = \mathbf{P}(\mathbb{R} \times \mathbb{R})$ which admit a fixed homogeneous hyperplane.

As the technology progressed, clinical MRI scanners started to pulse the linear magnetic field gradients instead of applying them with continuously changing slope. In this way, the ramps of the transvectional G-action could be sequenced. Additionally, the duration of the transmitted radiofrequency pulse was used to control the bandwidth of the pulses so that the width of the tomographic slices could be selected and varied by the frequency modulation G-action.

Let E denote a real vector space of finite dimension $n \geq 1$. Then E operates faithfully and transitively on itself by translations. Therefore E will be considered as a pointed affine space of the same dimension. In order to study the quantized calculus approach to clinical MRI which is based on the geometrical analysis of transvections implemented by the Heisenberg group G and operating as homologies on the three-dimensional superencoded projective space $\mathbf{P}(\mathbb{R} \times \mathrm{Lie}(G)^\star)$, it is convenient to consider E as the vector space of translations of an affine space A of dimension $n \in \{2, 3\}$ attached to the *direction* E. Then the additive group of the vector space E of translations which operates faithfully and transitively on A is isomorphic to the normal Abelian subgroup $\mathbf{SA}(A) \hookrightarrow \mathbf{GA}(A)$ of affine transvections. Let

$$u \colon A \longrightarrow A$$

denote an affine linear transformation. The vectorization of the affine space A attached to the direction E is performed by choosing an origin in A. This leads to a linear mapping

$$u_o : E \longrightarrow E$$

associated with u such that u_o and u commute with the group action of the direction E on A. More precisely, for each translation $t_1 \in E$ there exists a translation $t_2 \in E$ such that the diagram

$$
\begin{array}{ccc}
E & \xrightarrow{\;u_o\;} & E \\
t_1 \downarrow & & \downarrow t_2 \\
A & \xrightarrow{\;u\;} & A
\end{array}
$$

is commutative. The diagram implies the decomposition

$$u_o = t_2^{-1} \circ u \circ t_1 .$$

Because each linear mapping u_o coincides with its associated linear mapping $(u_o)_o$, the factorization

$$t_2 \circ u_o = u_o \circ t_1$$

holds. Specifically, $u : A \longrightarrow A$ is a bijective affine linear transformation if and only if the associated linear mapping $u_o : E \longrightarrow E$ forms an automorphism of the direction E. In this case, the translation $t_1 \in E$ and the affine linear transformation u uniquely determine the translation $t_2 \in E$. The inverse $u^{-1} : A \longrightarrow A$ of u is also an affine linear transformation with associated linear mapping $u_o^{-1} : E \longrightarrow E$. The correspondence $u \rightsquigarrow u_o$ between a bijective affine linear transformation $u : A \longrightarrow A$ and its associated linear mapping $u_o : E \longrightarrow E$ gives rise to a surjective homomorphism from the affine linear group $\mathbf{GA}(A)$ of A onto the linear group $\mathbf{GL}(E)$ of collineations of the direction E. The kernel of the group epimorphism

$$\mathbf{GA}(A) \longrightarrow \mathbf{GL}(E)$$

is the normal Abelian subgroup $\mathbf{SA}(A)$, isomorphic to the additive group of the translation space E. It follows that all affine linear transformations u of A which admit $u_o \in \mathbf{GL}(E)$ as their associated linear mapping are obtained by the formulas

$$u = u_o \circ t \qquad (t \in E)$$

or

$$u = t' \circ u_o \qquad (t' \in E).$$

The translations $t \in E$ and $t' \in E$ are uniquely determined. Since the affine linear transformations of A which leave the origin invariant are simply the maps $t^{-1} \circ u_o \circ t$, where u_o is an endomorphism of E, the bijective mapping

$$u_o \rightsquigarrow t^{-1} \circ u_o \circ t$$

allows for a translation of any property of endomorphisms of E into a corresponding property of affine linear transformations of A.

Let H_0 denote a homogeneous hyperplane in E and let $\mathbf{GL}(E; H_0)$ be the subgroup of the linear group $\mathbf{GL}(E)$ of E consisting of all collineations of E fixing pointwise every vector of the immersed vector space $H_0 \hookrightarrow E$. By taking the hyperplane H_0 as the projective hyperplane at infinity $\{0\} \times H_0$, the linear group

$$\mathbf{GL}(E; H_0) = \{u_o \in \mathbf{GL}(E) \mid u_o | H_0 = \mathrm{id}_{H_0}\}$$

can be envisaged as acting in the natural way on the $(n-1)$-dimensional real projective space

$$\mathbf{P}(E) = \mathbf{P}(\mathbb{R} \times H_0).$$

- In the line bundle model, the projective completion $\mathbf{P}(E)$ of H_0 consists of all lines of the n-dimensional real vector space $\mathbb{R} \times H_0$ with the origin removed.

The collineations of E belonging to $\mathbf{GL}(E; H_0)$ form the group $H(E)$ of all projective homologies of the real projective space $\mathbf{P}(E)$ containing $\{0\} \times H_0$ as its projective plane at infinity:

- The group $\mathbf{GL}(E; H_0)$ is Abelian if and only if the real projective space $\mathbf{P}(E)$ has dimension $n = 1$.

If a homogeneous line L_0 of $\mathbb{R} \times H_0$ is not contained in H_0, it is transversal to H_0 and meets the affine hyperplane

$$H_1 = \{1\} \times H_0$$

of direction $\{0\} \times H_0$ in a single point. The affine hyperplane H_1 provides the point model of the real projective space $\mathbf{P}(E)$:

- The unit is aligned with the affine scale $\mathbb{R} - \{0\}$ due to which the generic affine hyperplane H_1 is immersed into the projective completion $\mathbf{P}(E)$ of H_0 by $\mathbb{R}$.

Conversely, through any point of the generic affine hyperplane H_1 there exists a unique homogeneous line L_0 in E. This assignment of the point model of the real projective space $\mathbf{P}(E)$ defines the canonical injection

$$\phi : H_0 \longrightarrow \mathbf{P}(E)$$

which allows one to identify H_0 with its image $\phi(H_0) \hookrightarrow \mathbf{P}(E)$. The image under ϕ of any linear affine variety of dimension $p \leq n - 1$ in H_0 coincides with the restriction to $\phi(H_0)$ of that unique linear projective variety of the *same* dimension p, generated by its image under ϕ. Saying that two linear affine varieties in H_0 admit the same direction translates into the condition that their images under ϕ should generate linear projective varieties in the projective completion $\mathbf{P}(E)$ of H_0, which intersect the projective hyperplane at infinity $\{0\} \times H_0$ in the same subset.

For any vector $v \in E$ not belonging to H_0, the internal direct sum decomposition

$$E = \mathbb{R}v \oplus H_0$$

holds so that

$$u_o(v) = \alpha v + h$$

where $\alpha \in \mathbb{R}$ and $h \in H_0$. It should be noticed that the scalar $\alpha \neq 0$ is independent of the particular choice of the vector $v \notin H_0$. Indeed, the relation

$$\mathrm{codim}_{\mathbb{R}} H_0 = \dim_{\mathbb{R}} E/H_0 = 1$$

implies that every vector $v' \in E$ such that $v' \notin H_0$ can be written as $v' = \lambda v + k$ where $\lambda \neq 0$ and $k \in H_0$. For the image of v' under u_o it follows that $u_o(v') = \alpha v' + h'$, where $h' = (1 - \alpha)k + \lambda h$ is an element of H_0. Explicitly, the scalar $\alpha \in \mathbb{R}$ is given by

$$\alpha = \det u_o$$

and is therefore independent of the choice of the vector $v \notin H_0$. The identity

$$u_o(v') - \alpha v' = (1 - \alpha)k + \lambda h$$

suggests two different cases ([70], [147]):

- $\det u_o \neq 1$, and
- $\det u_o = 1$.

In the first case, the *diagonalizable* case $\det u_o \neq 1$, the choices $k = h$ and $\lambda = \alpha - 1$ imply $u_o(v') - \alpha v' = 0$. Let $w = (\alpha - 1)v + h$ in E. Then $u_o(w) = \alpha w$ and $u_o(v') = \alpha v'$ if and only if v' is an element of the homogeneous line $L_0' = \mathbb{R}w$ spanned by the vector $w \notin H_0$ in E. Hence L_0' is *transversal* to H_0, and $E = L_0' \oplus H_0$. The supplementary line $L_0' \hookrightarrow E$ forms, together with the homogeneous lines inside H_0, the unique line globally invariant under the collineation $u_o \in \mathbf{GL}(E; H_0)$. Because u_o induces on H_0 the identity and on the supplementary line L_0' the homothetic linear mapping of ratio $\alpha \neq 0$, it is called a *dilation* of E of ratio α with axis L_0' and fixed hyperplane H_0 ([70]):

- For tomographic slice selection, the axis L_0', which is supplementary to H_0, has the direction of the center Larmor frequency scale.

The polarity of u_o is given by the sign of its determinant, sign α. If a basis of E is constructed by adjoining $w \notin H_0$ to an arbitary basis of $H_0 \hookrightarrow E$, the dilation $u_o : E \longrightarrow E$ admits the block matrix

$$\begin{pmatrix} \alpha & 0 & \cdots & 0 \\ 0 & 1 & \cdots & 0 \\ 0 & 0 & \ddots & 0 \\ 0 & 0 & \cdots & 1 \end{pmatrix}.$$

It actually follows from this result by elementary row and column operations that the linear group $\mathbf{GL}(E)$ of collineations is generated by dilations of E. A necessary and sufficient condition for the nontrivial dilation $u_o \in \mathbf{GL}(E; H_0)$ with axis L_0' to commute in $\mathbf{GL}(E)$ with the nontrivial dilation $u_o' \in \mathbf{GL}(E; H_0')$ with axis L_0'' is that either $H_0 = H_0'$ and $L_0' = L_0''$ or $L_0' \subseteq H_0''$ and $L_0'' \subseteq H_0'$.

The concept of dilation $u_o \in \mathbf{GL}(E; H_0)$ can be extended to the concept of affine dilation of an affine space A attached to the translation space E. The affine dilation $u : A \longrightarrow A$ of ratio $\alpha \neq 0$ with the homogeneous line L_0' transversal to the homogeneous hyperplane H_0 in E, fixing pointwise each vector of the affine hyperplane H_1 of A of direction H_0. In the special case $\alpha = -1$, the affine dilation u of A forms the symmetry with respect to H_1 parallel to L_0'. In particular, each affine dilation of A forms an affine bijection:

- The solvable affine Lauterbur encoding technique of Fourier MRI processing using the temporal switching of linear magnetic field gradients is based on the control of transvections by the action of affine dilations inside the superencoded projective space.

In the second case, the *nondiagonalizable* case $\det u_o = 1$, it follows that $u_o(v) = v + h$ so that $u_o \neq \mathrm{id}_E$ implies $h \neq 0$. The identity

$$u_o(v') - v' = \lambda \left[(\alpha - 1)v + h \right]$$

implies that each vector $v' = \lambda v + k$ in E admits the image $u_o(v') = v' + \lambda h$. It is convenient to introduce the linear form $\lambda \neq 0$ on E so that

$$\lambda \in E^\star$$

is an element of the dual vector space $E^\star$ of E and $\lambda = \lambda(v')$. Then

$$H_0 = \ker(\lambda),$$

and the vector $h \in H_0$ satisfying

$$\lambda(h) = 0$$

is uniquely determined by the automorphism

$$u_o = \mathrm{id}_E + \lambda \otimes h$$

of E. Because the linear mapping $u_o - \mathrm{id}_E$ has rank 1, its image, the homogeneous line $L_0 = \mathbb{R}h$ spanned by the vector $h \in H_0$, in E is uniquely determined by

$u_o \neq \mathrm{id}_E$ and therefore independent of the particular equation $\lambda\left(v'\right) = 0$ taken for the homogeneous hyperplane $H_0 \hookrightarrow E$. The collineation $u_o \in \mathbf{GL}(E; H_0)$ is called the *transvection*, or elation in the terminology of Sophus Lie (1842–1899), of E with homogeneous baseline $L_0 \hookrightarrow H_0$ and fixed hyperplane $H_0 \hookrightarrow E$ ([70]). Conversely, for any linear form $\lambda \neq 0$ in $E^\star$ such that $H_0 = \ker(\lambda)$ and any fixed vector $h \neq 0$ in E, the prescription

$$u_o\left(v'\right) = v' + \lambda\left(v'\right)h,$$

where $v' \in E$, defines a transvection with inverse transvection

$$u_o^{-1}\left(v'\right) = v' - \lambda\left(v'\right)h,$$

both belonging to $\mathbf{GL}(E; H_0)$. Due to the intrinsic transvectional structure of the Heisenberg group G, the Kepplerian inversion of transvections by reflection of their baseline, in conjunction with the harmonic analysis of the solvable Lie group $\mathbf{GA}(\mathbb{R})$ of homologies of the projective real line $\mathbf{P}_1(\mathbb{R}) = \mathbf{P}(\mathbb{R} \times \mathbb{R})$, is of pivotal importance for the rephasing processing:

- The inversion of transvections can be implemented by a change of the dilation polarity $\lambda \rightsquigarrow -\lambda$ in the transvection control.
- The inversion of transvections can also be implemented by a reflection $h \rightsquigarrow -h$ of the homogeneous baseline $L_0 \hookrightarrow H_0$.

The scalar 1 is the only eigenvalue of u_o and $H_0 \hookrightarrow E$ forms the corresponding eigenspace. The only homogeneous lines globally invariant under the action of u_o are the lines inside H_0 which are left pointwise fixed by u_o. A necessary and sufficient condition for a vector subspace of E to be globally invariant under the action of u_o is that either it is contained in H_0 or it contains the homogeneous baseline $L_0 \hookrightarrow H_0$. The inner automorphism associated with the collineation $g \in \mathbf{GL}(E)$ transforms the transvection u_o of E with baseline $L_0 \hookrightarrow H_0$ and fixed hyperplane $H_0 \hookrightarrow E$ onto the conjugate transvection

$$g \circ u_o \circ g^{-1} = \mathrm{id}_E + \lambda \circ g^{-1} \otimes g(h)$$

of E with baseline $g(L_0) \hookrightarrow g(H_0)$ in the fixed hyperplane $g(H_0) \hookrightarrow E$:

- If the collineation $u_o \in \mathbf{GL}(E; H_0)$ is different from id_E and if there exists a specific vector $v' \in E$ such that $v' \notin H_0$ and $u_o\left(v'\right) - v' \in H_0$, then u_o is a transvection with the hyperplane $H_0 \hookrightarrow E$ of fixed points, and the inclusion $u_o\left(v'\right) - v' \in H_0$ holds for all vectors $v' \in E$. Otherwise u_o is a dilation of E.

Indeed, the identity $v' = \lambda v + k$, where $k \in H_0$ and $\lambda \neq 0$, implies $(\alpha - 1)v \in H_0$ and therefore $\alpha = 1$ due to $v \notin H_0$. So u_o forms a transvection. Otherwise $\alpha \neq 1$, and u_o is a dilation. As a corollary it follows that:

- For $u_o \neq \mathrm{id}_E$ the relation $\det u_o \neq 1$ implies that the collineation $u_o \in \mathbf{GL}(E; H_0)$ forms a dilation, and $\det u_o = 1$ implies that the collineation u_o forms a transvection of E.

When a basis of E is constructed by replacing in an arbitrary basis one of its elements by the vector $h \neq 0$ in H_0, then u_o admits the elementary block matrix

$$\begin{pmatrix} 1 & \lambda & \cdots & 0 \\ 0 & 1 & \cdots & 0 \\ 0 & 0 & \ddots & 0 \\ 0 & 0 & \cdots & 1 \end{pmatrix}.$$

Conversely, any linear mapping $u_o : E \longrightarrow E$ which admits a matrix with respect to a basis of E which is the unit matrix and only one element $\lambda \neq 0$ outside the main diagonal defines a transvection of E. Because multiplying an arbitrary element of the special linear group $\mathbf{SL}(E)$ by elementary matrices on the right and on the left corresponds to elementary row and column operations, it follows that the linear group $\mathbf{SL}(E)$ is generated by transvections of E. Due to the fact that any element of $\mathbf{GL}(E)$ factors in a product of a transvection and a dilation, it follows that the linear group $\mathbf{GL}(E)$ of collineations of E is generated by dilations, as previously mentioned:

- Each transvection of fixed hyperplane $H_0 \hookrightarrow E$ is the composition of two dilations of leaving the same hyperplane H_0 pointwise fixed, the axis and ratio of one of the dilations being chosen arbitrarily.

A necessary and sufficient condition for the nontrivial transvection

$$u_o \in \mathbf{GL}(E; H_0)$$

with baseline $L_0 \hookrightarrow H_0$ to commute in $\mathbf{GL}(E)$ with the nontrivial transvection $u'_o \in \mathbf{GL}(E; H'_0)$ with baseline $L'_0 \hookrightarrow H'_0$ is that either $H_0 = H'_0$ or $L_0 \subseteq H'_0$ and $L'_0 \subseteq H_0$. Indeed, for $H_0 \neq H'_0$ and a vector $v' \in H_0$ such that $v' \notin H'_0$, it follows that

$$u'_o\big(u_o(v')\big) = u'_o\big(v'\big) = u_o\big(u'_o(v')\big)$$

so that $u'_o(v') \in H_0$. Since the plane spanned in E by the vectors v' and $u'_o(v')$ contains L'_0, it follows that $L'_0 \subseteq H_0$, and in a similar way that $L_0 \subseteq H'_0$, too. As a consequence, it follows that:

- The set $\Theta\left(E; H_0\right)$ of transvections of the real vector space E leaving the same hyperplane $H_0 \hookrightarrow E$ pointwise fixed forms a subgroup of $\mathbf{GL}\left(E; H_0\right)$ which is isomorphic to the additive group of H_0.

Thus $\Theta\left(E; H_0\right)$ forms an Abelian subgroup of $\mathbf{GL}\left(E; H_0\right)$. The mapping obtained by preserving the first two row and column vectors of the elementary block matrices

$$\begin{pmatrix} 1 & \lambda & \cdots & 0 \\ 0 & 1 & \cdots & 0 \\ 0 & 0 & \ddots & 0 \\ 0 & 0 & \cdots & 1 \end{pmatrix} \rightsquigarrow \begin{pmatrix} 1 & \lambda \\ 0 & 1 \end{pmatrix}$$

defines a faithful group representation of $\Theta(E; H_0)$ in the plane $\mathbb{R} \oplus \mathbb{R}$. The group $\Theta(E; H_0)$ is the kernel of the group homomorphism

$$\det: \mathbf{GL}(E; H_0) \longrightarrow \mathbb{R} - \{0\}$$

and therefore a normal Abelian subgroup of $\mathbf{GL}(E; H_0)$. In particular, the quotient group $\mathbf{GL}(E; H_0)/\Theta(E; H_0)$ is isomorphic to the multiplicative group $\mathbb{R}^{\times} = \mathbb{R} - \{0\}$ and hence disconnected:

- The transvections in E with a given homogeneous baseline L_0 and variable hyperplane $H_0 \supseteq L_0$ form an Abelian subgroup $\Theta'(E; L_0)$ of the linear group $\mathbf{GL}(E)$ of collineations of E.

The group of transvections $\Theta'(E; L_0)$ is at the basis of the multiple-angle, variable-interval, nonorthogonal (MAVIN) technique of selecting independently each slice angle of obliquity and interslice interval in a single multislice pulse sequence ([280]). The acquisition of clinical MRI scans in oblique scans requires precise control of individual gradient coils. Any nonlinearity of the gradients results in degradation of the image quality. To avoid local loss of signal along the baseline $L_0 \hookrightarrow H_0$, scan planes are chosen so that L_0 is away from the ROI.

Similar to the case of dilations, the concept of transvection can be extended to the concept of affine transvection $u: A \longrightarrow A$. Let λ denote an affine linear form on the affine space A of direction E. Then λ belongs to the affine dual of E, and $u = \mathrm{id}_A + \lambda \otimes h$ defines an affine transvection of A fixing pointwise the affine hyperplane $\ker(\lambda) \hookrightarrow A$. The vector $h \neq 0$, which belongs to the direction $H_0 \hookrightarrow E$ of $\ker(\lambda)$, spans the line $L_0 \hookrightarrow H_0$. Each affine transvection $u: A \longrightarrow A$ forms an affine bijection of A.

The classification of the projective homologies of real projective spaces allows for a simple unifying interpretation of the dilations and transvections. Stepping the dimension by adjoining a transversal line to E, the homologies of the n-dimensional real projective space $\mathbf{P}(\mathbb{R} \times E)$ form the group $H(E)$ of bijections $\mathbf{P}(\mathbb{R} \times E) \longrightarrow \mathbf{P}(\mathbb{R} \times E)$ which transform each projective line onto a projective line and, if different from the mapping $\mathrm{id}_{\mathbf{P}(\mathbb{R} \times E)}$, leave fixed the single points of a projective hyperplane. Obviously, the projective hyperplane of fixed points can be located at the projective hyperplane at infinity $\{0\} \times E \hookrightarrow \mathbf{P}(\mathbb{R} \times E)$ so that $H(E)$ can be considered as a subgroup of $\mathbf{GA}(A)$. Its complement in $\mathbf{P}(\mathbb{R} \times E)$ is the affine space A of direction E:

- The affine dilations are those transformations in the affine linear group $\mathbf{GA}(A)$ which transport each line of $\mathbf{P}(\mathbb{R} \times E)$ onto a parallel line. Then both lines have the same intersection with the projective hyperplane $\{0\} \times E$ at infinity.
- The affine transvections form the normal Abelian subgroup $\mathbf{SA}(A) \hookrightarrow \mathbf{GA}(A)$ of the affine space A. It is isomorphic to the additive group of the translation space E.
- The quotient group $\mathbf{GA}(A)/\mathbf{SA}(A)$ is isomorphic to the multiplicative group $\mathbb{R}^{\times} = \mathbb{R} - \{0\}$.

- Any transformation in the group $H(E) \hookrightarrow \mathbf{GA}(A)$ of the homologies of the real projective space $\mathbf{P}(\mathbb{R} \times E)$ induces a dilation or a transvection on the linear affine variety A which is complementary to the plane at infinity $\{0\} \times E$.
- The involutions of the group $H(E)$ of projective homologies induce a reflection on the complement A to the projective hyperplane at infinity $\{0\} \times E$.

Some of the consequences of the classification of the projective homologies of $\mathbf{P}(\mathbb{R} \times E)$ which are relevant for the clinical MRI modality should be emphasized:

- Every transvection admits a factorization into the product of dilations of the same fixed hyperplane, the ratio of one being arbitrary.
- The factorization of a transvection acting on a symplectic affine plane gives rise to the Mellin transformation along an affine Lagrangian line.

Due to the slice selection by affine dilations, the baselines of the coadjoint orbits $\mathbf{P}(\mathbb{R} \times \mathcal{O}_\nu) \hookrightarrow \mathbf{P}(\mathbb{R} \times \mathrm{Lie}(G)^\star)$ $(\nu \neq 0)$ of the Heisenberg group G are parallel lines. Due to the intrinsic transvectional structure of G, it becomes obvious that a Lebesgue measure defines a Haar measure of G. The reflections of the homogeneous line $L_0 \hookrightarrow A$ are induced by a change of gradient polarity, while the reflections of the homogeneous baseline $L_0 \hookrightarrow A$ are induced by phase conjugation.

Group representation theory is so beautiful and so central to mathematics that it tends to draw authors like honey draws flies.

—Barry Simon (1996)

It is not easy to get into representation theory.... The experts have been writing for each other for so long that the literature is somewhat labyrinthine.

—Serge Lang (1974)

Variations on a theme by Kepler.

—Victor W. Guillemin and Shlomo Sternberg (1990)

2.4 GRADIENT ECHOES AND THE AFFINE WAVELET TRANSFORM

From the mathematical point of view, the generation of wavelets from the same mother wavelet in the case of affine wavelet sets ([135]) with average width parameter $\alpha \neq 0$ and synchronization parameter β on the Fourier transform side can be looked at as a $\mathbf{GA}(\mathbb{R})$ orbit of the disconnected affine solvable Lie group $\mathbf{GA}(\mathbb{R})$ of the real line $\mathbb{R}$. The exponential Lie group $\mathbf{GA}(\mathbb{R})$ is given by the set of matrices

$$\mathbf{GA}(\mathbb{R}) = \left\{ \begin{pmatrix} \alpha & \beta \\ 0 & 1 \end{pmatrix} \,\middle|\, \alpha \neq 0, \beta \in \mathbb{R} \right\}$$

with respect to the two-dimensional laboratory coordinate frame of reference. The affine bijections represented by the elements of $\mathbf{GA}(\mathbb{R})$ are transvections for $\alpha = 1$ and dilations of ratio $\alpha \neq 0$ for $\beta = 0$. The elements

$$\begin{pmatrix} \alpha & 1 \\ 0 & 1 \end{pmatrix} \in \mathbf{GA}(\mathbb{R})$$

form the *linear gradient* matrices for the generation of the affine linear Larmor scales or linear frequency ramps at the *generic* global Larmor frequency $\nu = 1$.

The multiplication law of $\mathbf{GA}(\mathbb{R})$ reads

$$\begin{pmatrix} \alpha_1 & \beta_1 \\ 0 & 1 \end{pmatrix} \begin{pmatrix} \alpha_2 & \beta_2 \\ 0 & 1 \end{pmatrix} = \begin{pmatrix} \alpha_1 \alpha_2 & \beta_1 + \alpha_1 \beta_2 \\ 0 & 1 \end{pmatrix}$$

so that $\mathbf{GA}(\mathbb{R})$ forms the semidirect product of the additive group $\mathbb{R}$ with the multiplicative group $\mathbb{R}^{\times}$. Performing the inverse within $\mathbf{GA}(\mathbb{R})$ adopts the form

$$\begin{pmatrix} \alpha & \beta \\ 0 & 1 \end{pmatrix}^{-1} = \begin{pmatrix} \dfrac{1}{\alpha} & -\dfrac{\beta}{\alpha} \\ 0 & 1 \end{pmatrix}.$$

Because a dilation never commutes with a transvection unless one or both are the identity map, the commutator subgroup is given by the transvections

$$[\mathbf{GA}(\mathbb{R}), \mathbf{GA}(\mathbb{R})] = \left\{ \begin{pmatrix} 1 & \beta \\ 0 & 1 \end{pmatrix} \,\middle|\, \beta \in \mathbb{R} \right\}.$$

In contrast to the Heisenberg group G, the center of $\mathbf{GA}(\mathbb{R})$ is trivial. Let $\mathbf{GA}^+(\mathbb{R})$ denote the connected affine ($'\alpha t + \beta'$) solvable Lie group of real matrices

$$\mathbf{GA}^+(\mathbb{R}) = \left\{ \begin{pmatrix} \alpha & \beta \\ 0 & 1 \end{pmatrix} \,\middle|\, \alpha > 0, \beta \in \mathbb{R} \right\}$$

with respect to the two-dimensional laboratory coordinate frame of reference. Then $\mathbf{GA}^+(\mathbb{R})$ forms a connected component of $\mathbf{GA}(\mathbb{R})$. It is not hard to show that, up to isomorphy, this is the only connected non-Abelian Lie group of dimension 2. To determine the unitary dual of the Lie group which encodes the structural and geometrical properties of wavelets, notice that in the affine case the connected affine solvable Lie group $\mathbf{GA}^+(\mathbb{R}) \hookrightarrow \mathbf{GA}(\mathbb{R})$ of the real line $\mathbb{R}$ admits the left and right Haar measures

$$\frac{d\alpha \otimes d\beta}{\alpha^2}, \qquad \frac{d\alpha \otimes d\beta}{\alpha},$$

respectively. Thus the affine Lie group $\mathbf{GA}^+(\mathbb{R})$ is not unimodular. Indeed, left multiplication stretches or compresses point sets localized on horizontal lines of the two-dimensional laboratory coordinate frame by moving these sets, whereas right multiplication does not stretch or compress sets localized on horizontal lines. Actually, $\mathbf{GA}^+(\mathbb{R})$ is the prototype of a non-unimodular Lie group. The modular group homomorphism of $\mathbf{GA}^+(\mathbb{R})$ onto the multiplicative group $\mathbb{R}_+^\times$ of strictly positive real numbers is given by the function

$$\begin{pmatrix} \alpha & \beta \\ 0 & 1 \end{pmatrix} \rightsquigarrow \det\begin{pmatrix} \alpha & \beta \\ 0 & 1 \end{pmatrix}^{-1} = \frac{1}{\alpha}.$$

Due to the identity

$$\exp_{\mathbf{GA}^+(\mathbb{R})}\left(t \begin{pmatrix} a & b \\ 0 & 0 \end{pmatrix} \right) = \begin{pmatrix} e^{ta} & t(e^{ta} - 1)b \\ 0 & 0 \end{pmatrix}$$

which holds for the parameter values $t \in \mathbb{R}$, the real Lie groups $\mathbf{GA}^+(\mathbb{R})$ and $\mathbf{GA}(\mathbb{R})$ admit the same Lie algebra of line matrices

$$\mathrm{Lie}\big(\mathbf{GA}^+(\mathbb{R})\big) = \mathrm{Lie}\big(\mathbf{GA}(\mathbb{R})\big) = \left\{ \begin{pmatrix} a & b \\ 0 & 0 \end{pmatrix} \,\middle|\, a, b \in \mathbb{R} \right\}.$$

In particular, the mapping $\exp_{\mathbf{GA}^+(\mathbb{R})} : \mathrm{Lie}\big(\mathbf{GA}^+(\mathbb{R})\big) \longrightarrow \mathbf{GA}^+(\mathbb{R})$ is surjective, so that

$$\exp_{\mathbf{GA}^+(\mathbb{R})} \big(\mathrm{Lie}\big(\mathbf{GA}^+(\mathbb{R})\big)\big) = \mathbf{GA}^+(\mathbb{R})$$

holds. Hence $\exp_{\mathbf{GA}^+(\mathbb{R})}$ is a diffeomorphism which does *not* take Lebesgue measure of $\mathrm{Lie}\big(\mathbf{GA}^+(\mathbb{R})\big)$ onto Haar measure of $\mathbf{GA}^+(\mathbb{R})$.

The Lie bracket $[\,\cdot\,,\cdot\,]$ of $\mathrm{Lie}(\mathbf{GA})$ is given by the linear commutator

$$\left[\begin{pmatrix} a & b \\ 0 & 0 \end{pmatrix}, \begin{pmatrix} a' & b' \\ 0 & 0 \end{pmatrix} \right] = \begin{pmatrix} 0 & \det\begin{pmatrix} a & a' \\ b & b' \end{pmatrix} \\ 0 & 0 \end{pmatrix}.$$

In terms of the canonical basis $\{X, Y\}$ of $\mathrm{Lie}(\mathbf{GA}^+(\mathbb{R}))$ consisting of the matrices

$$X = \begin{pmatrix} 1 & 0 \\ 0 & 0 \end{pmatrix}, Y = \begin{pmatrix} 0 & 1 \\ 0 & 0 \end{pmatrix},$$

the commutation relation in $\mathrm{Lie}(\mathbf{GA}^+(\mathbb{R}))$ reads

$$[X, Y] = Y.$$

The preceding identity characterizes the Lie algebra $\mathrm{Lie}(\mathbf{GA}^+(\mathbb{R}))$. For the associated derivation of $\mathrm{Lie}(\mathbf{GA}^+(\mathbb{R}))$ it follows that

$$\mathrm{ad}_{\mathrm{Lie}(\mathbf{GA}^+(\mathbb{R}))} \begin{pmatrix} a & b \\ 0 & 0 \end{pmatrix} = \begin{pmatrix} 0 & 0 \\ -b & a \end{pmatrix}.$$

In order to determine the coadjoint orbit visualization $\mathrm{Lie}(\mathbf{GA}^+(\mathbb{R}))^\star / \mathbf{GA}^+(\mathbb{R})$ of the unitary dual $\widehat{\mathbf{GA}}^+(\mathbb{R})$, it should be observed that the adjoint action $\mathrm{Ad}_{\mathbf{GA}^+(\mathbb{R})}$ of $\mathbf{GA}^+(\mathbb{R})$ operates by forming the conjugate in $\mathrm{Lie}(\mathbf{GA}^+(\mathbb{R}))$. Then

$$\mathrm{Ad}_{\mathbf{GA}^+(\mathbb{R})} \circ \exp_{\mathbf{GA}^+(\mathbb{R})} = \exp_{\mathbf{GA}^+(\mathbb{R})} \circ \mathrm{ad}_{\mathrm{Lie}(\mathbf{GA}^+(\mathbb{R}))},$$

and $\mathrm{Ad}_{\mathbf{GA}^+(\mathbb{R})}$ admits as an automorphism of $\mathrm{Lie}(\mathbf{GA}^+(\mathbb{R}))$ with respect to the canonical basis $\{X, Y\}$ of $\mathrm{Lie}(\mathbf{GA}^+(\mathbb{R}))$ the matrix

$$\mathrm{Ad}_{\mathbf{GA}^+(\mathbb{R})} \begin{pmatrix} \alpha & \beta \\ 0 & 1 \end{pmatrix} = \begin{pmatrix} 1 & 0 \\ -\beta & \alpha \end{pmatrix}.$$

In terms of the adjoint action, the modular function of $\mathbf{GA}^+(\mathbb{R})$ takes the previously encountered form

$$\begin{pmatrix} \alpha & \beta \\ 0 & 1 \end{pmatrix} \rightsquigarrow \det \mathrm{Ad}_{\mathbf{GA}^+(\mathbb{R})} \left(\begin{pmatrix} \alpha & \beta \\ 0 & 1 \end{pmatrix}^{-1} \right) = \frac{1}{\alpha}.$$

The real vector space dual of $\mathrm{Lie}(\mathbf{GA}^+(\mathbb{R}))$ may be realized as the real vector space of column matrices

$$\mathrm{Lie}(\mathbf{GA}^+(\mathbb{R}))^\star = \mathrm{Lie}(\mathbf{GA}(\mathbb{R}))^\star = \left\{ \begin{pmatrix} x & 0 \\ y & 0 \end{pmatrix} \,\middle|\, x, y \in \mathbb{R} \right\}.$$

The pairing between the matrices of $\mathrm{Lie}(\mathbf{GA}^+(\mathbb{R}))$ and $\mathrm{Lie}(\mathbf{GA}^+(\mathbb{R}))^\star$ is given by taking the trace of products. Hence

$$\left(\begin{pmatrix} a & b \\ 0 & 0 \end{pmatrix}, \begin{pmatrix} x & 0 \\ y & 0 \end{pmatrix} \right) \rightsquigarrow \mathrm{tr}\left[\begin{pmatrix} a & b \\ 0 & 0 \end{pmatrix} \begin{pmatrix} x & 0 \\ y & 0 \end{pmatrix} \right] = ax + by.$$

By transition to the contragredient of the adjoint action $\mathrm{Ad}_{\mathbf{GA}^+(\mathbb{R})}$, the coadjoint action $\mathrm{CoAd}_{\mathbf{GA}^+(\mathbb{R})}$ of $\mathbf{GA}^+(\mathbb{R})$ in the real vector space dual $\mathrm{Lie}(\mathbf{GA}^+(\mathbb{R}))^\star$ of

$\mathrm{Lie}\left(\mathbf{GA}^{+}(\mathbb{R})\right)$ with respect to the dual basis $\left\{X^{\star}, Y^{\star}\right\}$ consisting of the matrices

$$X^{\star} = \begin{pmatrix} 1 & 0 \\ 0 & 0 \end{pmatrix}, \quad Y^{\star} = \begin{pmatrix} 0 & 0 \\ 1 & 0 \end{pmatrix}$$

admits as an automorphism of $\mathrm{Lie}\left(\mathbf{GA}^{+}(\mathbb{R})\right)^{\star}$ the matrix

$$\mathrm{CoAd}_{\mathbf{GA}^{+}(\mathbb{R})} \begin{pmatrix} \alpha & \beta \\ 0 & 1 \end{pmatrix} = \begin{pmatrix} 1 & \dfrac{\beta}{\alpha} \\ 0 & \dfrac{1}{\alpha} \end{pmatrix}.$$

Thus the image $\mathrm{CoAd}_{\mathbf{GA}^{+}(\mathbb{R})}(L)$ of the linear form $L = xX^{\star} + yY^{\star}$ under the coadjoint action of $\mathbf{GA}^{+}(\mathbb{R})$ adopts the coordinates (x', y') with respect to $\left\{X^{\star}, Y^{\star}\right\}$, where

$$x' = x + \frac{\beta}{\alpha}y,$$

$$y' = \frac{1}{\alpha}y.$$

Therefore the connected affine solvable Lie group $\mathbf{GA}^{+}(\mathbb{R})$ admits only two nontrivial, noninteractive, coadjoint orbits $\left\{\mathcal{O}_{+}, \mathcal{O}_{-}\right\}$ which are represented by complementary open half-planes $y > 0$ and $y < 0$, respectively,

$$\mathcal{O}_{+} = \left\{ \begin{pmatrix} x & 0 \\ y & 0 \end{pmatrix} \,\middle|\, x \in \mathbb{R}, y > 0 \right\}, \quad \mathcal{O}_{-} = \left\{ \begin{pmatrix} x & 0 \\ y & 0 \end{pmatrix} \,\middle|\, x \in \mathbb{R}, y < 0 \right\},$$

and single-point orbits

$$\left\{ \begin{pmatrix} r & 0 \\ 0 & 0 \end{pmatrix} \,\middle|\, r \in \mathbb{R} \right\}$$

located on the horizontal line $y = 0$ with respect to the two-dimensional laboratory coordinate frame of reference. Thus the decomposition

$$\mathrm{Lie}\left(\mathbf{GA}^{+}(\mathbb{R})\right)^{\star}/\mathbf{GA}^{+}(\mathbb{R}) = \mathbb{R} \cup \mathcal{O}_{+} \cup \mathcal{O}_{-}$$

holds:

- The nonsingular coadjoint orbits $\mathcal{O}_{\pm}$ of the affine linear group $\mathbf{GA}^{+}(\mathbb{R})$ merge to the projectively completed, symplectic affine coadjoint orbits $\mathbf{P}\left(\mathbb{R} \times \mathcal{O}_{\nu}\right)(\nu \neq 0)$ of the Heisenberg group G by resonance.

The elements of the unitary dual $\widehat{\mathbf{GA}}^{+}(\mathbb{R})$ associated with the trivial orbit

$$\left\{ \begin{pmatrix} r & 0 \\ 0 & 0 \end{pmatrix} \,\middle|\, r \in \mathbb{R} \right\}$$

are just the unitary characters

$$\chi_r : \begin{pmatrix} \alpha & \beta \\ 0 & 1 \end{pmatrix} \rightsquigarrow e^{2\pi i r \log \alpha} = \alpha^{2\pi i r} \qquad (r \in \mathbb{R})$$

of $\mathbf{GA}^+(\mathbb{R})$. This follows from the fact that the continuous group homomorphism

$$\begin{pmatrix} \alpha & \beta \\ 0 & 1 \end{pmatrix} \rightsquigarrow \alpha$$

of $\mathbf{GA}^+(\mathbb{R})$ onto the multiplicative group $\mathbb{R}_+^\times$ of strictly positive real numbers has as its kernel the derived group of $\mathbf{GA}^+(\mathbb{R})$, which is, due to the commutator identity,

$$\left[\begin{pmatrix} \alpha_1 & \beta_1 \\ 0 & 1 \end{pmatrix}, \begin{pmatrix} \alpha_2 & \beta_2 \\ 0 & 1 \end{pmatrix} \right] = \begin{pmatrix} 1 & \beta_1 - \beta_2 + \alpha_1\beta_2 - \beta_1\alpha_2 \\ 0 & 1 \end{pmatrix},$$

given by the closed normal subgroup of unipotent matrices

$$N = \left[\mathbf{GA}^+(\mathbb{R}), \mathbf{GA}^+(\mathbb{R}) \right] = \left\{ \begin{pmatrix} 1 & \beta \\ 0 & 1 \end{pmatrix} \,\middle|\, \beta \in \mathbb{R} \right\}.$$

There are two non-one-dimensional irreducible unitary linear representations $U^\pm$ of $\mathbf{GA}^+(\mathbb{R})$ associated with the coadjoint orbits $\mathcal{O}_\pm$. They are unitarily induced from N by the unitary characters

$$\chi_\pm : \begin{pmatrix} 1 & \beta \\ 0 & 1 \end{pmatrix} \rightsquigarrow e^{\pm 2\pi i \beta}$$

and are therefore *contragredient* to each other:

$$U^\pm = L^2 - \mathrm{Ind}_{\underset{N}{\uparrow}}^{\mathbf{GA}^+(\mathbb{R})} \chi_\pm \ .$$

Of course, $\mathbf{GA}^+(\mathbb{R})$ is the semi-direct product of N and the one-parameter subgroup of $\mathbf{GA}^+(\mathbb{R})$ determined by X and formed by the diagonal matrices

$$A = \left\{ \begin{pmatrix} \alpha & 0 \\ 0 & 1 \end{pmatrix} \,\middle|\, \alpha \in \mathbb{R}_+^\times \right\},$$

where $\alpha = e^t$ and $t = \log \alpha$ for $t \in \mathbb{R}$. Thus the unitarily induced representations $U^\pm$ of $\mathbf{GA}^+(\mathbb{R})$ can be explicitly realized on the standard complex Hilbert space $L_\mathbb{C}^2(\mathbb{R})$ according to the action

$$U^\pm \begin{pmatrix} \alpha & \beta \\ 0 & 1 \end{pmatrix} \psi(t) = e^{(\pm 2\pi i \beta e^t)} \psi(t + \log \alpha)$$

for $\psi \in L_\mathbb{C}^2(\mathbb{R})$ and $t \in \mathbb{R}$. It follows that the irreducible unitary representations $U^\pm$ of $\mathbf{GA}^+(\mathbb{R})$ are square integrable. Because the mapping

$$\mathbf{GA}^+(\mathbb{R}) \ni \begin{pmatrix} \alpha & \beta \\ 0 & 1 \end{pmatrix} \rightsquigarrow \log \alpha \in \mathbb{R}$$

is a surjective homomorphism of $\mathbf{GA}^+(\mathbb{R})$ onto the additive group of the reals and the diffeomorphism

$$\log : \mathbb{R}_+^\times \longrightarrow \mathbb{R}$$

provides the transition

$$\text{Fourier transform} \implies \text{Mellin transform},$$

it follows that the irreducible unitary representations $U^\pm$ of $\mathbf{GA}^+(\mathbb{R})$ act faithfully by the Mellin transform on the standard complex Hilbert space $L_\mathbb{C}^2(\mathbb{R})$.

The punchline of the mathematical model of clinical MRI is to include the stratigraphic time line $\mathbb{R}$ into the coadjoint orbit visualization of the Heisenberg Lie group G in order to bind the temporal switching of linear gradients into the foliated geometry of the superencoding space $\mathbf{P}(\mathbb{R} \times \mathrm{Lie}^\star(G))$ by means of *homogeneous* coordinates:

- Due to the factorization of transvections into dilations, the filter banks of the projectively completed coadjoint orbits $\mathbf{P}(\mathbb{R} \times \mathcal{O}_\nu)$ ($\nu \neq 0$) can be homogeneously coordinatized by the Mellin transform of coexisting linear magnetic field gradients which are temporally switched in the laboratory frame of reference.
- The projective completion $\mathbf{P}(\mathbb{R} \times \mathrm{Lie}(G)^\star)$ of the dual $\mathrm{Lie}(G)^\star$ by the stratigraphic time line $\mathbb{R}$ incorporates the time dependence of the linear gradient coordinatization along affine Lagrangian lines.

The transform coding that is implemented by $\mathbf{GA}^+(\mathbb{R}) \hookrightarrow \mathbf{GA}(\mathbb{R})$ is the Mellin transform coding. On the Fourier transform side $\alpha \neq 0$ denotes the average width parameter and β is the sychronization parameter of the rotating coordinate frame of reference.

The Mellin transform allows the identification of the real Lie algebra of the multiplicative group $\mathbb{R}_+^\times$ with the stratigraphic time line $\mathbb{R}$. Of course, the open negative half-line $\mathbb{R}_-^\times$ is defined by reflection:

- The tracial reflection of matrix

$$\begin{pmatrix} -1 & 0 \\ 0 & 1 \end{pmatrix} \in \mathbf{O}(2, \mathbb{R}) - \mathbf{SO}(2, \mathbb{R})$$

  is at the basis of the gradient echo technique. It allows the elimination of the dispersive component in the spectrum of the free induction decay generated by the temporal switching of linear gradients in the laboratory frame of reference.

The isometry associated with the tracial reflection admits the block matrix

$$\left(\begin{array}{cc|c} -1 & 0 & 0 \\ 0 & 1 & 0 \\ \hline 0 & 0 & 1 \end{array} \right).$$

Gradient echo techniques generate quantum holograms in the same way as conventional pulse sequences for standard spin echo imaging with two exceptions. The first is that the initial RF excitation pulse of flip angle $\theta = \frac{1}{2}\pi$ in each repetition of the spin echo pulse sequence is replaced in gradient echo sequences by an initial pulse that can be of smaller flip angle θ. Thus the (T_1, T_2) spin–relaxation decomposition of the contact one-form κ governs also the image contrast enhancement in gradient echo imaging.

The second difference is that during the repetition period T_R the gradient echo techniques use only one RF excitation pulse for spin manipulation via resonance. The rephasing is performed by rewinding the linear gradients which spatially encode the transverse plane:

- The spatially encoding linear gradients define the dual code in the transverse plane to the temporal code of the spin echo pulse sequences.

Because these transverse linear gradients implement the two-dimensional laboratory coordinate frame of reference inside the projectively completed, symplectic affine plane $\mathbf{P}(\mathbb{R} \times \mathcal{O}_\nu)$, their reflection generates a spatial refocusing effect in dissipative spin systems and therefore does not globally compensate the inhomogeneities of the external magnetic field.

In pulsed Fourier MRI, the applications of linear gradients are included in all kinds of pulse sequences for frequency encoding, differential phase encoding, and slice selection. Therefore they are not specific for gradient echo techniques. A specific feature of these techniques, however, is the application of reverse linear gradients for compensation of signal losses by linear gradient rewinding.

Multiple echoes can be produced by repeatedly reversing the read-out gradient direction, but any inhomogeneity of the flux density of the external magnetic field will produce a cumulative dephasing of the free induction decay of the spin isochromats.

Gradient echo techniques permit the use of pulse flip angles $\theta < \frac{1}{2}\pi$ for the RF excitation pulses. Appropriate choice of pulse flip angle $\theta < \frac{1}{3}\pi$ in the STAGE (small tip angle gradient echo) method allows for an efficient control of soft tissue morphology contrast enhancement by an additional image protocol parameter. Actually the RF excitation pulse flip angle has a major effect on image contrast. While the terminology used in the areas of spin echo and inversion recovery techniques is generally accepted, the terminology in the area of gradient echo techniques is heterogeneous and depends upon the manufacturer's specific choice.

Gradient echo techniques incorporate a whole family of different RF pulse sequences which rely on a reduced flip angle and how the transverse magnetization component within the select planar coadjoint orbit $\mathbf{P}(\mathbb{R} \times \mathcal{O}_\nu)$ $(\nu \neq 0)$ is controlled between the measurement of the NMR trace filter response and the start of the next excitation pulse sequence ([324]). As an example, the pulse sequence for FLASH (fast low-angle shot) or SPGR (spoiled gradient recalled acquisition in the steady state) consists of a selective excitation to define the tomographic planar slice with the RF excitation pulse flip angle θ selectable to be in the interval $[0, \pi]$. This is followed by a differential phase twist period to temporally encode one spatial direction, a switched linear gradient to induce a gradient echo, and read-out in the presence of an orthogonal in-plane linear gradient. The read-out process is then followed by dephasing gradients of constant amplitudes which spoil by stimulus-evoked desynchronization any residual transverse magnetization component of the dissipative spin system within the select planar tomographic slice $\mathbf{P}(\mathbb{R} \times \mathcal{O}_\nu)$ ($\nu \neq 0$). With this sequence, image contrast can be varied by varying the RF excitation pulse flip angle $\theta \in [0, \pi]$ and repetition period T_R.

There are several methods to destroy the residual transverse magnetization component within the selected planar slice $\mathbf{P}(\mathbb{R} \times \mathcal{O}_\nu)$. Besides the application of spoiler gradients, another way is to apply short RF bursts at the resonant frequency $\nu = (1/2\pi)\dot{\vartheta}$ for destructive interference originating in stimulus-evoked desynchronization. The ultrafast version of the FLASH modality, called Turbo-FLASH, allows for reduction of the repetition time T_R to 3 ms and the image acquisition time T_A to the subsecond range without loss of resolution of about 1 mm. An advantage of the Turbo-FLASH technique is that it eliminates the risk of flow imaging artifacts and motion-related image artifacts ([136], [324]). Because conventional abdominal Fourier MRI suffers from artifacts as a consequence of peristaltic and respiratory motion, the Turbo-FLASH modality can improve the diagnostic quality and the capability of detection of pathology in the arena of abdominal imaging. Combined with the rapid intravenous bolus administration of an exogenous paramagnetic contrast enhancing agent, Turbo-FLASH allows for dynamic tomo-angiographic visualization of great vessels in various oblique planes, such as the thoracic aorta and pulmonary artery, as vascular structures of high NMR trace filter response compared to surrounding tissue.

The FISP (fast imaging with steady precession), GRASS (gradient recalled acquisition in the steady state), and FAST (Fourier acquired steady state technique) sequence modalities again use linear magnetic field gradient echoes. Whereas FLASH and SPGR dephase residual transverse magnetization of the dissipative spin system by switching spoiling gradients between the measurement of the gradient echo and the start of the next pulse sequence, these techniques are based on the refocusing of an existing transverse magnetization within the selected tomographic slice $\mathbf{P}(\mathbb{R} \times \mathcal{O}_\nu)$ ($\nu \neq 0$). The rewinder gradients of constant amplitudes are switched between the measurement of the NMR trace filter response wavelet and the start of the next excitation pulse sequence. Acting as local rephasing gradients, the purpose of the rewinder gradients is to rewind the Heisenberg helices of the logitudinal axis that is aligned with the direction of the external magnetic flux density.

The SSGE (steady state gradient field echo) imaging modalities preserve transverse magnetization and provide an increased response intensity by feeding it back into the longitudinal magnetization on the next RF excitation pulse ([105], [141], [145], [324], [348], [366]). Combined with the fast-scan procedure STAGE, this technique leads to the ultrafast EPI modality ([215], [216], [366]).

For the differentiated form of $U^\pm$ at the canonical basis of $\mathrm{Lie}(\mathbf{GA}^+(\mathbb{R}))$, it follows that

$$U^\pm(X) = \frac{\mathrm{d}}{\mathrm{d}t}, \quad U^\pm(Y) = \pm 2\pi i e^t \times$$

with the maximal domain as skew-adjoint operators. If χ is any unitary character of A, then the unitary representation

$$L^2 - \mathrm{Ind}_{\underset{A}{\uparrow}}^{\mathbf{GA}^+(\mathbb{R})} \chi$$

is isomorphic to the Hilbert sum representation $U^+ \oplus U^-$ of $\mathbf{GA}^+(\mathbb{R})$. Hence $U^+ \oplus U^-$ is the full story about reducibility.

Starting from the irreducible unitary linear representation $\left(U^+, L^2_{\mathbb{C}}(\mathbb{R}^\times_+)\right)$ of $\mathbf{GA}^+(\mathbb{R})$, the next step is to consider the holomorphic discrete series of the special linear group $\mathbf{SL}(2, \mathbb{R}) \hookrightarrow \mathbf{GL}^+(2, \mathbb{R})$ labeled by the spin $n \in \frac{1}{2}\mathbb{N}^\times$. The Iwasawa decomposition

$$\mathbf{SL}(2, \mathbb{R}) = \mathrm{K}.\mathrm{S}^+$$

gives rise to the maximal compact subgroup $\mathrm{K} \hookrightarrow \mathbf{SL}(2, \mathbb{R})$ which can be identified with the special orthogonal group $\mathbf{SO}(2, \mathbb{R})$ of planar rotations

$$\mathrm{K} = \left\{ \begin{pmatrix} \cos 2\pi\vartheta & \sin 2\pi\vartheta \\ -\sin 2\pi\vartheta & \cos 2\pi\vartheta \end{pmatrix} \;\middle|\; \vartheta \in \left[-\tfrac{1}{2}, +\tfrac{1}{2}\right] \right\}.$$

The maximal torus group K serves as synchronization reference for the linear gradients temporally switched in the laboratory frame of reference when the nonsingular coadjoint orbits $\mathcal{O}_\pm$ of $\mathbf{GA}^+(\mathbb{R})$ are merged by resonance to the projectively completed, symplectic affine coadjoint orbits $\mathbf{P}(\mathbb{R} \times \mathcal{O}_\nu)$ $(\nu \neq 0)$ of G.

The infinitesimal generator of K is formed by the alternating matrix

$$-J = \begin{pmatrix} 0 & 1 \\ -1 & 0 \end{pmatrix}$$

belonging to the Lie algebra $\mathrm{Lie}\left(\mathbf{SL}(2, \mathbb{R})\right)$ of traceless real matrices. The solvable Lie group $\mathrm{S}^+ \hookrightarrow \mathbf{SL}(2, \mathbb{R})$ consists of triangular matrices

$$\mathrm{S}^+ = \left\{ \begin{pmatrix} a & b \\ 0 & \dfrac{1}{a} \end{pmatrix} \;\middle|\; a > 0, b \in \mathbb{R} \right\}.$$

More generally, the Iwasawa decomposition gives rise to a unique factorization of the elements of $\mathbf{GL}^+(2, \mathbb{R})$ according to the recipe

$$\begin{pmatrix} a & b \\ c & d \end{pmatrix} = \begin{pmatrix} r & 0 \\ 0 & r \end{pmatrix} \begin{pmatrix} y & x \\ 0 & 1 \end{pmatrix} \begin{pmatrix} \cos 2\pi\vartheta & \sin 2\pi\vartheta \\ -\sin 2\pi\vartheta & \cos 2\pi\vartheta \end{pmatrix},$$

where

$$\det \begin{pmatrix} a & b \\ c & d \end{pmatrix} = ad - bc > 0, \quad r > 0, \quad y > 0,$$

and

$$\vartheta \in \left[-\frac{1}{2}, +\frac{1}{2}\right].$$

Let the open upper complex half-plane of $\mathbb{C}$ be identified with the coadjoint orbit

$$\mathcal{O}_+ = \{w \in \mathbb{C} \mid w = x + iy, \Im w = y > 0\}$$

of $\mathbf{GA}^+(\mathbb{R})$ and the phase conjugate lower complex half-plane with $\mathcal{O}_-$. Then the diagonal matrix

$$\begin{pmatrix} r & 0 \\ 0 & r \end{pmatrix}$$

of the factorization above is identified with the scalar $r \in \mathbb{R}_+^\times$, the matrix

$$\begin{pmatrix} y & x \\ 0 & 1 \end{pmatrix} \in \mathbf{GA}^+(\mathbb{R})$$

is identified with the complex number $w = x + iy = (1/r)e^{2\pi i\vartheta}(ai + b) \in \mathcal{O}_+$, and the rotation

$$\begin{pmatrix} \cos 2\pi\vartheta & \sin 2\pi\vartheta \\ -\sin 2\pi\vartheta & \cos 2\pi\vartheta \end{pmatrix} \in \mathbf{SO}(2, \mathbb{R})$$

is identified with $e^{2\pi i\vartheta} = (1/r)(d - ic) \in K$. Clearly, for the spin label $n \in \frac{1}{2}\mathbb{N}^\times$, every function f which is defined on $\mathcal{O}_+$ can be lifted to a function

$$\begin{pmatrix} r & 0 \\ 0 & r \end{pmatrix}\begin{pmatrix} y & x \\ 0 & 1 \end{pmatrix}\begin{pmatrix} \cos 2\pi\vartheta & \sin 2\pi\vartheta \\ -\sin 2\pi\vartheta & \cos 2\pi\vartheta \end{pmatrix} \rightsquigarrow f(x + iy)y^{n+1/2}\chi_{2n+1}(\vartheta)$$

on the group $\mathbf{GL}^+(2, \mathbb{R})$ by means of the unitary character

$$\chi_{2n+1} : \begin{pmatrix} \cos 2\pi\vartheta & \sin 2\pi\vartheta \\ -\sin 2\pi\vartheta & \cos 2\pi\vartheta \end{pmatrix} \rightsquigarrow e^{2\pi i(2n+1)\vartheta} = \chi_{2n+1}(\vartheta)$$

of K. Let $\mathcal{O}_+$ be equipped with the differential two-form

$$\frac{dx \wedge dy}{y^2} = \frac{i}{2y^2} dw \wedge d\bar{w}$$

associated with the left Haar measure of $\mathbf{GA}^+(\mathbb{R}) \hookrightarrow \mathbf{GL}^+(2, \mathbb{R})$. Then the half-plane $\mathcal{O}_+$ carries the measure

$$\mu = \frac{dx \otimes dy}{y^2}$$

which is invariant under the holomorphic and transitive group action by fractional linear transformations

$$\begin{pmatrix} a & b \\ c & d \end{pmatrix} w = \frac{aw + b}{cw + d}$$

of $\mathbf{SL}(2,\mathbb{R}) \hookrightarrow \mathbf{GL}^+(2,\mathbb{R})$ on $\mathcal{O}_+$ satisfying

$$\det \begin{pmatrix} a & b \\ c & d \end{pmatrix} = ad - bc = 1.$$

Clearly, the preceding action is inherited from the natural action of $\mathbf{SL}(2,\mathbb{R})$ on the *projective* real line $\mathbf{P}_1(\mathbb{R})$. The group of diagonal matrices

$$\begin{pmatrix} r & 0 \\ 0 & r \end{pmatrix} \in \mathbf{GL}^+(2,\mathbb{R})$$

operates trivially. Due to the identity

$$\frac{i\cos 2\pi\vartheta + \sin 2\pi\vartheta}{-i\sin 2\pi\vartheta + \cos 2\pi\vartheta} = i,$$

the stabilizer of the point $w = i$ is the subgroup $\mathrm{K} \hookrightarrow \mathbf{SL}(2,\mathbb{R})$. It follows from the decomposition

$$\mathbf{SL}(2,\mathbb{R}) = \mathrm{S}^+\mathrm{K}$$

that the homogeneous manifold $\mathbf{SL}(2,\mathbb{R})/\mathrm{K}$ is the open upper half-plane $\mathcal{O}_+$, and the homogeneous manifold $\mathbf{SL}(2,\mathbb{R})/\mathrm{S}^+$ is the compact unit circle $\mathbb{S}_1$. Thus the Poincaré half-plane allows for the representation

$$\mathcal{O}_+ = \mathbf{SL}(2,\mathbb{R})/\mathrm{K}$$

and the matrix

$$\begin{pmatrix} \sqrt{y} & \dfrac{x}{\sqrt{y}} \\ 0 & \dfrac{1}{\sqrt{y}} \end{pmatrix} \in \mathrm{S}^+$$

transports the point i into $w \in \mathcal{O}_+$. The unitary character $\bar{\chi}_{2n+1}$ of K induces on $\mathbf{SL}(2,\mathbb{R})$ the unitary linear representation

$$T^n = \mathrm{Ind}_{\mathrm{K}}^{\mathrm{S}^+\mathrm{K}} \bar{\chi}_{2n+1}$$

which irreducibly acts on the complex Hilbert space $H_n^2(\mathcal{O}_+)$ of complex-valued functions f which are holomorphic on the open half-plane $\mathcal{O}_+$ such that the function

$$w \rightsquigarrow y^{2n+1}|f(w)|^2$$

is integrable with respect to the measure μ of $\mathcal{O}_+$. The lift of spin label n provides a unitary isomorphism of T^n onto the holomorphic discrete series representation of $\mathbf{SL}(2,\mathbb{R})$ whose action on $f \in H_n^2(\mathcal{O}_+)$ for $n \in \frac{1}{2}\mathbb{N}^\times$ reads

$$T^n \begin{pmatrix} a & b \\ c & d \end{pmatrix} f(w) = \frac{1}{(cw-a)^{2n+1}} f\left(\frac{b-dw}{cw-a}\right)$$

where $w \in \mathcal{O}_+$. In a similar way, for $n \leq -\frac{1}{2}$ the antiholomorphic discrete series representation of $\mathbf{SL}(2, \mathbb{R})$ can be defined. It irreducibly acts on the complex Hilbert space $H_n^2(\mathcal{O}_-)$ of complex-valued functions g which are anti-holomorphic on the open half-plane $\mathcal{O}_+$ such that the function

$$w \rightsquigarrow y^{2|n|+1}|g(w)|^2$$

is integrable with respect to the measure μ of $\mathcal{O}_+$ and therefore is contragredient to the holomorphic discrete series representation of $\mathbf{SL}(2, \mathbb{R})$, which will be identified with T^n.

From the action of the holomorphic discrete series representation T^n of $\mathbf{SL}(2, \mathbb{R})$, the affine wavelet transform obtains by transfer to the positive real half-line $\mathbb{R}_+^\times$ via the Mellin transform. For $\psi \in L_{\mathbb{C}}^2(\mathbb{R}_+^\times)$ and $w = x + iy \in \mathbb{C}$, the affine wavelet transform reads, in the two-dimensional laboratory coordinate frame of reference,

$$\psi \rightsquigarrow \left(w \rightsquigarrow y^{2n+1} \int_{\mathbb{R}_+^\times} e^{(2\pi i xy - y^2)t'} t'^n \psi(t') \, dt' \right)$$

for the spin label $n \in \frac{1}{2}\mathbb{N}^\times$ with $y = \Im w$.

Recall that for $\alpha > -1$ the Laguerre polynomials L_m^α of degree $m \geq 0$ are orthogonal with respect to the measure of density $t \rightsquigarrow t^\alpha e^{-t}$ on the positive real half-line $\mathbb{R}_+$ equipped with Lebesgue measure dt. The cases $\alpha = \pm \frac{1}{2}$ are of particular importance. Up to normalization constants, $L_m^{-1/2}(t^2)$ provides the Hermite polynomial $H_{2m}(t)$ of even degree, and $t L_m^{1/2}(t^2)$ provides the Hermite polynomial $H_{2m+1}(t)$ of odd degree. Then the harmonic oscillator wave functions $(h_m)_{m \geq 0}$ admit the Gaussian density with respect to the Hermite polynomials H_m of degree $m \geq 0$. The group-theoretic background of these functions is the metaplectic representation T of the metaplectic group $\mathbf{Mp}(2, \mathbb{R})$:

- For spin label $n \in \frac{1}{2}\mathbb{N}^\times$ the phase factor along an affine Lagrangian line introduces a desynchronization effect into the affine wavelet transform with an off-resonance attenuation factor.
- The radial Laguerre functions

$$\sqrt{\frac{2^{2|m|+1}(j - |m|)!}{\Gamma(j + |m| + 1)}} \left(2\pi |\nu| r^2\right)^{|m|} e^{-2\pi r^2} L_{j-|m|}^{2|m|}\left(4\pi r^2\right) \quad (j \in \mathbb{N}, |m| \leq j, \nu \neq 0)$$

  can be lifted off resonance to the weak spectral transform of the left-invariant sub-Laplacian differential operator $\mathcal{L}_G$ of G with absolutely continuous spectrum.
- The eigenvalue associated with the normalized radial Laguerre function is given by $(2j + 1)|\nu| + 2m\nu$.

Switching from the holomorphic discrete series representations to the antiholomorphic discrete series representations of $\mathbf{SL}(2, \mathbb{R})$ leads, by nonlinear phase conjugation

$$\mathcal{O}_+ \rightsquigarrow \mathcal{O}_-$$

within the complex plane $\mathbb{C}$, to the wavelet transform on $L^2_{\mathbb{C}}(\mathbb{R}^{\times}_-)$. In clinical MRI scanners, the switching is performed by linear magnetic gradient reversal with respect to the laboratory frame. Due to the Fourier inversion formula, inversion of the gradient polarity allows for elimination of the dispersion spectrum generated by the application of linear magnetic gradients which impart a phase shift or phase warp on the precessing spins:

- The wavelet transform models the line broadening contribution of linear gradient encoding and the phase conjugation refocusing of the phase spread out by bipolar linear magnetic gradient application.

The interference capability of wavelets, which is of fundamental importance for nonalgorithmic analog computing, is not preserved by digitization, used for the algorithmic evaluation of affine wavelets.

For a gyromagnetic ratio $\gamma = \gamma_{1H} = 42.575$ MHz/T the read-out linear gradient of 3.125 mT/m is needed. It follows that short echo times T_E and high spatial resolution simultaneously can be realized only by application of high magnetic gradient flows. Presently the standard values are 10 mT/m, so that an echo time of $T_E = 10$ ms provides a spatial resolution of 0.25 mm in the direction of the laboratory frame of reference determined by the read-out linear gradient.

The typical sampling rates are up to 100 kHz, and the typical switching periods for the magnetic linear gradients are 1 ms. It is the temporal switching on and off of the linear gradients and the rapidly changing magnetic field which cause vibrations of the gradient coils against the cryostat and make the noise associated with MRI scanning.

The EPI modality, however, requires gradients which are at least twice as strong as those of conventional MRI scanners, and their switching speed should be 5 to 10 times that of conventional gradients (Figure 25). Modern clinical MRI scanners use high-powered electronic switches to enable the gradient switching rate to be varied and hence allow flexible adjustment to the extrinsic synchronized timing parameters. High-powered EPI gradient hardware is capable of operating up to peripheral nerve stimulation levels.

In most modern MRI scanners, the NMR trace filter response wavelet is sampled 512 times per echo, even though the display resolution in the frequency-encode direction is usually taken to be 256. Because this task is accomplished by merely increasing the digitizing rate of the sampling circuitry, it imposes no imaging time penalty. In addition to oversampling, the spin echo signal is also routinely passed through a steep bandpass filter, further eliminating spurious high-frequency components. The sampling time interval in the direction of differential phase-encoding determined by swapping through the alternating matrix J is on the order of seconds since essentially all phase-locked rows of the quantum hologram generated by the traces of the Heisenberg helices must be collected to obtain the complete raw data set for the FFT reconstruction of the image.

Most gross physiological motions such as respiration, swallowing, and cardiac pulsation occur over a hundred milliseconds to several seconds. Because these mo-

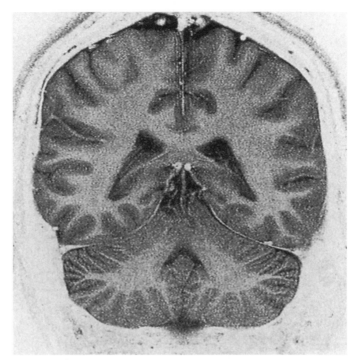

Figure 25. High resolution EPI acquisition of a transverse section of the cerebrum in less than 100 ms. In 1977, the data acquisition of the first FONAR transverse MRI scan took 4 h 45 min.

tions are slow in relation to the frequency-encode sampling interval, they produce only a small amount of spatial blurring locally in the frequency-encode direction. Conversely, since the phase sampling interval is generally equal to or longer than the period of most physiological motions, artifacts are more prominent in this direction. Furthermore, these artifacts are propagated in the phase-encode direction regardless of whether the physiological motion has occurred in the frequency-encode, phase-encode, or slice-select direction ([145], [146]).

In many ways spin dynamics are the theoretician's dream come true.
—Narayanan Chandrakumar (1986)

In the literature especially elegant formulas are given in the four dimensional case. These formulas can be obtained by using $\mathbf{SU}(2, \mathbb{C})$ as a group acting transitively on $\mathbb{S}_3$.
—Ronald R. Coifman and Guido Weiss (1968)

Magnetic resonance embraces a large number of academic and industrial disciplines between which there is often little communication. Each discipline has its own jargon and thought processes which, by evolution, may be well adapted to its own development, but which also tend to hinder attempts to penetrate the subject from without. However, a common language which unites these disciplines may be used, with due care and attention, to facilitate entry. If we were to exclude the biological sciences from the assembly, then such a lingua franca *would undoubtedly be mathematics.*
—Chen Ching-Nien and David I. Hoult (1989)

2.5 PHASE-COHERENT WAVELET GEOMETRY AND SPHERICAL VOLUME SHIMS

The generic planar coadjoint orbit $\mathbf{P}(\mathbb{R} \times \mathcal{O}_1)$ of G forms a cross section in the tangent bundle $T\mathbb{S}_2$ of the compact unit sphere $\mathbb{S}_2$ of the real Euclidean vector space $\mathbb{R}^3$. There exists a noncanonical bijection between the set of all symplectic coordinate frames at a point of the base manifold $\mathbb{S}_2$ and the linear structure group $\mathbf{Sp}(2, \mathbb{R})$ of the principal fiber bundle sitting over $\mathbb{S}_2$. Of course, this set includes the rotating coordinate frame of reference revolving through azimuth angle ϑ at the Larmor reference frequency $\nu = (1/2\pi)\dot{\vartheta} = 1$ of synchronized spin precession and the two-dimensional laboratory coordinate frame which is implemented by transverse in-plane linear gradients at the isocenter (x, y) of the superconducting magnet inside the symplectic manifold $\mathbf{P}(\mathbb{R} \times \mathcal{O}_1)$.

From the quantum mechanical point of view, the trace filter response wavelets represent G-coherent states ([245]). The natural dual pair $(\mathbf{Mp}(2, \mathbb{R}), \mathbf{O}(3, \mathbb{R}))$ inside the symplectic subgroup $\mathbf{Sp}(4, \mathbb{R})$ of the special linear group $\mathbf{SL}(4, \mathbb{R})$ determines, by the decomposition of the unitary projective oscillator representation T of $\mathbf{Sp}(4, \mathbb{R})$ into discrete series representations as a special case, the coordinate frame bundle of computer-controlled in-plane linear gradients along affine Lagrangian lines. In this context, duality means that each group of the dual pair inside $\mathbf{Sp}(4, \mathbb{R})$ forms the centralizer of the other one ([161], [241]). Due to the transcendental version of the theory of spherical harmonics, the duality more generally gives rise to a natural decomposition of $S_{\mathbb{C}}(\mathbb{R}^3) \hookrightarrow L^2_{\mathbb{C}}(\mathbb{R}^3)$ into tensor products of vector subspaces of rotationally invariant functions and harmonic polynomials, which are irreducible under the action of the unitary projective oscillator representation T.

Notice that the automorphism group $\mathbf{SL}(2, \mathbb{C}) = \mathbf{Sp}(4, \mathbb{R})$ of the complexified Heisenberg Lie group letting its center be pointwise fixed admits the simply connected Lie group $\mathbf{SU}(2, \mathbb{C})$ as a maximal compact subgroup. The corresponding maximal subgroup $\mathbf{SO}(2, \mathbb{R})$ of $\mathbf{Sp}(2, \mathbb{R}) = \mathbf{SL}(2, \mathbb{R})$ generates the stroboscopic lattice from the projection of the discrete Heisenberg subgroup on the individual hologram plane.

The rows of the stroboscopic lattice represent the time-domain differential phase encoding steps acquired by the scan. Hence, their number equals the number of repetitions which determines the spatial resolution of the quantum hologram. The display FOV determines the size of the planar two-dimensional torus $\mathbb{T} \times \mathbb{T}$ which forms the base manifold of the compact Heisenberg nilmanifold $\Gamma \backslash G$. The Poisson lift

$$p_1 \colon \psi \rightsquigarrow \left[\begin{pmatrix} 1 & x & z \\ 0 & 1 & y \\ 0 & 0 & 1 \end{pmatrix} \rightsquigarrow \sum_{n \in \mathbb{Z}} e^{2\pi i(z+ny)} \psi(n - x) \right]$$

embeds $S_{\mathbb{C}}(\mathbb{R})$ into the complex vector space $C^{\infty}(\Gamma \backslash G)$ by Γ-periodization and defines a unitary isomorphism of the linear Schrödinger representation $\left(U^1, L^2_{\mathbb{C}}(\mathbb{R}) \right)$ of G with projectively completed coadjoint orbit $\mathbf{P}\left(\mathbb{R} \times \mathcal{O}_1 \right)$ onto the right translation operator δ_1 of $\Gamma \backslash G$. Thus

$$p_1 \circ U^1 = \delta_1 \circ p_1 .$$

It is important to observe that the Poisson lift $p_1 \colon S_{\mathbb{C}}(\mathbb{R}) \hookrightarrow C^{\infty}(\Gamma \backslash G)$ permits a filter bank family interpretation ([4]) of the holographic transform coding $(\psi, \varphi) \rightsquigarrow H_1(\psi, \varphi; \cdot, \cdot)$. Due to the universality of the circle maps ([93]), the principal circle bundle $\Gamma \backslash G$ forms the natural geometrical foundation for a stimulus-evoked synchronized cooperative interaction model in synchronized network organizations based on phase-coupled circle maps. The computer simulation of phase correlation by coupled circle maps within the Feigenbaum scenario is more efficient than by differential equations and is valid even when the phase-coherent wavelet of the single neuron is chaotic ([2]). The technique of circle maps to simulate deterministic chaos can also be applied to study the dynamics of Josephson junctions ([22]).

An application of the intertwining operator $T_J = \bar{\mathcal{F}}_{\mathbb{R}}$ associated with the alternating matrix $J \in \mathbf{SO}(2, \mathbb{R})$ through the azimuth angle $\vartheta = \frac{1}{2}\pi$ yields the symplectic form of the Poisson summation formula

$$e^{\pi ixy} \sum_{n \in \mathbb{Z}} e^{2\pi i(z+ny)} \psi(n + x) = e^{-\pi ixy} \sum_{n \in \mathbb{Z}} e^{2\pi i(z-nx)} \bar{\mathcal{F}}_{\mathbb{R}} \psi(n + y)$$

for $\psi \in S_{\mathbb{C}}(\mathbb{R})$ and $(x, y) \in \mathbb{R} \oplus \mathbb{R}$. Ignoring a common phase factor by putting $z = 0$ in order to implement the canonical projection

$$G \longrightarrow G/C$$

of G onto its polarized cross section G/C, the preceding reasoning shows that the symplectic form of the Poisson summation formula which Godfrey Harold Hardy (1877–1947) used to give in his lectures ([33]) actually has a group-theoretic foundation. In particular, the identity

$$\sum_{n \in \mathbb{Z}} \psi(n) = \sum_{n \in \mathbb{Z}} \bar{\mathcal{F}}_{\mathbb{R}} \psi(n) \qquad [\psi \in S_{\mathbb{C}}(\mathbb{R})]$$

follows so that the counting measure associated with the Dirac comb $\sum_{n \in \mathbb{Z}} \varepsilon_n$ of the lattice $\mathbb{Z} \hookrightarrow \mathbb{R}$ is invariant under the Fourier transformation $\mathcal{F}_{\mathbb{R}}$ of the real line $\mathbb{R}$.

The importance of the Poisson summation formula goes beyond the application to the EPI modality. The counting measure of the two-dimensional lattice

$$\Gamma = \{\varepsilon_n \otimes \varepsilon_p \mid (n, p) \in \mathbb{Z} \oplus \mathbb{Z}\}$$

is invariant with respect to the action of the Fourier transformation $\mathcal{F}_{\mathbb{R}}$. Because the invariance holds up to a multiplicative constant, the invariace of the Gaussian

$$\mathcal{F}_{\mathbb{R}}\left(e^{-\pi t^2}\right)(x) = e^{-\pi x^2} \qquad (x \in \mathbb{R})$$

with respect to $\mathcal{F}_{\mathbb{R}}$ allows to normalize the constant to 1 and to establish for the theta function

$$\vartheta(t) = \sum_{n \in \mathbb{Z}} e^{-\pi n^2 t} \qquad (t > 0)$$

the useful functional equation due to Carl Gustav Jacob Jacobi (1804–1851),

$$\vartheta(t) = \frac{1}{\sqrt{t}} \vartheta\left(\frac{1}{t}\right) \qquad (t > 0).$$

In particular, the function

$$\theta(t) = \sum_{n \geq 1} e^{-\pi n^2 t} \qquad (t > 0)$$

satisfies $\vartheta = 1 + 2\theta$ and therefore the functional equation

$$\theta(t) = -\frac{1}{2} + \frac{1}{2\sqrt{t}} + \frac{1}{\sqrt{t}} \theta\left(\frac{1}{t}\right) \qquad (t > 0).$$

The Mellin transform of the function θ at $s \in \mathbb{C}$, where $\Re s > 1$, combined with the Riemann zeta function $\zeta(s) = \sum_{n \geq 1} n^{-s}$, which can be extended to the complex plane $\mathbb{C}$ as a meromorphic function with one simple pole at $s = 1$, and Euler's gamma function $\Gamma(s) = \int_0^\infty e^{-t} t^{s-1}\, dt$, adopts the form

$$\int_0^\infty \theta(t)\, t^{s-1}\, dt = \pi^{-s} \sum_{n \geq 1} n^{-2s} \int_0^\infty e^{-t} t^{s-1}\, dt = \pi^{-s} \Gamma(s)\, \zeta(2s) \qquad (\Re s > 1).$$

The decomposition of the integral along the positive half-line $\mathbb{R}_+^\times$ according to $\int_0^\infty = \int_0^1 + \int_1^\infty$ yields, for $\Re s > 1$,

$$\pi^{-s/2} \Gamma\left(\frac{s}{2}\right) \zeta(s) = \int_0^1 \theta(t)\, t^{s/2-1}\, dt + \int_1^\infty \theta(t)\, t^{s/2-1}\, dt.$$

The functional equation of the function θ implies the identity

$$\pi^{-s/2}\,\Gamma\left(\frac{s}{2}\right)\,\zeta(s) = \frac{1}{2}\int_0^1\left(\frac{1}{\sqrt{t}}-1\right)t^{s/2-1}\,dt + \int_0^1\theta\left(\frac{1}{t}\right)t^{(s-3)/2}\,dt$$
$$+ \int_1^\infty\theta(t)\,t^{s/2-1}\,dt\,.$$

The change of the integration variable

$$t \rightsquigarrow \frac{1}{t}$$

implies, for $\Re s > 1$, the identity

$$\pi^{-s/2}\,\Gamma\left(\frac{s}{2}\right)\,\zeta(s) = \frac{s-1}{s(s-1)} + \int_1^\infty\left(t^{s/2}+t^{(1-s)/2}\right)\theta(t)\,\frac{dt}{t}\,.$$

The invariance of the right side with respect to the reflection

$$s \rightsquigarrow (1-s)$$

gives rise to the functional equation of the ζ function,

$$\pi^{-s/2}\,\Gamma\left(\frac{s}{2}\right)\,\zeta(s) = \Gamma\left(\frac{1-s}{2}\right)\pi^{-(1-s)/2}\,\zeta(1-s) \qquad (\Re s > 1)\,.$$

The preceding proof of the functional equation of the ζ function has been designed in the spirit of Keppler's.

Let $r > 0$ denote the radius of the Keppler circle serving as a synchronization reference. The radial tempered distribution

$$r^{-s} = e^{-s\log r} \qquad (\Re s > 0)\,,$$

which is defined in the open right complex half-plane $\{s \in \mathbb{C}|\Re s > 0\}$, admits for $\Re s \in\,]0, 1[$ the Fourier transform in the dual Schwartz space $S'_{\mathbb{C}}(\mathbb{R})$,

$$\mathcal{F}_{\mathbb{R}}\,r^{-s} = 2^{1/2-s}\,\frac{\Gamma[(1-s)/2]}{\Gamma(s/2)}r^{s-1}\,.$$

Thus Riemann's functional equation yields the identity

$$\frac{(2\pi)^{s/2}}{\zeta(s)}\,\mathcal{F}_{\mathbb{R}}\,r^{-s} = \frac{(2\pi)^{(1-s)/2}}{\zeta(1-s)}r^{s-1} \qquad (0 < \Re s < 1)\,.$$

An application of Euler's complementary formula of the meromorphic Γ function $\Gamma(s)$, extended to the whole complex plane $\mathbb{C}$ with simple poles at $s = -n$, $n \in \mathbb{N}$, and the duplication formula of $\Gamma(s)$ due to Adrien–Marie Legendre (1752–1833) yields

$$\Gamma\left(\frac{1-s}{2}\right)\Gamma\left(\frac{1+s}{2}\right) = \frac{\pi}{\sin[(1-s)\pi/2]}$$

and

$$\Gamma\left(\frac{s}{2}\right)\Gamma\left(\frac{1+s}{2}\right) = 2^{1-s}\sqrt{\pi}\,\Gamma(s).$$

Multiplication of both sides with the factor $\Gamma[(1+s)/2]$ yields the functional equation of the zeta function

$$\zeta(s) = \prod_p \frac{1}{1-p^{-s}}$$

in the form

$$\zeta(1-s) = 2^{1-s}\pi^{-s}\left(\cos\frac{\pi s}{2}\right)\zeta(s) \qquad (\Re s > 1).$$

The symplectic form of the Poisson summation formula is equivalent to the Whittaker-Shannon sampling theorem of digital signal processing. Thus the display FOV determines the Nyquist sampling rate according to the prescription of the sampling theorem ([290], [291]). Unfolding of the planar compact two-dimensional torus $\mathbb{T} \times \mathbb{T}$ which forms the base of the principal circle bundle $\Gamma\backslash G$ shows that wrap-around image artifacts ([210]) are based on the Γ-periodization implemented by the Feigenbaum scenario within the Heisenberg nilmanifold $\Gamma\backslash G$. They may occur in the differential phase or local frequency encoding direction or both when parts of the object spatially extend beyond the bandwidth of the display FOV, for instance, in abdominal MRI ([284]). The resulting artifact appears in $\mathbf{P}(\mathbb{R} \times \mathcal{O}_\nu)$ as a translation δ_1 of the portions of the anatomy from outside the display FOV into the image and therefore appears at artifactual locations of the image plane. In tomographic coronal and sagittal body imaging where the direction of the local frequency encoding is along the body axis, aliasing is very disturbing and adaptively filtering by the magnetic spin echo hologram filter bank family alone is not effective for completely removing this artifact. An effective remedy is oversampling the response wavelet by the ADC to avoid the wrap-around aliasing image artifacts. In this case, the data acquisition sampling rate is doubled and the acquisition FOV is expanded by a factor of 2. In the no-phase-wrap and no-frequency-wrap imaging options, twice as many samples are collected in the differential phase or local frequency encoding direction where aliasing occurs, in the same sampling time. The data set outside the display FOV are discarded after reconstruction.

Another important consequence of the symplectic form of the Poisson summation formula which is based on the vortex lattice of hard superconductors as implemented by the compact Heisenberg nilmanifold $\Gamma\backslash G$ is the diffraction effect of Josephson tunnel junctions ([19]). In a junction of rectangular cross section with a magnetic flux density B_0 applied in the plane of the junction of thickness d, normal to an edge of width w, the current is given by

$$j = j_0 \text{sinc} \left(\frac{wdeB_0}{hc} \right),$$

where j_0 denotes the maximum zero-voltage current that can be passed by the Josephson junction, c denotes the velocity of light, and as usual in the Whittaker–Shannon sampling theorem,

$$\text{sinc: } t \rightsquigarrow \begin{cases} \dfrac{\sin \pi t}{\pi t} & t \neq 0 \\ 1 & t = 1 \end{cases}$$

denotes the *sinus cardinalis*. It is the Fourier transformed version of the discontinuous spline of compact support $[-\frac{1}{2}, +\frac{1}{2}]$. The diffraction effect is beyond the original Josephson effect, which is a consequence of the cohomological index identity. The Josephson junction forms the central part of the highly sensitive superconducting quantum interference devices (SQUIDs), which allow for contactless noninvasive measurement of the spatiotemporal clusters of biomagnetic signals from nerves, muscles, the cardiac muscle, and the brain ([246]). Multichannel magnetocardiography forms a promising approach to the three–dimensional localization of electrical sources within the heart. In particular, SQUID imaging supports neurofunctional MRI of the brain in correlating cerebral anatomy *in vivo* and the function of the somatosensory cortex and the cortex cerebralis auditorius ([40]). A prominent feature of the visual cortex is the arrangement of cells having like-orientation preference into columns or bands. Specifically in the visual cortex, simultaneous neurophysiological multiple microelectrode extracellular recordings and multichannel SQUID experiments indicate that neurons exhibit wavelet responses which are able to synchronize across spatially separate columns ([125]) and even between different cortical areas ([74]) if elicited by external local stimuli sharing coherent features. Although fast MRI methods have a temporal resolution in the subsecond range, the invasive neurophysiological multiple microelectrode techniques are currently the only simultaneous recording methods available to respond rapidly enough so that their nanosecond information can compete with the interaction between different areas of the brain on the millisecond time scale. Corresponding to the canonical projection

$$G \longrightarrow G/C$$

of the Heisenberg Lie group G onto its polarized cross section G/C given by the epimorphism

$$\begin{pmatrix} 1 & x & z \\ 0 & 1 & y \\ 0 & 0 & 1 \end{pmatrix} \rightsquigarrow \begin{pmatrix} 1 & x & 0 \\ 0 & 1 & y \\ 0 & 0 & 1 \end{pmatrix},$$

a common phase factor within the simultaneous neurophysiological extracellular recordings of the array of microelectrodes is ignored ([187]):

- The temporary long-range synchronization of wavelet responses of spatially distributed neuron assemblies serves the formation of transiently cooperating synchronized cell clusters even in different cortical areas. The stimulus-evoked interareal synchronized cooperative interaction of neural cell assemblies can be explained neither by far field volume conduction nor by a direct entrainment by frequency components contained in the common stimulus.

Therefore a neuron assembly may be defined as a cluster of neurons that transiently cooperate in order to perform, by synchronization, a specific computation for a specific task, such as the solution of the object binding problem in visual perception ([84], [307]). It follows that phase coherence of neural wavelets is a basic feature of cerebral functional self-organization ([75], [76], [85], [108], [113], [126], [187], [301], [316]–[319]). Apart from the multichannel recording of evoked local field potentials too brief to be detected by a fast MRI modality, magnetencephalography (MEG) admits clinical applications in the localization of epileptic foci and the study of stroke. Stroke is actually a lay term denoting a sudden loss of neurological function. Because it is, especially in the acute phase, a dynamic process which is associated with both local and distant alterations in cerebral or spinal cord function, a better approach is to elucidate precisely the cause of the neurological deficit by neurofunctional imaging ([174]). The contactless, noninvasive multichannel approach to the measurement of evoked cerebral potentials by the SQUID promises to replace the conventional EEG in the near future.

Let the compact simply connected manifold $\mathbf{SU}(2, \mathbb{C})$ of dimension 3 be identified with the compact unit sphere $\mathbb{S}_3 \hookrightarrow \mathbb{R}^4$ under the homeomorphism

$$\mathbb{S}_3 \ni (x_1, x_2, x_3, x_4) \rightsquigarrow -i \begin{pmatrix} -x_3 + ix_4 & x_1 + ix_2 \\ x_1 - ix_2 & x_3 + ix_4 \end{pmatrix} \in \mathbf{SU}(2, \mathbb{C})$$

which maps the normalized Haar measure of $\mathbf{SU}(2, \mathbb{C})$ onto the canonical Liouville measure of $\mathbb{S}_3$. In this way $\mathbf{SU}(2, \mathbb{C})$ is embedded into the linear group $\mathbf{SO}(4, \mathbb{R})$ of orientation preserving rotations of the real Euclidean vector space $\mathbb{R}^4$. In order to express the natural action of the real Lie group $\mathbf{SU}(2, \mathbb{C})$ by rotations on the three-dimensional homogeneous hyperplane $x_4 = 0$ of $\mathbb{R}^4$, it is advantageous to introduce the three Pauli spin matrices

$$\varepsilon_1 = \begin{pmatrix} 0 & -i \\ -i & 0 \end{pmatrix}, \quad \varepsilon_2 = \begin{pmatrix} 0 & 1 \\ -1 & 0 \end{pmatrix}, \quad \varepsilon_3 = \begin{pmatrix} i & 0 \\ 0 & -i \end{pmatrix}$$

which span the hyperplane $x_4 = 0$ of $\mathbb{R}^4$. In terms of the standard basis $\{e_+, e_-, h\}$ of $\mathrm{Lie}(\mathbf{SL}(2, \mathbb{R}))$, the Pauli spin matrices adopt the form

$$\varepsilon_1 = i(e_+ + e_-), \qquad \varepsilon_2 = e_+ - e_-, \qquad \varepsilon_3 = ih.$$

The rotations induce the adjoint representation $\text{Ad}_{\mathbf{SU}(2,\mathbb{C})}$ of $\mathbf{SU}(2, \mathbb{C})$ on its Lie algebra $\text{Lie}(\mathbf{SU}(2, \mathbb{C}))$. Because

$$\varepsilon_4 = \begin{pmatrix} 1 & 0 \\ 0 & 1 \end{pmatrix}$$

is the neutral element of $\mathbf{SU}(2, \mathbb{C})$, this Lie algebra is formed by the anti-Hermitian traceless matrices

$$\text{Lie}(\mathbf{SU}(2, \mathbb{C})) = \left\{ -i \begin{pmatrix} -x_3 & x_1 + ix_2 \\ x_1 - ix_2 & x_3 \end{pmatrix} \middle| x_1, x_2, x_3 \in \mathbb{R} \right\}$$

and therefore isomorphic to the vector space $\mathbb{R}^3$. Indeed, the cyclic relations for the Pauli spin matrices

$$\varepsilon_1 \varepsilon_2 = \varepsilon_3 , \quad \varepsilon_2 \varepsilon_3 = \varepsilon_1 , \quad \varepsilon_3 \varepsilon_1 = \varepsilon_2$$

imply the commutator relations

$$[\varepsilon_1, \varepsilon_2] = 2\varepsilon_3, \quad [\varepsilon_2, \varepsilon_3] = 2\varepsilon_1, \quad [\varepsilon_3, \varepsilon_1] = 2\varepsilon_2 ,$$

so that

$$\left(\tfrac{1}{2} \varepsilon_k \right)_{1 \leq k \leq 3}$$

forms a cyclic basis of $\text{Lie}(\mathbf{SU}(2, \mathbb{C}))$ over $\mathbb{R}$. By letting

$$x_1 = 1, \quad x_2 = 0, \quad x_3 = 0,$$
$$x_1 = 0, \quad x_2 = 1, \quad x_3 = 0,$$
$$x_1 = 0, \quad x_2 = 0, \quad x_3 = 1,$$

one establishes that the cyclic basis of $\text{Lie}(\mathbf{SU}(2, \mathbb{C}))$ corresponds to the canonical basis of the vector space $\mathbb{R}^3$. Notice the identities

$$\varepsilon_k^2 = -\varepsilon_4 \quad (1 \leq k \leq 3),$$

which are known as the standard basis relations of the four-dimensional division algebra $\mathbb{H}$ of real quaternions. Moreover

$$\varepsilon_2 = J \in \mathbf{SO}(2, \mathbb{R}).$$

In the spin analog of the boson theory of flux quantization in superconductivity ([19]), the columns of the Pauli spin matrix ε_2 correspond to the Zeeman states spin down and spin up, respectively. Let the real vector space $\text{Lie}(\mathbf{SU}(2, \mathbb{C}))$ be identified with its own dual $\text{Lie}(\mathbf{SU}(2, \mathbb{C}))^\star$ by the $\mathbf{SU}(2, \mathbb{C})$-invariant Killing form. Notice that the Killing form is a multiple of the standard scalar product of the Euclidean vector space

$\mathbb{R}^3$. The adjoint representation $\mathrm{Ad}_{\mathbf{SU}(2,\mathbb{C})}$ of $\mathbf{SU}(2,\mathbb{C})$ in $\mathrm{Lie}(\mathbf{SU}(2,\mathbb{C}))$ is a rotation of $\mathbb{R}^3$ under the parametrization by the Euler angles of a polar coordinate sytem introduced into $\mathbb{R}^3$. Therefore it preserves the function

$$-i \begin{pmatrix} -x_3 & x_1 + ix_2 \\ x_1 - ix_2 & x_3 \end{pmatrix} \rightsquigarrow \det\left(-i \begin{pmatrix} -x_3 & x_1 + ix_2 \\ x_1 - ix_2 & x_3 \end{pmatrix} \right) = x_1^2 + x_2^2 + x_3^2 .$$

- The coadjoint representation $\mathrm{CoAd}_{\mathbf{SU}(2,\mathbb{C})}$ acts by rotations on $\mathrm{Lie}(\mathbf{SU}(2,\mathbb{C}))^{\star}$. The nontrivial coadjoint orbits of $\mathbf{SU}(2,\mathbb{C})$ in $\mathrm{Lie}(\mathbf{SU}(2,\mathbb{C}))^{\star}$ are compact spheres S^r of radius $r > 0$ in the Euclidean vector space $\mathbb{R}^3$:

$$S^r = \left\{ (x_1, x_2, x_3) \in \mathbb{R}^3 \mid x_1^2 + x_2^2 + x_3^2 = r^2 \right\} \hookrightarrow \mathbb{R}^3.$$

Actually, $\mathrm{CoAd}_{\mathbf{SU}(2,\mathbb{C})}$ defines a surjective mapping of $\mathbf{SU}(2,\mathbb{C})$ onto the rotation group $\mathbf{SO}(3,\mathbb{R})$ which admits as its kernel the center of $\mathbf{SU}(2,\mathbb{C})$, the diagonal matrices $\{\varepsilon_4, -\varepsilon_4\}$, so that $\mathbf{SU}(2,\mathbb{C})$ forms a twofold covering group of $\mathbf{SO}(3,\mathbb{R})$. Thus the exact sequence

$$1 \longrightarrow \mathbb{Z}/2\mathbb{Z} \longrightarrow \mathbf{SU}(2,\mathbb{C}) \longrightarrow \mathbf{SO}(3,\mathbb{R}) \longrightarrow 1$$

holds in analogy to the metaplectic group $\mathbf{Mp}(2,\mathbb{R})$ which doubly covers the special linear group $\mathbf{SL}(2,\mathbb{R})$. The transitive group action of $\mathbf{SU}(2,\mathbb{C})$ on the compact unit sphere $\mathbb{S}_3 \hookrightarrow \mathbb{R}^4$ allows to identify the image $\mathbb{S}_2$ of $\mathbb{S}_3$ under the Hopf projector with a compact $\mathbf{SU}(2,\mathbb{C})$-homogeneous manifold, where a closed subgroup K leaves $\varepsilon_3 \in \mathbb{S}_3$ fixed. The Hopf projector consists of keeping the declination angle $\theta \in [0, \pi]$ and azimuth angle $\vartheta \in [-\pi, +\pi[$ for tomographic sagittal and transaxial slice imaging and forgetting about the third Euler angle. The subgroup K is the stabilizer with respect to the north pole

$$-i \begin{pmatrix} -1 & 0 \\ 0 & 1 \end{pmatrix}$$

of the unit sphere $\mathbb{S}_3 \hookrightarrow \mathbb{R}^4$:

- The compact $\mathbf{SU}(2,\mathbb{C})$ homogeneous manifold $\mathbb{S}_2 \hookrightarrow \mathbb{R}^3$ does not carry any Lie group structure.

To optimize the homogeneity of the external magnetic flux density aligned with the longitudinal direction of the cylindrical bore

$$\Omega = \mathbb{R} \times \mathbb{S}_1$$

of the superconducting magnet by spherical volume shims, which is particularly crucial in high resolution nuclear MRS, spatially localized MRI, MRM, and MRA visualization of small vessels, the transcendental version of the theory of spherical harmonics, which is based on the theory of semisimple compact connected Lie groups, can be applied to generate tensor product decompositions.

The dual of $\mathbf{SU}(2, \mathbb{C})$ is isomorphic to the set $\mathbb{N}$. Thus the isomorphy classes of irreducible linear representations of $\mathbf{SU}(2, \mathbb{C})$ can be parametrized by the set of nonnegative half-integers

$$\ell \in \tfrac{1}{2}\mathbb{N}.$$

Then $\mathbf{SU}(2, \mathbb{C})$ acts by the restriction of the standard representation L^{ℓ} of the simply connected Lie group $\mathbf{SL}(2, \mathbb{C})$ in the complex vector space $\mathbb{C}^2$ under its usual Hermitian scalar product. Let $\mathcal{P}(\mathbb{C}^2)$ denote the complex vector space of polynomials in two complex indeterminates. Then $\mathbf{SU}(2, \mathbb{C})$ acts in the complex vector subspace $\mathcal{P}^{(2\ell)}(\mathbb{C}^2) \hookrightarrow \mathcal{P}(\mathbb{C}^2)$ of complex polynomials on $\mathbb{C}^2$, homogeneous of degree 2ℓ, by the linear representation of highest weight ℓ. Note that

$$\dim_{\mathbb{C}} \mathcal{P}^{(2\ell)}(\mathbb{C}^2) = 2\ell + 1.$$

In this description, $\ell = 0$ yields the trivial representation of $\mathbf{SU}(2, \mathbb{C})$. The irreducible representations of the group of rotations $\mathbf{SO}(3, \mathbb{R})$ underlying the quaternion group $\mathbf{SU}(2, \mathbb{C})$ are in bijective correspondence with the irreducible representations L^{ℓ} of $\mathbf{SU}(2, \mathbb{C})$ in which $-\varepsilon_4$ acts as the identity. Because $-\varepsilon_4$ acts as multiplication by $(-1)^{2\ell}$ on $\mathcal{P}^{(2\ell)}(\mathbb{C}^2)$, it follows that the pairs $(L^{2\ell}, \mathcal{P}^{(4\ell)}(\mathbb{C}^2))$ yield the irreducible linear representations of the compact group $\mathbf{SO}(3, \mathbb{R})$ of orientation preserving rotations of $\mathbb{R}^3$.

In analogy to the Cartan decomposition of the simply connected Lie group $\mathbf{SL}(2, \mathbb{C})$, which serves to introduce spherical coordinates, the compact simply connected Lie group $\mathbf{SU}(2, \mathbb{C})$ admits the Euler half-angle decomposition

$$\mathbf{SU}(2, \mathbb{C}) = \mathrm{KAK},$$

which serves to introduce spherical coordinates into $\mathbb{S}_3 \hookrightarrow \mathbb{R}^4$. The one-parameter subgroup K of infinitesimal generator $\frac{1}{2}\varepsilon_3$ takes the form of diagonal matrices of pairs of rotations (ζ_1, ζ_2) through the azimuth half-angles $\{-\frac{1}{2}\vartheta, +\frac{1}{2}\vartheta\}$ with opposing orientation. The pairs $(\zeta_1, \zeta_2) \in \mathbf{U}(1, \mathbb{C}) \times \mathbf{U}(1, \mathbb{C})$ are coupled by the condition

$$\zeta_1 \zeta_2 = 1.$$

In the Euler azimuth half-angle parametrization, the maximal connected Abelian subgroup of diagonal matrices

$$\mathrm{K} = \left\{ \begin{pmatrix} e^{i\vartheta/2} & 0 \\ 0 & e^{-i\vartheta/2} \end{pmatrix} \,\middle|\, \vartheta \in [-2\pi, +2\pi] \right\}$$

satisfying the coupling condition

$$\det \mathrm{K} = 1$$

forms a maximal torus of $\mathbf{SU}(2, \mathbb{C})$ isomorphic to the one-dimensional compact torus group

$$\mathbf{U}(1, \mathbb{C}) = \mathbb{S}_1 = \mathbb{T} = \mathbb{R}/\mathbb{Z}$$

and hence to $\mathbf{SO}(2, \mathbb{R})$. Any subgroup of $\mathbf{SU}(2, \mathbb{C})$ may be conjugated to become a subgroup of K. The Weyl group $W\big(\mathbf{SU}(2, \mathbb{C}), K\big)$ relative to K is the symmetric group $S(2)$ on two letters permuting the rotations through the set of azimuth half–angles $\{-\frac{1}{2}\vartheta, +\frac{1}{2}\vartheta\}$ of opposite orientation by means of the alternating matrix $J \in W\big(\mathbf{SU}(2, \mathbb{C}), K\big)$. Indeed,

$$JKJ^{-1} = \bar{K} = K,$$

and therefore,

$$W\big(\mathbf{SU}(2, \mathbb{C}), K\big) = S(2).$$

The two-dimensional compact homogeneous manifold $\mathbf{SU}(2, \mathbb{C})/K$ is diffeomorphic to the projective plane $\mathbf{P}_1(\mathbb{C})$ and $\mathbf{SO}(3, \mathbb{R})/\mathrm{Ad}_{\mathbf{SU}(2,\mathbb{C})}(K)$ is homeomorphic to the compact unit sphere $\mathbb{S}_2$. The Riemann sphere $\mathbb{S}_2$ projects stereographically from the north pole $(0, 0, 1)$ of $\mathbb{S}_2$, which corresponds to ε_3, onto the tomographic transaxial plane $x_1 = 0$, which is diffeomorphic, to the transverse coadjoint orbit $\mathbf{P}\big(\mathbb{R} \times \mathcal{O}_1\big)$ of G. Thus one has the principal sphere bundle

$$
\begin{array}{ccc}
\mathbb{S}_1 & \longrightarrow & \mathbb{S}_3 \\
 & & \Big\downarrow \\
 & & \mathbb{S}_2
\end{array}
$$

which forms the Hopf fibration of $\mathbb{S}_3 \hookrightarrow \mathbb{R}^4$. The canonical Liouville measure of $\mathbb{S}_2$ is the projection of the normalized Haar measure of $\mathbf{SO}(3, \mathbb{R})$.

By subducing onto the maximal torus group K of $\mathbf{SU}(2, \mathbb{C})$, the standard representation L^ℓ provides as tracial character of L^ℓ on $\mathbf{SU}(2, \mathbb{C})$ the real-valued function

$$\mathrm{tr}\, L^\ell : \vartheta \rightsquigarrow U_{2\ell}(\cos \vartheta),$$

where, as usual, tr denotes the trace functional. It can be expressed in terms of the Čebysev polynomial of the second kind,

$$U_{2\ell}(X) \in \mathbb{R}[X],$$

of degree $2\ell \in \mathbb{N}$, with weight function

$$w_U : [-1, +1] \ni r \rightsquigarrow \sqrt{1 - r^2}$$

and Rodrigues formula

$$U_{2\ell}(X) = \frac{(-1)^{2\ell}(2\ell + 1)\sqrt{\pi}}{w_U(X)2^{2\ell+1}\Gamma(2\ell + \frac{3}{2})} \frac{\mathrm{d}^{2\ell}}{\mathrm{d}X^{2\ell}}\left(\left(1 - X^2\right)^{2\ell+1/2}\right).$$

The subduced adjoint representation $\mathrm{Ad}_{\mathbf{SU}(2,\mathbb{C})}|K$ in $\mathbf{SO}(3, \mathbb{R})$ provides the rotation in the transaxial coadjoint orbit $\mathbf{P}\big(\mathbb{R} \times \mathcal{O}_1\big)$ of G through the azimuth angle ϑ of the matrix

$$\begin{pmatrix} \boxed{\begin{matrix} \cos \vartheta & \sin \vartheta \\ -\sin \vartheta & \cos \vartheta \end{matrix}} & \begin{matrix} 0 \\ 0 \end{matrix} \\ \begin{matrix} 0 & 0 \end{matrix} & 1 \end{pmatrix}$$

and infinitesimal generator $\varepsilon_2 = J$. The box $\square$ with $\vartheta = 2\pi t$ corresponds to the circular ray traces of the Heisenberg helices.

In the parametrization by the Euler declination half-angles, the one-parameter subgroup A of infinitesimal generator $\frac{1}{2}\varepsilon_1$ takes the form

$$A = \left\{ \begin{pmatrix} \cos \dfrac{\theta}{2} & -i \sin \dfrac{\theta}{2} \\ -i \sin \dfrac{\theta}{2} & \cos \dfrac{\theta}{2} \end{pmatrix} \;\middle|\; \theta \in [0, \pi] \right\}.$$

The subduced adjoint representation $\mathrm{Ad}_{\mathbf{SU}(2,\mathbb{C})}|A$ in $\mathbf{SO}(3, \mathbb{R})$ provides the rotation through the declination angle θ in a plane parallel to the tomographic sagittal plane N of matrix

$$\begin{pmatrix} 1 & 0 & 0 \\ 0 & \cos \theta & -\sin \theta \\ 0 & \sin \theta & \cos \theta \end{pmatrix}.$$

The matrix coefficients of the standard representation L^ℓ evaluated at the elements

$$-i \begin{pmatrix} i \cos \dfrac{\theta}{2} & \sin \dfrac{\theta}{2} \\ \sin \dfrac{\theta}{2} & i \cos \dfrac{\theta}{2} \end{pmatrix} \in A$$

with respect to the basis

$$e_n \colon \mathbb{C}^2 \ni (z_1, z_2) \rightsquigarrow \frac{1}{\sqrt{(\ell + n)!(\ell - n)!}} z_1^{\ell-n} z_2^{\ell+n} \quad (-\ell \le n \le +\ell, \ \ell - n \in \mathbf{Z})$$

of the complex vector space $\mathcal{P}^{(2\ell)}(\mathbb{C}^2)$ and its standard scalar product $< \cdot | \cdot >$ read

$$\theta \rightsquigarrow \; < L^\ell \left(-i \begin{pmatrix} i \cos \dfrac{\theta}{2} & \sin \dfrac{\theta}{2} \\ \sin \dfrac{\theta}{2} & i \cos \dfrac{\theta}{2} \end{pmatrix} \right) e_n \big| e_m > .$$

They form a symmetric matrix $\left(P^\ell_{(m,n)}\right)_{m,n}$ where the subscripts are running in the symmetric range

$$m, n \in \{-\ell, -\ell + 1, \ldots, \ell - 1, \ell\}.$$

The matrix coefficients give rise to a local trigonometric series expansion of the magnetic flux density inside the bore Ω of the superconducting magnet in terms of spherical harmonics

$$[0\,,\,\pi] \times [-\pi\,,\,+\pi[\,\ni\,(\theta,\vartheta) \rightsquigarrow P^{\ell}_{(m,n)}(\cos\theta)\chi_m(\vartheta)\,.$$

An application of Taylor's formula shows that the coefficient functions $P^{\ell}_{(m,n)}$ of these local trigonometric series expansions are given by the Rodrigues type formula

$$P^{\ell}_{(m,n)}(x) = \frac{i^{n-m}}{2^{\ell+m}} \cdot \sqrt{\frac{(\ell+m)!}{(\ell-m)!(\ell+n)!(\ell-n)!}} \cdot (1+x)^{-(n+m)/2}(1-x)^{(n-m)/2}$$

$$\times \frac{d^{\ell-m}}{dx^{\ell-m}}\left[(x-1)^{\ell-n}(x+1)^{\ell+n}\right]\,.$$

Therefore the function

$$[0\,,\,\pi] \ni \theta \rightsquigarrow P^{\ell}_{(m,n)}(\cos\theta)$$

differs by a factor from the classical Jacobi polynomial

$$P^{(\alpha,\beta)}_{k}(X) \in \mathbb{R}[X]$$

in the variable $X = \cos\theta$ of degree

$$k = \ell - m$$

and Jacobi weights

$$\alpha = m - n, \qquad \beta = m + n\,.$$

Indeed, because $P^{(\alpha,\beta)}_{k}(X)$ satisfies the Rodrigues formula

$$P^{(\alpha,\beta)}_{k}(X) = \frac{(-1)^k}{2^k k!}(1-X)^{-\alpha}(1+X)^{-\beta}\frac{d^k}{dX^k}\left[(1-X)^{k+\alpha}(1+X)^{k+\beta}\right]\,,$$

it follows for the declination angle $\theta \in [0\,,\,\pi]$ that

$$P^{\ell}_{(m,n)}(\cos\theta) = \frac{1}{2^m}i^{m-n}\sqrt{\frac{(\ell+m)!(\ell-m)!}{(\ell+n)!(\ell-n)!}}\left(\sin\frac{\theta}{2}\right)^{\alpha}\left(\cos\frac{\theta}{2}\right)^{\beta}P^{(\alpha,\beta)}_{k}(\cos\theta)\,.$$

Identifying $\mathbb{S}_2$ with the compact homogeneous manifold $\mathbf{SU}(2,\mathbb{C})/K$, the implementation of the $\mathbf{SO}(3,\mathbb{R})$-invariant Hopf projector

$$\mathbf{SU}(2,\mathbb{C}) \longrightarrow \mathbb{S}_2$$

implies that the matrix coefficients of the representations L^{ℓ} of highest weight

$$\ell \in \mathbb{N}$$

with index $n = 0$ and index $m \in \mathbb{Z}$ such that

$$|m| \le \ell \qquad (\ell \in \mathbb{N})$$

are actually sufficient to construct a Hilbert basis of the complex Hilbert space $L^2_{\mathbb{C}}(\mathbb{S}_2)$ with respect to the canonical Liouville measure of the compact unit sphere $\mathbb{S}_2 \hookrightarrow \mathbb{R}^3$. Consequently, in this Hilbert basis only the ultraspherical weights

$$\alpha = \beta = m \in \mathbb{Z}$$

occur. To construct the classical spherical harmonics

$$[0, \pi] \times [-\pi, +\pi[\ni (\theta, \vartheta) \rightsquigarrow P^{\ell}_{(m,0)}(\cos \theta)\chi_m(\vartheta),$$

it is therefore sufficient to concentrate on the Legendre polynomials

$$P_k(X) = P^0_k(X) = P^{(0,0)}_k(X) \in \mathbb{R}[X]$$

of degree $k \in \mathbb{N}$ with zonal weight function

$$w_P = 1$$

and Rodrigues formula

$$P_k(X) = \frac{(-1)^k}{2^k k!} \frac{\mathrm{d}^k}{\mathrm{d}X^k} \left[(1 - X^2)^k \right]$$

and the associated Legendre functions of order $p \in \mathbb{Z}$,

$$P^p_k(x) = \frac{2^p (k + p)!}{k!}(1 - x^2)^{-p/2} P^{(-p,-p)}_{k+p}(x),$$

where $|p| \le k$, and Rodrigues formula

$$P^p_k : x \rightsquigarrow \frac{(-1)^{p+k}}{2^k k!}(1 - x^2)^{p/2} \frac{\mathrm{d}^{p+k}}{\mathrm{d}x^{p+k}} \left[(1 - x^2)^k \right].$$

Thus the Legendre identities

$$P^p_k(x) = (-1)^p (1 - x^2)^{p/2} \frac{\mathrm{d}^p}{\mathrm{d}x^p} P_k(x)$$

hold for $x \in \mathbb{R}$. It follows that the basic building block for the current controlled generation of zonal spherical harmonics is a toroidal channel, coaxial with the axis of the cylinder Ω. The associated Legendre functions P^p_k satisfy the reflection identities

$$P^p_k(-x) = (-1)^{k+p} P^p_k(x)$$

for $x \in \mathbb{R}$, which reduce to the identities

$$P_k(-x) = (-1)^k P_k(x)$$

for $p = 0$. It follows for $\ell \in \mathbb{N}$ and $0 \le m \le \ell$ that

$$P^{\ell}_{(m,0)} = i^m \sqrt{\frac{(\ell + m)!}{(\ell - m)!}} P^{-m}_{\ell}.$$

In view of the identity

$$P^{-m}_{\ell} = (-1)^m \frac{(\ell - m)!}{(\ell + m)!} P^m_{\ell} \qquad (m \ge 1),$$

it is sufficient to compute the Legendre polynomials $P_k(x)$ and the associated Legendre functions $P^m_k(x)$ of degree $k \in \mathbb{N}$ and order $m \in \mathbb{N}$, where

$$1 \le m \le k,$$

to calculate the coefficients of the classical spherical harmonics expansion of the magnetic flux density inside the bore Ω of the superconducting magnet in the variable

$$x = \cos \theta \qquad (\theta \in [0, \pi])$$

and tesseral weight function

$$(1 - x^2)^{m/2} = (\sin \theta)^m \qquad (m \ge 1).$$

See Table 2.1 and Table 2.3.

The radial part of the classical spherical harmonics expansion of the magnetic flux density inside the spheres

$$S^r \hookrightarrow \Omega \qquad (r > 0)$$

can be explicitly calculated in terms of tensor products with spherical Bessel functions by the transcendental version of the theory of spherical harmonics.

The lowest weight module decomposition establishes that the vector subspace of rotationally invariant functions in the complex vector space $S_{\mathbb{C}}(\mathbb{R}) \hookrightarrow L^2_{\mathbb{C}}(\mathbb{R})$ is the unique $\mathbf{Mp}(2, \mathbb{R})$ lowest weight module $\mathcal{M}_{1/2}$ of lowest weight $\frac{1}{2}$:

- The $\mathrm{Lie}\big(\mathbf{SL}(2, \mathbb{R})\big)$ action commutes with the $\mathbf{O}(3, \mathbb{R})$ action. Therefore the linear groups mutually determine their spectral decompositions.

Table 2.1. Legendre Polynomials

k	$P_k(\cos \theta)$
0	1
1	$\cos \theta$
2	$\frac{1}{2}\left(3(\cos \theta)^2 - 1\right)$
3	$\frac{1}{2}\left(5(\cos \theta)^3 - 3\cos \theta\right)$
4	$\frac{1}{8}\left(35(\cos \theta)^4 - 30(\cos \theta)^2 + 3\right)$
5	$\frac{1}{8}\left(63(\cos \theta)^5 - 70(\cos \theta)^3 + 15\cos \theta\right)$
6	$\frac{1}{16}\left(231(\cos \theta)^6 - 315(\cos \theta)^4 + 105(\cos \theta)^2 - 5\right)$

Table 2.2. Magic Angles (deg)

k	$\theta^{(k)}$		
1	90.00		
2	54.74		
3	39.23	90.00	
4	30.56	70.12	
5	25.02	57.42	90.00
6	21.18	48.61	76.19

In view of the preceding dual-pair argument, the complex vector spaces $\mathcal{P}^{(2\ell)}(\mathbb{C}^2)$ have to be endowed with the lowest weight vector h_0, then tensored by the module $\mathcal{M}_{\ell+1/2}$, and finally completed in order to obtain the decomposition of $S_{\mathbb{C}}(\mathbb{R}^3) \hookrightarrow L^2_{\mathbb{C}}(\mathbb{R}^3)$ into irreducible $\mathbf{O}(3, \mathbb{R})$-invariant vector subspaces

$$\mathcal{P}^{(2\ell)}(\mathbb{C}^2) h_0(r) \otimes \mathcal{M}_{\ell+1/2} \quad (\ell \in \mathbb{N}).$$

The tesseral components of the local trigonometric series expansion associated with the sphere S^r can be calculated by Bochner's formula for the Fourier transform in terms of the Hankel transform of order

$$\ell + \tfrac{3}{2} - 1 = \ell + \tfrac{1}{2} \quad (\ell \in \mathbb{N}).$$

Denoting by $J_{(\ell+1/2)}$ the Bessel function of half-integral weight associated with the lowest weight $\ell + \tfrac{1}{2}$, the components read

$$(r, \theta, \vartheta) \rightsquigarrow \frac{1}{\sqrt{r}} J_{(\ell+1/2)}(r) P^\ell_{(m,0)}(\cos \theta) \chi_m(\vartheta) \quad (|m| \le \ell),$$

where $(r, \theta, \vartheta) \in \mathbb{R}^\times_+ \times [0, \pi] \times [-\pi, +\pi[$.

In the longitudinal direction of Ω, the zonal components take the form

$$\mathbb{R}^\times_+ \times [0, \pi] \ni (r, \theta) \rightsquigarrow \frac{1}{\sqrt{r}} J_{(k+1/2)}(r) P_k(\cos \theta) \quad (k \in \mathbb{N}).$$

The magic angles $\theta^{(k)}$ averaging the declination of $k + 1$ spinning directions give rise to a cone with apex angle $2\theta^{(k)}$ and are characterized by the equation (Table 2.2)

$$P_k\left(\cos \theta^{(k)}\right) = 0.$$

For the design of linear gradient coil systems the following remark is of importance:

- The linear gradients of magnetic flux densities at the isocenter (x, y, z) of the superconducting magnet inside the spherical volume shim form zonal spherical harmonics of degree $k = 1$ which are produced by opposing current controlled toroidal channels.

Zonal correcting coil systems can be used as magnetic flux density linear gradient coil systems along the longitudinal direction. Corresponding to the fact that $\mathbf{SU}(2, \mathbb{C})$ forms a twofold covering group of the rotation group $\mathbf{SO}(3, \mathbb{R})$, the coil systems consist of pairs of current controlled toroidal channels wound on the cylinder Ω. The orientation of the toroidal channels follows from the reflection identities of the Legendre polynomials. In this context, the cylindrical surface of Ω represents the bore of the superconducting magnet. The turn of linear gradient coil systems displays the azimuth angle $\vartheta = \frac{1}{2}\pi$ corresponding to the alternating matrix $J \in \mathbf{W}\big(\mathbf{SU}(2, \mathbb{C}), \mathbf{K}\big)$.
It follows that:

- According to the natural decomposition of $S_{\mathbb{C}}(\mathbb{R}^3) \hookrightarrow L^2_{\mathbb{C}}(\mathbb{R}^3)$, the magnetic field corrections broken down into mutual orthogonal components of zonal and tesseral surface spherical harmonics of degree $k \geq 0$ determine the geometry of

Table 2.3. Associated Legendre Functions

k	$P_k^m(\cos\theta) \qquad (1 \leq m \leq k)$
1	$\sin\theta$
2	$3\sin\theta\cos\theta$
	$3(\sin\theta)^2$
3	$\frac{3}{2}\sin\theta\big[5(\cos\theta)^2 - 1\big]$
	$15(\sin\theta)^2\cos\theta$
	$15(\sin\theta)^3$
4	$\frac{5}{2}\sin\theta\big[7(\cos\theta)^3 - 3\cos\theta\big]$
	$\frac{15}{2}(\sin\theta)^2\big[7(\cos\theta)^2 - 1\big]$
	$105(\sin\theta)^3\cos\theta$
	$105(\sin\theta)^4$
5	$\frac{15}{8}\sin\theta\big[21(\cos\theta)^4 - 14(\cos\theta)^2 + 1\big]$
	$\frac{105}{2}(\sin\theta)^2\big[3(\cos\theta)^3 - \cos\theta\big]$
	$\frac{105}{2}(\sin\theta)^3\big[9(\cos\theta)^2 - 1\big]$
	$945(\sin\theta)^4\cos\theta$
	$945(\sin\theta)^5$
6	$\frac{21}{8}\sin\theta\big[33(\cos\theta)^5 - 30(\cos\theta)^3 + 5\cos\theta\big]$
	$\frac{105}{8}(\sin\theta)^2\big[33(\cos\theta)^4 - 18(\cos\theta)^2 + 1\big]$
	$\frac{315}{2}(\sin\theta)^3\big[11(\cos\theta)^3 - 3\cos\theta\big]$
	$\frac{345}{2}(\sin\theta)^4\big[11(\cos\theta)^2 - 1\big]$
	$10395(\sin\theta)^5\cos\theta$
	$10395(\sin\theta)^6$

the current controlled toroidal and saddle shim and linear gradient surface coil systems sitting as pairs of circular arcs of current on the cylindrical bore Ω of the superconducting magnet of the clinical MRI scanner. The second coil system is rotated about the longitudinal axis through the azimuth angle $\vartheta = \frac{1}{2}\pi$. In this way, an approximate homogeneity in spherical volume of the external magnetic flux density at the isocenter of the superconducting magnet can be achieved.

Specifically, Maxwell pairs, Golay coils, and quadrupole sets, for example ([104]), are designed in terms of the Euler half-angle decomposition KAK of $\mathbf{SU}(2, \mathbb{C})$ by zonal and tesseral surface spherical harmonics, and hence by Legendre polynomials and associated Legendre functions. The strategy underlying the particular designs of opposing current pairs of electrical shim and linear gradient coil systems is primarily the elimination of all degrees less than that desired and of the next highest degree of the same order. A typical value for the magnetic field homogeneity is ± 3.0 ppm over 40 cm diameter of spherical volume (dsv). The values guaranteed by vendors of whole-body scanners is ± 5.0 ppm over 50 cm dsv and ± 1.5 ppm over 20 cm dsv and allow for design of open-access clinical MRI scanners with the potential for interventional MRI at the isocenter of the superconducting magnet.

A consequence of the mutual orthogonality of the zonal and tesseral surface spherical harmonics in the complex Hilbert space $L^2_{\mathbb{C}}(\mathbb{S}_2)$ is that current controlled shim coil systems which generate spherical harmonics provide, by the natural decomposition of $S_{\mathbb{C}}(\mathbb{R}^3) \hookrightarrow L^2_{\mathbb{C}}(\mathbb{R}^3)$, components of magnetic field corrections which are noninteractive. The property of noninteractivity is particularly useful in high resolution nuclear MRS where magnetic field corrections up to the degree $k = 12$ are commonly applied for current controlled room temperature shims. According to the fact that $\mathbf{SU}(2, \mathbb{C})$ forms a twofold covering group of $\mathbf{SO}(3, \mathbb{R})$, the coil system consists of pairs of toroidal and circular arc channels on the cylindrical bore Ω. As emphasized before, the coil systems are turned through the azimuth angle $\vartheta = \frac{1}{2}\pi$ corresponding to the alternating matrix $J \in W\big(\mathbf{SU}(2, \mathbb{C}), K\big)$.

There are four sources of heat leaks into a cryostat: direct thermal conduction along the supports of the magnet, residual gas conduction, infrared radiation from higher to low temperatures, and joule heating from eddy currents. These currents are induced in metallic portions of the cryostat by pulsing of the linear gradient coils during imaging. The first three types of heat leak are minimized by proper cryostat design. Classical spherical harmonics play also an important role in eddy current compensation by combination of the big bore superconducting magnet with the shielded gradient coil system. Whenever fields which change the flux lines of a small bore magnet are changed rapidly, as is the case with the computer controlled linear gradient switching in an imaging experiment, eddy currents create an array of spherical harmonic fields which affect image quality. With a suitable calibration, each spherical harmonic can be corrected by the appropriate time-dependent current control in the shim coils, each unit of which is designed to generate a specific spherical harmonic. Such a compensation procedure is routinely implemented on commercial clinical MRI scanners. Composite filamentary wire is used, with the main magnet winding and the active-shield winding being connected in series.

A clinical MRI scanner set may contain 10 to 15 separate coils in each set, but those corresponding to low-order spherical harmonics, the shim coils that adjust the main field and the linear gradient shims, are the most crucial to image quality. A typical superconducting magnet has a total of about 17,000 turns of niobium–titanium wire wound on coil forms of about 0.65 m radius. The total length of the superconducting wire will be on the order of 65 km. This total length of wire must be constructed without any interruption of its superconducting properties in order to achieve persistent operation and adequate temporal stability. The total weight of the wire and its supporting structures is on the order of 3 tons.

Apart from the current controlled room temperature spherical volume shims and the computer controlled local magnetic flux density linear gradient strategy for the macroscopic quantum field phenomenon of superconductivity, harmonic analysis of the natural dual pair $(\mathbf{SL}(2, \mathbb{R}), \mathbf{O}(d, \mathbb{R}))$ provides the singular value decomposition of the rapidly decreasing Radon transform $\mathcal{R}_d$ of the projection–reconstruction method in the d-dimensional real Euclidean vector space $\mathbb{R}^d$ in terms of Laguerre polynomials $L_{\ell-m}^{|m|+\frac{d}{2}-1}(X)$ of order $|m| + \frac{1}{2}d - 1$ and degree $\ell - m$ and oscillator wave functions $h_{2\ell}$ of degree 2ℓ on the real line $\mathbb{R}$, respectively, tensored with the surface spherical harmonics of degree $|m|$ ([292]).

In the simplest case of dimension $d = 2$, the singular value decomposition of the compactly supported Radon transform

$$\mathcal{R}_2 : L_{\mathbb{C}}^2(D) \to L_{w_U^{-1}}^2(\Omega)$$

mapping the complex Hilbert space of square integrable complex-valued functions on the compact unit disk

$$D = \{z \in \mathbb{C} \,|\, |z| \le 1\}$$

into the complex Hilbert space of square integrable functions on the compact unit cylinder

$$\Omega = [-1, +1] \times \mathbb{S}_1 \hookrightarrow \mathbb{R}^3$$

with respect to the reciprocal Čebysev weight function $w_U^{-1} \ge 0$ reduces to the system of Zernike polynomials:

$$z \rightsquigarrow \begin{cases} \sqrt{\dfrac{\ell+1}{\pi}} |z|^{|m|} P_{\ell-m}^{(0,|m|)}(2|z|^2 - 1)\chi_{|m|}(\arg z) & z \in D, \\ 0 & z \in \mathbb{C} - D \end{cases}$$

and functions

$$(r, \vartheta) \rightsquigarrow \begin{cases} \dfrac{1}{\pi} w_U(r) U_{2\ell}(r)\chi_{|m|}(\vartheta) & |r| \le 1, \\ 0 & |r| > 1, \end{cases}$$

where $2\sqrt{\pi/(\ell+1)}$ is the associated singular value of $\mathcal{R}_2$. As a consequence, it follows that:

- The compactly supported Radon transform $\mathcal{R}_2$ is an ill-posed transform of order $\frac{1}{2}$.

Recently the CT-like projection–reconstruction method of zeugmatography has undergone a revival for use with fast short echo time imaging, where the RF excitation pulse flip angle $\theta \in [0, \pi]$ is kept small. Thus the natural duality between symplectic and orthogonal linear groups links the theory of automorphic forms and quadratic reciprocity ([167], [367]) to the generation of phase-coherent wavelets in electrical engineering and neurophysiology and underpins the holographic transform coding with a stringlike theory.

Mathematicians are like Frenchman: Whatever you say to them they translate into their own language and forthwith it is something completely different.

                    —Johann Wolfgang von Goethe (1749–1832)

Harmonic analysis usually begins with a group but, sometimes, conceptually, more appropriately starts with a geometric object attached to the group.

                    —Carl Herz (1994)

2.6   THE TRANSVECTIONAL ENCODING PROCEDURE

Let U^ν denote the linear Schrödinger representation of G acting in the standard complex Hilbert space $L^2_{\mathbb{C}}(\mathbb{R})$. The isomorphy class of U^ν is associated with the planar coadjoint orbit $\mathbf{P}(\mathbb{R} \times \mathcal{O}_\nu)$ $(\nu \neq 0)$ of G under the Kirillov bijection. Then U^ν subduces the one-dimensional representation χ_ν on the center C of G:

$$U^\nu \,|\, C = \chi_\nu \,,$$

and $(U^\nu, L^2_{\mathbb{C}}(\mathbb{R}))$ forms the quantization associated with the coadjoint orbit $\mathbf{P}(\mathbb{R} \times \mathcal{O}_\nu)$ $(\nu \neq 0)$ of G and uniquely determined up to unitary isomorphy. The complex vector space of smooth vectors $L^2_{\mathbb{C}}(\mathbb{R})^\infty$ for U^ν is the Schwartz space $S_{\mathbb{C}}(\mathbb{R})$ of infinitely differentiable complex-valued functions on the real line $\mathbb{R}$ that, along with their derivatives, are rapidly decaying at infinity. Its complex topological vector space dual $S'_{\mathbb{C}}(\mathbb{R})$, with respect to the canonical Fréchet space topology of $S_{\mathbb{C}}(\mathbb{R})$, is formed by the tempered distributions on $\mathbb{R}$. The Heisenberg Lie group G is the semidirect product of the closed normal subgroup

$$N = \left\{ \begin{pmatrix} 1 & 0 & z \\ 0 & 1 & y \\ 0 & 0 & 1 \end{pmatrix} \,\middle|\, y \in \mathbb{R}, z \in \mathbb{R} \right\}$$

which forms the direction of the tomographic sagittal planes and the closed subgroup

$$T = \left\{ \begin{pmatrix} 1 & x & 0 \\ 0 & 1 & 0 \\ 0 & 0 & 1 \end{pmatrix} \,\middle|\, x \in \mathbb{R} \right\}$$

of transvections having N as their homogeneous fixed-point plane transversal to the line T. Obviously,

$$C \hookrightarrow N \hookrightarrow G \,,$$

and the action by conjugation of $T \in \Theta(G, N) \cap G$ on N is given by the identity

$$\begin{pmatrix} 1 & x & 0 \\ 0 & 1 & 0 \\ 0 & 0 & 1 \end{pmatrix} \begin{pmatrix} 1 & 0 & z \\ 0 & 1 & y \\ 0 & 0 & 1 \end{pmatrix} \begin{pmatrix} 1 & x & 0 \\ 0 & 1 & 0 \\ 0 & 0 & 1 \end{pmatrix}^{-1} = \begin{pmatrix} 1 & 0 & z + xy \\ 0 & 1 & y \\ 0 & 0 & 1 \end{pmatrix} .$$

The irreducible unitary linear representation U^ν of G is induced by the unitary character

$$\chi_{(0,\beta,\nu)} = \chi_\nu^N : N \ni \begin{pmatrix} 1 & 0 & z \\ 0 & 1 & y \\ 0 & 0 & 1 \end{pmatrix} \rightsquigarrow e^{2\pi i(\beta y + \nu z)} \quad (\nu \neq 0)$$

which extends the central unitary character χ_ν from C to N. This follows from the identities

$$\chi_\nu = \chi_{(0,0,\nu)} = \chi_{(0,\beta,\nu)} \mid C = \chi_\nu^N \mid C$$

and the fact that the two-dimensional Lie subalgebra

$$\mathrm{Lie}(N) = \left\{ \begin{pmatrix} 0 & 0 & c \\ 0 & 0 & b \\ 0 & 0 & 0 \end{pmatrix} \mid b, c \in \mathbb{R} \right\}$$

of $\mathrm{Lie}(G)$ is a totally isotropic vector subspace with respect to the symplectic form $[\,\cdot\,,\,\cdot\,]$ on $\mathrm{Lie}(G)/\mathbb{R}I$, hence a *polarization* associated with $I^\star$ and subordinated ([291]) to the $\mathbb{R}$-linear form

$$L_{(0,\beta,\nu)} = \beta Q^\star + \nu I^\star \in \mathrm{Lie}(N)^\star$$

on $\mathrm{Lie}(N)$, where $L_{(0,\beta,\nu)}$ satisfies the condition

$$L_{(0,\beta,\nu)}(I) = \nu \neq 0.$$

Indeed, the total isotropy condition

$$L_{(0,\beta,\nu)}\big(\big[\mathrm{Lie}(N), \mathrm{Lie}(N) \big] \big) = 0$$

and the identity

$$\chi_{(0,\beta,\nu)} \left[\exp_N \begin{pmatrix} 0 & 0 & c \\ 0 & 0 & b \\ 0 & 0 & 0 \end{pmatrix} \right] = \exp \left[2\pi i L_{(0,\beta,\nu)} \begin{pmatrix} 0 & 0 & c \\ 0 & 0 & b \\ 0 & 0 & 0 \end{pmatrix} \right]$$

are easily verified. Due to the factorization of the elements of

$$G = TN$$

by elements of T and N according to

$$\begin{pmatrix} 1 & x & z \\ 0 & 1 & y \\ 0 & 0 & 1 \end{pmatrix} = \begin{pmatrix} 1 & x & 0 \\ 0 & 1 & 0 \\ 0 & 0 & 1 \end{pmatrix} \begin{pmatrix} 1 & 0 & z - xy \\ 0 & 1 & y \\ 0 & 0 & 1 \end{pmatrix},$$

the geometrical construction of induced representations of unimodular Lie groups from closed normal subgroups, by representing G on the square integrable cross sections of a Hilbert bundle sitting over the quotient group G/N, implies that for

$\beta \in \mathbb{R}$, $\nu \in \mathbb{R}$, $\nu \neq 0$, the irreducible unitary linear representation

$$\left(U^{\nu}, L^{2}_{\mathbb{C}}(\mathbb{R})\right) = L^{2} - \operatorname{Ind}^{G}_{\underset{N}{\uparrow}} \chi_{(0,\beta,\nu)} = L^{2} - \operatorname{Ind}^{G}_{\underset{N}{\uparrow}} \chi_{\nu}$$

of G acts on the elements $\psi \in S_{\mathbb{C}}(\mathbb{R})$ by translation and modulation with respect to the projected time variable

$$T \ni \begin{pmatrix} 1 & t & 0 \\ 0 & 1 & 0 \\ 0 & 0 & 1 \end{pmatrix} \rightsquigarrow t \in \mathbb{R}$$

of the Lagrangian line T in G as follows:

$$U^{\nu} \begin{pmatrix} 1 & x & z \\ 0 & 1 & y \\ 0 & 0 & 1 \end{pmatrix} \psi(t) = e^{2\pi i \nu(z+yt)} \psi(t+x) \qquad (t \in \mathbb{R}).$$

Thus the following Hilbert bundle diagram holds:

$$L^{2}_{\mathbb{C}}(\mathbb{R}) \quad \longrightarrow \quad L^{2}_{\mathbb{C}}(G)^{\chi_{(0,\beta,\nu)}}$$
$$\downarrow$$
$$G/N,$$

where the complex Hilbert spaces $L^{2}_{\mathbb{C}}(G)^{\chi_{(0,\beta,\nu)}}$ and $L^{2}_{\mathbb{C}}(T)$ are isomorphic under the cross-sectional unitary linear operator.

The initial central phase shift performed by the action of U^{ν} is stationary. For $\nu \neq 0$, the directional differentiation yields as linear gradients the linear Schrödinger operators acting on the complex vector space $S_{\mathbb{C}}(\mathbb{R})$ and satisfying the canonical commutation relation:

$$U^{\nu}(P) \quad = \quad \frac{\mathrm{d}}{\mathrm{d}s} U^{\nu}(\exp_{G}(sP))\Big|_{s=0} \quad = \quad 2\pi i \nu t,$$

$$U^{\nu}(Q) \quad = \quad \frac{\mathrm{d}}{\mathrm{d}s} U^{\nu}(\exp_{G}(sQ))\Big|_{s=0} \quad = \quad \frac{\mathrm{d}}{\mathrm{d}t},$$

$$U^{\nu}(I) \quad = \quad \frac{\mathrm{d}}{\mathrm{d}s} U^{\nu}(\exp_{G}(sI))\Big|_{s=0} \quad = \quad 2\pi i \nu.$$

The preceding equations are an expression of the fundamental Lauterbur $\tau o \xi v \gamma \mu \alpha$ link in terms of holographic transform encoding. They help establish that the trans-vections-implemented Heisenberg nilpotent real Lie group G define the structure group of the spin isochromats which are the dissipative spin systems naturally associated with the Fourier MRI modality.

For notational simplicity, let us concentrate on the generic irreducible unitary linear representation U^{1} of G in $L^{2}_{\mathbb{C}}(\mathbb{R})$ associated with the prototype $\mathbf{P}(\mathbb{R} \times \mathcal{O}_{1})$ of the coadjoint orbits of G sitting inside the projectively completed, real vector space dual $\mathbf{P}(\mathbb{R} \times \mathrm{Lie}(G)^{\star})$ of $\mathrm{Lie}(G)$. Recall that $\mathbf{P}(\mathbb{R} \times \mathcal{O}_1)$ is equipped with the canonical exterior differential two-form $\omega_1 = \mathrm{d}x \wedge \mathrm{d}y$ and measure μ. Let

$$\bar{\mathcal{F}}^2_{\mathbb{R} \oplus \mathbb{R}} : S'_{\mathbb{C}}(\mathbb{R} \oplus \mathbb{R}) \to S'_{\mathbb{C}}(\mathbb{R} \oplus \mathbb{R})$$

be the two-dimensional inverse partial Fourier transform with respect to the second spatial variable. It maps by duality ([308], [309]) the complex vector space $S'_{\mathbb{C}}(\mathbb{R} \oplus \mathbb{R})$ onto itself. The Schwartz kernel K_f on $\mathbf{P}(\mathbb{R} \times \mathcal{O}_1)$ associated with the extension

$$U^1(f) \in S'_{\mathbb{C}}(\mathbb{R} \oplus \mathbb{R})$$

of U^1 by temporal phase averaging modulo C over the tempered distribution $f \in S'_{\mathbb{C}}(\mathbb{R} \oplus \mathbb{R})$ is given in terms of synchronized spatial coordinates of the rotating coordinate frame of reference inside the tomographic slice $\mathbf{P}(\mathbb{R} \times \mathcal{O}_1) \hookrightarrow \mathbf{P}(\mathbb{R} \times \mathrm{Lie}(G)^{\star})$ by

$$K_f(x, y; 1) = \bar{\mathcal{F}}^2_{\mathbb{R} \oplus \mathbb{R}}(f)(x - y, y).$$

The linear mapping

$$K_1 : S'_{\mathbb{C}}(\mathbb{R} \oplus \mathbb{R}) \ni f \rightsquigarrow K_f \in S'_{\mathbb{C}}(\mathbb{R} \oplus \mathbb{R})$$

defines an isomorphism which restricts according to the Stone–von Neumann theorem ([291]) to an isometric isomorphism of $L^2_{\mathbb{C}}(\mathbb{R} \oplus \mathbb{R})$ onto the complex Hilbert space $L^2_{\mathbb{C}}(\mathbb{R}) \hat{\otimes}_2 L^2_{\mathbb{C}}(\mathbb{R})$ of Hilbert–Schmidt endomorphisms of $L^2_{\mathbb{C}}(\mathbb{R})$ under its canonical scalar product. In view of the Zecman order, the resonance isomorphism K_1 is at the center of pulse Fourier MRI reconstruction.

Note that the isometric isomorphy to the Hilbert–Schmidt operators on $L^2_{\mathbb{C}}(\mathbb{R})$ is a geometrical consequence of the flatness of the coadjoint orbit $\mathbf{P}(\mathbb{R} \times \mathcal{O}_1)$. Due to the unicity result of the Stone–von Neumann theorem ([291]), the linear Schrödinger representation of G in the complex Hilbert space $L^2_{\mathbb{C}}(\mathbb{R})$ can be extended to a unitary *projective* or ray representation of the semidirect product of G with the symplectic group $\mathbf{Sp}(2, \mathbb{R}) = \mathbf{SL}(2, \mathbb{R})$ by the fundamental covariance identity

$$T_g \circ U^1 \begin{pmatrix} 1 & x & z \\ 0 & 1 & y \\ 0 & 0 & 1 \end{pmatrix} \circ T_{g^{-1}} = U^1 \left(\begin{pmatrix} 1 & x & z \\ 0 & 1 & y \\ 0 & 0 & 1 \end{pmatrix} g \right).$$

In the preceding covariance identity, the unitary projective oscillator representation ([292])

$$T : g \rightsquigarrow T_g$$

of $\mathbf{SL}(2, \mathbb{R})$ in $L^2_{\mathbb{C}}(\mathbb{R})$ acts trivially on the elements of the center line C. It provides the intertwining operators between the unitarily isomorphic representations

$$\begin{pmatrix} 1 & x & z \\ 0 & 1 & y \\ 0 & 0 & 1 \end{pmatrix} \rightsquigarrow U^1 \begin{pmatrix} 1 & x & z \\ 0 & 1 & y \\ 0 & 0 & 1 \end{pmatrix} \qquad \begin{pmatrix} 1 & x & z \\ 0 & 1 & y \\ 0 & 0 & 1 \end{pmatrix} \rightsquigarrow U^1 \left(\begin{pmatrix} 1 & x & z \\ 0 & 1 & y \\ 0 & 0 & 1 \end{pmatrix} g \right)$$

of G in $L^2_{\mathbb{C}}(\mathbb{R})$ of central unitary character χ_1. The twofold covering group $\mathbf{Mp}(2, \mathbb{R})$ of $\mathbf{SL}(2, \mathbb{R})$ exists because the fundamental group of $\mathbf{SL}(2, \mathbb{R})$ is isomorphic to the group $\mathbb{Z}$. The metaplectic group $\mathbf{Mp}(2, \mathbb{R})$ implements the unique nonsplit group extension of $\mathbf{SL}(2, \mathbb{R})$ by $\mathbb{Z}/2\mathbb{Z}$ as displayed by the sequence

$$\mathbb{Z}/2\mathbb{Z} \lhd \mathbf{Mp}(2, \mathbb{R}) \longrightarrow \mathbf{SL}(2, \mathbb{R}).$$

It allows for a lifting of the unitary projective oscillator representation $T : g \rightsquigarrow T_g$ to a unitary representation

$$\tilde{g} \rightsquigarrow T_{\tilde{g}},$$

which is called the metaplectic representation of $\mathbf{Mp}(2, \mathbb{R})$ in $L^2_{\mathbb{C}}(\mathbb{R})$, such that the covariance identity is preserved and the exact sequence of Lie groups

$$1 \longrightarrow \mathbb{Z}/2\mathbb{Z} \longrightarrow \mathbf{Mp}(2, \mathbb{R}) \longrightarrow \mathbf{SL}(2, \mathbb{R}) \longrightarrow 1$$

arises. By a slight abuse of notation, the metaplectic representation of $\mathbf{Mp}(2, \mathbb{R})$ in the complex Hilbert space $L^2_{\mathbb{C}}(\mathbb{R})$ will also be denoted by T.

According to the explicit construction of the metaplectic group by the methods group cohomology ([242]), the elements of the nontrivial group extension $\mathbf{Mp}(2, \mathbb{R})$ admit the form of pairs

$$\tilde{g} = \big(g, \eta(g) \big) \in \mathbf{SL}(2, \mathbb{R}) \times \mathbb{T}.$$

Utilizing the mapping

$$\eta : \mathbf{SL}(2, \mathbb{R}) \longrightarrow \mathbb{T},$$

the group law of $\mathbf{Mp}(2, \mathbb{R})$ takes the form

$$\big(g, \eta(g) \big) \big(g', \eta(g') \big) = \big(gg', \eta(g)\eta(g')c(g, g')^{-1} \big),$$

where

$$\mathbf{SL}(2, \mathbb{R}) \times \mathbf{SL}(2, \mathbb{R}) \ni (g, g') \rightsquigarrow c(g, g') \in \mathbb{T}$$

denotes the 2-cocycle on $\mathbf{SL}(2, \mathbb{R})$ with values in $\mathbb{T}$ associated with the Maslov index ([207], [277], [367])

$$\mathbf{SL}(2, \mathbb{R}) \times \mathbf{SL}(2, \mathbb{R}) \ni (g, g') \rightsquigarrow \tau(g, g') \in \mathbb{Z}$$

as the *index of inertia* of a triplet of lines ([207], [278])

$$\tau(g, g') = \mathrm{Inert}(D, g^{-1}D, g'D)$$

in the orbit of $\mathbf{SL}(2, \mathbb{R})$ which naturally acts as a doubly transitive group on the set of lines D of G/C. It is easy to verify that the Maslov index $\tau(\cdot, \cdot)$ is actually independent of the choice of the Lagrangian line D in G/C. For each triple $(g_k)_{1 \leq k \leq 3}$ of elements of $\mathbf{SL}(2, \mathbb{R})$, the identity

$$c(g_1 g_2, g_3) c(g_1, g_2) = c(g_1, g_2 g_3) c(g_2, g_3)$$

holds. The natural projection of $\mathbf{Mp}(2, \mathbb{R})$ onto its first coordinate $\mathbf{SL}(2, \mathbb{R})$ form an epimorphism the kernel of which is isomorphic to $\mathbb{Z}/2\mathbb{Z}$.

In terms of the 2-cocycle c, the unitary projective oscillator representation T of $\mathbf{SL}(2, \mathbb{R})$ satisfies the functional equation of projective c-representations in $L^2_{\mathbb{C}}(\mathbb{R})$

$$T_{g \cdot g'} = c(g, g') \cdot T_g \circ T_{g'}$$

for all pairs $(g, g') \in \mathbf{SL}(2, \mathbb{R}) \times \mathbf{SL}(2, \mathbb{R})$. Moreover, the group cohomological index identity

$$c = e^{-(\pi/4)i\tau}$$

holds. The identity

$$c^2(g, g') = \eta(g)\eta(g')\eta(gg')^{-1}$$

for $(g, g') \in \mathbf{SL}(2, \mathbb{R}) \times \mathbf{SL}(2, \mathbb{R})$ implies the coboundary relation

$$c^2 = d\eta.$$

Thus the group cohomology associated with the metaplectic representation T of the nontrivial group extension $\mathbf{Mp}(2, \mathbb{R})$ implies a remarkable quantization of the wavelet phase. Notice that the special linear group $\mathbf{SL}(2, \mathbb{R})$ is generated in $\mathbf{GL}(2, \mathbb{R})$ by the set of matrices

$$\{J\} \cup \left\{ \begin{pmatrix} \alpha & 0 \\ 0 & \alpha^{-1} \end{pmatrix} \,\middle|\, \alpha \in \mathbb{R}, \, \alpha \neq 0 \right\} \cup \left\{ \begin{pmatrix} 1 & \beta \\ 0 & 1 \end{pmatrix} \,\middle|\, \beta \in \mathbb{R} \right\}$$

where $\alpha \in \mathbb{R}$, $\alpha \neq 0$, denotes the scale parameter of the diagonal matrices

$$\Delta = \begin{pmatrix} \alpha & 0 \\ 0 & \alpha^{-1} \end{pmatrix} \qquad (\alpha \neq 0)$$

in $\mathbf{SL}(2, \mathbb{R})$. The matrix $\Delta \in \mathbf{SL}(2, \mathbb{R})$ gives rise to the unitary scale operator

$$T_\Delta \psi : t \rightsquigarrow \frac{1}{\sqrt{|\alpha|}} \psi\left(\frac{t}{\alpha}\right)$$

acting on the phase-coherent wavelets $\psi \in S_{\mathbb{C}}(\mathbb{R}) \hookrightarrow L^2_{\mathbb{C}}(\mathbb{R})$. For the affine linear mapping of matrix

$$g = \begin{pmatrix} 1 & \beta \\ 0 & 1 \end{pmatrix} \in N,$$

where, as before,

$$N = \left[\mathbf{GA}^+(\mathbb{R}), \mathbf{GA}^+(\mathbb{R})\right]$$

denotes the derived group of $\mathbf{GA}^+(\mathbb{R})$, the contribution of the Maslov index pops up on the Fourier transform side. Indeed, the Fourier transform

$$t \rightsquigarrow \mathcal{F}_{\mathbb{R}}(T_g \psi)(t)$$

yields a modulation of $t \rightsquigarrow \mathcal{F}_{\mathbb{R}} \psi(t)$ by the chirp wavelet

$$\mathbb{R} \ni t \rightsquigarrow e^{\pi i \beta t^2} \underbrace{e^{-i(\pi/4)\mathrm{sgn}(\beta)}} \in \mathbb{T}$$

according to the group cohomological index identity, where

$$\mathrm{sgn}(\beta) = \frac{\beta}{|\beta|} \qquad (\beta \in \mathbb{R}, \beta \neq 0).$$

The Heisenberg group G is the semidirect product of the closed normal subgroup

$$M = \left\{ \begin{pmatrix} 1 & x & z \\ 0 & 1 & 0 \\ 0 & 0 & 1 \end{pmatrix} \middle| x \in \mathbb{R}, z \in \mathbb{R} \right\}$$

which forms the direction of the tomographic coronal planes and the closed subgroup

$$S = \left\{ \begin{pmatrix} 1 & 0 & 0 \\ 0 & 1 & y \\ 0 & 0 & 1 \end{pmatrix} \middle| y \in \mathbb{R} \right\}$$

of transvections having M as their homogeneous fixed-point plane transversal to the line S. Obviously,

$$C \hookrightarrow M \hookrightarrow G,$$

and the action by conjugation of $S \in \Theta(G, M) \cap G$ on M is given by the identity

$$\begin{pmatrix} 1 & 0 & 0 \\ 0 & 1 & y \\ 0 & 0 & 1 \end{pmatrix} \begin{pmatrix} 1 & x & z \\ 0 & 1 & 0 \\ 0 & 0 & 1 \end{pmatrix} \begin{pmatrix} 1 & 0 & 0 \\ 0 & 1 & y \\ 0 & 0 & 1 \end{pmatrix}^{-1} = \begin{pmatrix} 1 & x & z - xy \\ 0 & 1 & 0 \\ 0 & 0 & 1 \end{pmatrix}.$$

The irreducible unitary linear representation V^ν of G is induced by the unitary character

$$\chi_{(\alpha,0,\nu)} = \chi_\nu^M : M \ni \begin{pmatrix} 1 & x & z \\ 0 & 1 & 0 \\ 0 & 0 & 1 \end{pmatrix} \rightsquigarrow e^{2\pi i(\alpha x + \nu z)} \qquad (\nu \neq 0)$$

which extends the central unitary character χ_ν from C to M. This follows from the identities

$$\chi_\nu = \chi_{(0,0,\nu)} = \chi_{(\alpha,0,\nu)} \mid C = \chi_\nu^M \mid C$$

and the fact that the two-dimensional Lie subalgebra

$$\mathrm{Lie}(M) = \left\{ \begin{pmatrix} 0 & a & c \\ 0 & 0 & 0 \\ 0 & 0 & 0 \end{pmatrix} \;\middle|\; a, c \in \mathbb{R} \right\}$$

of $\mathrm{Lie}(G)$ is a totally isotropic vector subspace with respect to the symplectic form $[\,\cdot\,,\cdot\,]$ on $\mathrm{Lie}(G)/\mathbb{R}I$, hence a *polarization* associated with $I^\star$ and subordinated to the $\mathbb{R}$-linear form

$$L_{(\alpha,0,\nu)} = \alpha P^\star + \nu I^\star \in \mathrm{Lie}(N)^\star$$

on $\mathrm{Lie}(M)$, where $L_{(\alpha,0,\nu)}$ satisfies the condition

$$L_{(\alpha,0,\nu)}(I) = \nu \neq 0.$$

Indeed, the total isotropy condition

$$L_{(\alpha,0,\nu)}\big(\big[\mathrm{Lie}(M), \mathrm{Lie}(M)\big] \big) = 0$$

and the identity

$$\chi_{(\alpha,0,\nu)} \left[\exp_M \begin{pmatrix} 0 & a & c \\ 0 & 0 & 0 \\ 0 & 0 & 0 \end{pmatrix} \right] = \exp \left[2\pi i L_{(\alpha,0,\nu)} \begin{pmatrix} 0 & a & c \\ 0 & 0 & 0 \\ 0 & 0 & 0 \end{pmatrix} \right]$$

are easily verified. Due to the factorization of the elements of

$$G = SM$$

by elements of S and M according to

$$\begin{pmatrix} 1 & x & z \\ 0 & 1 & y \\ 0 & 0 & 1 \end{pmatrix} = \begin{pmatrix} 1 & 0 & 0 \\ 0 & 1 & y \\ 0 & 0 & 1 \end{pmatrix} \begin{pmatrix} 1 & x & z \\ 0 & 1 & 0 \\ 0 & 0 & 1 \end{pmatrix},$$

the geometrical construction of induced representations of unimodular Lie groups from closed normal subgroups by representing G on the square integrable cross-sections of a Hilbert bundle sitting over the quotient group G/M implies that, for $\alpha \in \mathbb{R}, \nu \in \mathbb{R}, \nu \neq 0$, the irreducible unitary linear representation

$$\left(V^\nu, L_\mathbb{C}^2(\mathbb{R})\right) = L^2 - \mathrm{Ind}^G_{\underset{M}{\uparrow}} \chi_{(\alpha,0,\nu)} = L^2 - \mathrm{Ind}^G_{\underset{M}{\uparrow}} \chi_\nu$$

of G acts on the elements $\psi \in S_{\mathbb{C}}(\mathbb{R})$ by translation and modulation with respect to the projected time variable

$$S \ni \begin{pmatrix} 1 & 0 & 0 \\ 0 & 1 & s \\ 0 & 0 & 1 \end{pmatrix} \rightsquigarrow s \in \mathbb{R}$$

of the Lagrangian line S in G as follows:

$$V^{\nu} \begin{pmatrix} 1 & x & z \\ 0 & 1 & y \\ 0 & 0 & 1 \end{pmatrix} \psi(t) = e^{2\pi i \nu(z + xs - xy)} \psi(s - y) \qquad (s \in \mathbb{R});$$

thus the Hilbert bundle diagram

$$L^2_{\mathbb{C}}(\mathbb{R}) \longrightarrow L^2_{\mathbb{C}}(G)^{\chi_{(\alpha,0,\nu)}}$$
$$\downarrow$$
$$G/M$$

holds, where the complex Hilbert spaces $L^2_{\mathbb{C}}(G)^{\chi_{(\alpha,0,\nu)}}$ and $L^2_{\mathbb{C}}(S)$ are isomorphic under the cross-sectional unitary linear operator (Table 2.4). In view of the fact that the elements of

$$G = STC$$

admit the factorization

$$\begin{pmatrix} 1 & x & z \\ 0 & 1 & y \\ 0 & 0 & 1 \end{pmatrix} = \begin{pmatrix} 1 & 0 & 0 \\ 0 & 1 & y \\ 0 & 0 & 1 \end{pmatrix} \begin{pmatrix} 1 & x & 0 \\ 0 & 1 & 0 \\ 0 & 0 & 1 \end{pmatrix} \begin{pmatrix} 1 & 0 & z \\ 0 & 1 & 0 \\ 0 & 0 & 1 \end{pmatrix},$$

Table 2.4. The $\left(U^{\nu}, V^{\nu}\right)$ Correspondence Associated with Coadjoint Orbit $\mathbf{P}\left(\mathbb{R} \times \mathcal{O}_{\nu}\right)$ $(\nu \neq 0)$ of G

U^{ν}	V^{ν}
$U^{\nu} \begin{pmatrix} 1 & x & 0 \\ 0 & 1 & 0 \\ 0 & 0 & 1 \end{pmatrix} \psi(t) = \psi(t + x)$	$V^{\nu} \begin{pmatrix} 1 & x & 0 \\ 0 & 1 & 0 \\ 0 & 0 & 1 \end{pmatrix} \psi(s) = e^{-2\pi i \nu x s} \psi(s)$
$U^{\nu} \begin{pmatrix} 1 & 0 & 0 \\ 0 & 1 & y \\ 0 & 0 & 1 \end{pmatrix} \psi(t) = e^{2\pi i \nu y t} \psi(t)$	$V^{\nu} \begin{pmatrix} 1 & 0 & 0 \\ 0 & 1 & y \\ 0 & 0 & 1 \end{pmatrix} \psi(s) = \psi(s - y)$
$U^{\nu} \begin{pmatrix} 1 & 0 & z \\ 0 & 1 & 0 \\ 0 & 0 & 1 \end{pmatrix} \psi(t) = e^{2\pi i \nu z} \psi(t)$	$V^{\nu} \begin{pmatrix} 1 & 0 & z \\ 0 & 1 & 0 \\ 0 & 0 & 1 \end{pmatrix} \psi(s) = e^{2\pi i \nu z} \psi(s)$

the rows of the matrix below establish that the Fourier cotransform

$$T_J = \bar{\mathcal{F}}_{\mathbb{R}}$$

associated with the alternating matrix J is a unitary isomorphism mapping U^1 onto V^1 as an intertwining unitary linear operator. From this result, the unitary isomorphy between U^ν and V^ν becomes explicit for $\nu \neq 0$. Thus the intertwiner

$$T_J : L^2_{\mathbb{C}}(\mathbb{R}) \longrightarrow L^2_{\mathbb{C}}(\mathbb{R})$$

provides the phase-sensitive quadrature detection of the transvectional encoding procedure.

The exponential maps $\exp_{\mathbf{SL}(2,\mathbb{R})}$ of $\mathrm{Lie}\big(\mathbf{SL}(2,\mathbb{R})\big)$ onto $\mathbf{SL}(2,\mathbb{R})$ and $\exp_{\mathbf{Mp}(2,\mathbb{R})}$ of $\mathrm{Lie}\big(\mathbf{SL}(2,\mathbb{R})\big)$ onto $\mathbf{Mp}(2,\mathbb{R})$ give rise to the tori

$$\mathbb{T} = \exp_{\mathbf{SL}(2,\mathbb{R})}(\mathbb{R}J)$$

and

$$\widetilde{\mathbb{T}} = \exp_{\mathbf{Mp}(2,\mathbb{R})}(\mathbb{R}J)$$

as the stratified images of the line $\mathbb{R}J$. The twofold covering $\widetilde{\mathbb{T}}$ of the torus group $\mathbb{T}$ corresponds to the antipodal spherical visualization of spin dynamics. The associated kernels are the discrete sets

$$\ker\big(\exp_{\mathbf{SL}(2,\mathbb{R})} \mid \mathbb{R}J\big) = 2\pi\mathbb{Z}J$$

and

$$\ker\big(\exp_{\mathbf{Mp}(2,\mathbb{R})} \mid \mathbb{R}J\big) = 4\pi\mathbb{Z}J .$$

In view of the identity

$$\mathrm{Lie}\big(\mathbf{Mp}(2,\mathbb{R})\big) = \mathrm{Lie}\big(\mathbf{SL}(2,\mathbb{R})\big) ,$$

for the isotropic presentation of G, an explicit computation establishes the identity

$$T_{\exp_{\mathbf{Mp}(2,\mathbb{R})}(-\vartheta J)} \circ U^1 \begin{pmatrix} 1 & x & 0 \\ 0 & 1 & y \\ 0 & 0 & 1 \end{pmatrix} \circ T_{\exp_{\mathbf{Mp}(2,\mathbb{R})}(\vartheta J)}$$

$$= U^1 \begin{pmatrix} 1 & x\cos\vartheta - y\sin\vartheta & 0 \\ 0 & 1 & x\sin\vartheta + y\cos\vartheta \\ 0 & 0 & 1 \end{pmatrix} .$$

For the polarized presentation of G this identity reads

$$T_{\exp_{\mathbf{Mp}(2,\mathbb{R})}(-\vartheta J)} \circ U^1 \begin{pmatrix} 1 & x & 0 \\ 0 & 1 & y \\ 0 & 0 & 1 \end{pmatrix} \circ T_{\exp_{\mathbf{Mp}(2,\mathbb{R})}(\vartheta J)}$$

$$= U^1 \begin{pmatrix} 1 & -y\sin\vartheta & x\cos\vartheta & 0 \\ 0 & 1 & 0 & x\sin\vartheta \\ 0 & 0 & 1 & y\cos\vartheta \\ 0 & 0 & 0 & 1 \end{pmatrix},$$

where the angle of rotation is given by $\vartheta = 2\pi t$, $t \in \mathbb{R}$:

- The symmetry group of the traces of the Heisenberg helices forming a circular grating in the coadjoint orbit $\mathbf{P}(\mathbb{R} \times \mathcal{O}_1)$ is given by its metaplectic representation $T_{\exp_{\mathbf{Mp}(2,\mathbb{R})}(\mathbb{R}J)}$.

The differentiated form of the metaplectic representation T establishes that the infinitesimal generator of $T_{\exp_{\mathbf{Mp}(2,\mathbb{R})}(\mathbb{R}J)}$ is formed by the harmonic oscillator Hamiltonian

$$U^1(\mathcal{L}_G) = \frac{\mathrm{d}^2}{\mathrm{d}t^2} - 4\pi^2 t^2.$$

It follows that the harmonic oscillator wave functions $(h_n)_{n \geq 0}$ can be expressed in terms of the raising and lowering operators

$$U^1\left(\tfrac{1}{2}(P + iQ)\right), \qquad U^1\left(\tfrac{1}{2}(P - iQ)\right)$$

of the Bargmann–Fock model of G. Note that these operators are obtained from the differentiated form of the linear Schrödinger representation U^1 of G by transversal rotations of the canonical basis $\{P, Q, I\}$ of $\mathrm{Lie}(G)$ through the angles

$$\left\{\tfrac{1}{4}\pi, \tfrac{3}{4}\pi\right\}.$$

Thus the differentiated form of the Schrödinger representation U^1, which is associated with the generic coadjoint orbit $\mathcal{O}_1$ of G, is evaluated on the octants:

- The location operator $\psi \rightsquigarrow 2\pi i t \psi(t)\, \mathrm{d}t$ is implemented by $U^1(P)$, and the momentum operator $\psi \rightsquigarrow \psi'(t)\, \mathrm{d}t$ is implemented by $U^1(Q)$.
- The weak eigenfunctions of the harmonic oscillator Hamiltonian $U^1(\mathcal{L}_G)$ of eigenvalue $-2\pi(n+1)$ are the normalized harmonic oscillator wave functions $(h_n)_{n \geq 0}$.
- The harmonic oscillator wave fuctions $(h_n)_{n \geq 0}$ admit the Gaussian density $t \rightsquigarrow e^{-\pi t^2}$ with respect to the Hermite polynomials $(H_n(t))_{n \geq 0}$.

Thus the metaplectic representation T of $\mathbf{Mp}(2, \mathbb{R})$ links the differentiated form of the generic linear Schrödinger representation U^1 evaluated on the left-invariant sub-Laplacian differential operators $\mathcal{L}_G$ to the torus group. The harmonic oscillator Hamiltonian $U^1\left(\mathcal{L}_G\right)$ is called the Ornstein–Uhlenbeck generator. In view of the fact that the Legendre transform of the principal symbol of $\mathcal{L}_G$ determines the left-invariant sub-Riemannian metric of G, the central role of the sub-Laplacian differential operator $\mathcal{L}_G$ for the mathematical foundations of MRI becomes obvious.

Rapid changes in the phase and frequency occur within synchronous events and multiple periods of synchrony invariably occur on each trial. These findings indicate that coherent oscillations between two relatively distant points in cortex develop, collapse, and reform on a rapid time scale during a single response period ranging from 500–1.500 ms.
                                                                    —Charles M. Gray (1992)

Stimulus-specific synchronization is a true neural self-organization process having degrees of freedom from stimulus in the frequency and phase of the oscillations.
                                                                    —Reinhard Eckhorn (1991)

2.7 PHASE–LOCKED SYNCHRONIZED NEURAL NETWORKS

Two types of variables are basically relevant to a biological neural network organization: neural signals and the interactivity connections of cerebral functional self-organization. According to the results of electrophysiology, phase-coherent wavelets represent the neural signals in phase-locked, synchronized neural networks.

To describe the interactivity connections in phase-locked, synchronized neural networks by the process of graph matching, let $\Gamma_{m,n}$ denote the complete bichromatic graph of $m + n$ vertices. Let $(c(\Gamma_{m,n}, \ell))_{0 \leq \ell \leq [\frac{m+n}{2}]}$ denote the matching coefficients ([159], [294], [357]) of $\Gamma_{m,n}$ with matching polynomial

$$\Phi_{m,n}(X) = \sum_{0 \leq \ell \leq [\frac{m+n}{2}]} (-1)^\ell c(\Gamma_{m,n}, \ell) X^{m+n-2\ell}$$

in the real algebra $\mathbb{R}[X]$ of polynomials in the indeterminate X. Due to $c(\Gamma_{m,n}, 0) = 1$ and the fact that $c(\Gamma_{m,n}, \ell)$ denotes the number of *choices* of $\ell \geq 1$ disjoint edges in $\Gamma_{m,n}$, a combinatorial argument which is based on the explicit expression of the Laguerre polynomials

$$L_n^\alpha(X) = \sum_{0 \leq k \leq n} \frac{(-1)^k}{k!} \binom{n + \alpha}{n - k} X^k \qquad (\alpha \geq -1)$$

in $\mathbb{R}[X]$ shows that the Laguerre polynomials occurring in the centerless matrix coefficients $\mathcal{H}_1$ of the generic linear Schrödinger representation $(U^1, L_\mathbb{C}^2(\mathbb{R}))$ of G with respect to the harmonic oscillator wave functions $(h_n)_{n \geq 0}$ in $S_\mathbb{C}(\mathbb{R})$ give rise to the matching polynomial functions

$$\Phi_{m,n}(v) = (-1)^n n! v^{m-n} L_n^{m-n}(|v|^2) \qquad (m \geq n \geq 0)$$

in terms of the complex variable $v = \sqrt{\pi}\, \bar{w}$ proportional to the complex conjugate of

$$w = x + iy \in \mathbb{C}.$$

Thus the linkage between quantum holography and the layered architecture of temporally encoded synchronized neural network organizations of stimulus-evoked synchronized response association ([293], [295], [296], [355], [356]) can be expressed in terms of the complete bichromatic graphs $\left(\Gamma_{m,n}\right)_{m\geq 0,n\geq 0}$ by the dynamical connectivity identity

$$\mathcal{H}_1\left(h_m, h_n; x, y\right) = \frac{(-1)^n}{\sqrt{m!n!}}e^{-(1/2)|v|^2}\Phi_{m,n}(v) \qquad (m \geq n \geq 0)$$

for the quantum holograms $(\mathcal{H}_1(h_m, h_n; \cdot, \cdot))_{m\geq 0,n\geq 0}$ of the harmonic oscillator wave functions.

The complete bichromatic graphs $\left(\Gamma_{m,n}\right)_{m\geq 0,n\geq 0}$ of the graph matching process are to be understood as the basic functional connectivity clusters generated by stimulus-evoked synchronized interaction ([181], [226]). An application of Schur's lemma ([36], [291], [314]) yields the dissonance conditions

$$< \mathcal{H}_\nu\left(\psi, \varphi; \cdot, \cdot\right)|\mathcal{H}_{\nu'}\left(\psi', \varphi'; \cdot, \cdot\right) > = 0 \qquad \left(\nu \neq \nu'\right)$$

associated with the pair of disjoint coadjoint orbits $\left(\mathbf{P}\left(\mathbb{R} \times \mathcal{O}_\nu\right), \left(\mathbf{P}\left(\mathbb{R} \times \mathcal{O}_{\nu'}\right)\right)\right.$ of G and $\psi, \varphi, \psi', \varphi' \in S_\mathbb{C}(\mathbb{R})$. For $\nu = \nu'$, the discrete series trace formula associated with $\mathbf{P}\left(\mathbb{R} \times \mathcal{O}_\nu\right) (\nu \neq 0)$ arises:

$$< \mathcal{H}_\nu(\psi, \varphi; \cdot, \cdot)|\mathcal{H}_\nu(\psi', \varphi'; \cdot, \cdot) > = \nu < \psi \otimes \varphi'|\psi' \otimes \varphi >$$

In the discrete series trace formula for the holographic transform $\mathcal{H}_\nu$, the scalar product is given by

$$< \psi \otimes \varphi'|\psi' \otimes \varphi > = < \psi|\psi' >< \varphi'|\varphi > .$$

The identity holds in the complex tensor product Hilbert space $L^2_\mathbb{C}(\mathbb{R})\hat{\otimes}_2 L^2_\mathbb{C}(\mathbb{R})$ of Hilbert–Schmidt endomorphisms of $L^2_\mathbb{C}(\mathbb{R})$ as isometrically realized according to the Stone–von Neumann theorem by $L^2_\mathbb{C}(\mathbb{R} \oplus \mathbb{R})$.

The discrete series trace formula for the holographic transform $\mathcal{H}_\nu$ can be used to prove a version of the Schwartz kernel or nuclear theorem ([308]). In analogy with massively parallel, nonalgorithmic, photonic neurocomputing, it follows as a conclusion:

- Quantum holograms are linear superpositions of the family of orthogonal quantum holograms associated with the generic coadjoint orbit $\mathbf{P}\left(\mathbb{R} \times \mathcal{O}_1\right) \hookrightarrow \mathbf{P}\left(\mathbb{R} \times \text{Lie}^\star(G)\right)$, $(\mathcal{H}_1(h_m, h_n; \cdot, \cdot))_{m\geq 0,n\geq 0}$, and define a synchronized neural network organization of response wavelets by the graph matching process. The edges of the superposition of the associated family of complete bichromatic graphs $\left(\Gamma_{m,n}\right)_{m\geq 0,n\geq 0}$ represent the transient clusters of synchronized dynamical interactivity connections per cell of neural network organizations which nonalgorithmically emulate the semantic association of tomographic images and emulate functional topographic image processing.

Specifically in the organization of the striate cortex by a transient array of synchronously tuned "metronomes" generated by the projection of the retinal coordinates and iso-orientation onto the cortical sheet under the retinotopic map, the connections of interactivity link cell assemblies activated by contours have the same orientation and are aligned colinearly. Selective dynamical links are formed between distant neural assemblies via reciprocal connections in a process called reentry in the theory of neuronal cluster selection ([77], [78]). Reentrant phase-coherent wavelets establish phase-sensitive temporal cross-correlations between cortical maps within or between different levels of the CNS. These quantized holograms act as adaptive filter bank families which are able to evaluate relationsships between spatially distributed features and to create image representations for particular, frequently occurring constellations of features. These representations in turn can be used for scene segmentation ([129]) to assign spatially distributed contours within the visual scene to particular objects, individual figures, and embedding background:

- The quantum holograms $\left(\mathcal{H}_1\left(h_m, h_n; \cdot, \cdot\right)\right)_{m \geq 0, n \geq 0}$ are radial functions on $\mathbb{R} \oplus \mathbb{R}$ if and only if they are tracial functions in the sense that the degrees of the harmonic oscillator wave functions are located on the diagonal $n = m$.

- In the trace case, sandwich symmetry of the generic coadjoint orbit $\mathbf{P}\left(\mathbb{R} \times \mathcal{O}_1\right)$ and its echo orbit $\mathbf{P}\left(\mathbb{R} \times \mathcal{O}_{-1}\right)$ occurs.

- The traces of the phase-locked synchronized neural network on the observation plane $\mathbf{P}\left(\mathbb{R} \times \mathcal{O}_\infty\right)$ provides the spin isochromat density $f \in L_{\mathbb{C}}^2(\mathbb{R} \oplus \mathbb{R}) \hookrightarrow S_{\mathbb{C}}'(\mathbb{R} \oplus \mathbb{R})$.

Because the traces of the Heisenberg helices form circular grating arrays, the spin echo technique defines a reentrant procedure to achieve a phase-locked synchronized neural network by an application of $^\vee$-pulse sequences. The group $\mathbf{SO}(2, \mathbb{R})$ and its image under the reflection

$$\begin{pmatrix} 1 & 0 \\ 0 & -1 \end{pmatrix} \in \mathbf{O}(2, \mathbb{R}) - \mathbf{SO}(2, \mathbb{R})$$

are operating on the homogeneous plane $x_3 = 0$ of $\mathbb{R}^3$ which is parametrized by the matrices

$$-i \begin{pmatrix} 0 & x_1 + ix_2 \\ x_1 - ix_2 & 0 \end{pmatrix}$$

of complex conjugate entries. Transferring the coordinate system to the projectively completed dual $\mathbf{P}\left(\mathbb{R} \times \text{Lie}(G)^\star\right)$, a practical consequence is the fact that gauging by rotating frames of counterpropagating orientations

$$\begin{pmatrix} 0 & x + iy \\ x - iy & 0 \end{pmatrix} \qquad [(x, y) \in \mathbb{R} \oplus \mathbb{R}]$$

of the generic planar coadjoint orbit $\mathbf{P}\left(\mathbb{R} \times \mathcal{O}_1\right)$ of G and its echo orbit $\mathbf{P}\left(\mathbb{R} \times \mathcal{O}_{-1}\right)$ associated with the central character χ_1 and is conjugate χ_{-1}. It allows to implement the quantum coherent phenomenon of non-linear phase conjugation refocusing of a disspitative spin system by $^\vee$-pulse inversion.

In a standard spin echo sequence, a $^\vee$-pulse follows after one-half of the spin echo time T_E to the RF excitation pulse of flip angle

$$\theta = \tfrac{1}{2}\pi$$

and central frequency ν, which turns the spins out of alignment with the external magnetic field of longitudinal direction into the planar coadjoint orbit $\mathbf{P}(\mathbb{R} \times \mathcal{O}_1)$ by inducing transversally an additional, temporally switched external magnetic flux density. The magnetic flux density, which actually flips the magnetization perturbation through the angles $\tfrac{1}{2}\pi$ and π according to its length, rotates through the azimuth angle ϑ at the Larmor reference frequency $\nu = (1/2)\pi\dot{\vartheta} = 1$ of synchronized spin precession and is therefore stationary with respect to the rotating coordinate frame. The $^\vee$-pulse of central frequency $\nu = 1$ which globally rephases the response wavelet by the reflection within the rotating coordinate frame

$$^- : x + iy \rightsquigarrow x - iy$$

therefore produces in $\mathbf{P}(\mathbb{R} \times \mathcal{O}_1)$ a spin echo centered at time T_E after the application of the RF excitation pulse of flip angle $\theta = \tfrac{1}{2}\pi$. From the Euler half-angle decomposition $\mathbf{SU}(2, \mathbb{C}) = \mathrm{KAK}$ displayed above, it follows:

- The refocusing $^\vee$-pulse of pulse flip angle $\theta = \pi$ performs the reflection $^-$ of spin echo generation by the Pauli spin matrix

$$\varepsilon_1 = \begin{pmatrix} 0 & -i \\ -i & 0 \end{pmatrix}$$

  which is the infinitesimal generator of the one-parameter subgroup A of $\mathbf{SU}(2, \mathbb{C})$.

Frequency encoding of an in-plane direction of $\mathbf{P}(\mathbb{R} \times \mathcal{O}_1)$ is accomplished by turning on the frequency encoding gradient at two separate times during each imaging cycle. The first application of the frequency encoding gradient, which is called the *dephase lobe*, transiently changes the local frequency of pixels from each column of the grating array of synchronously tuned traces of Heisenberg helices according to its location within that gradient. When the gradient is turned off, nuclear spins residing in pixel columns that experienced the frequency encoding gradient have gained phase compared with spins that had not experienced the frequency encoding gradient. The $^\vee$-pulse inverts this spatially dependent distribution of phases. To refocus the filter response wavelet into a spin echo, the frequency encoding gradient must be turned on a second time to act as the read-out gradient. The read-out lobe has twice the duration of the dephase lobe, allowing for full spin echo to be refocused. The peak of the echo occurs at the center of the read-out lobe at time T_E when complete rephasing occurs.

Because the decoding of the magnetic spin echo holograms is performed by a digital computer which realizes the symplectic Fourier transform by a two-dimensional FFT algorithm, it follows ([300]):

- Clinical MRI scanners form temporally encoded analog quantum neurocomputers for massively parallel nonalgorithmic computation combined with digital computers to solve the visual object binding problem of tomographic visualization by stimulus-evoked synchronized response association. At the interface of the analog and digital computer domains are magnetic spin echo holograms which non-algorithmically emulate the semantic association of tomographic images. Acting as adaptive filter bank families, magnetic spin echo holograms dynamically perform microvascular functional topographic neuroimaging of cognitive processing.

Accordingly, the required functions of a clinical MRI scanner are divided into analog and digital computer domains. The analog functions include linear gradient and RF power amplifiers, the RF transceiver, probes, and the big superconducting magnet itself. The digital functions include computer operations needed to exert control over the massively parallel analog functions:

- Examples of control functions are the programmed pulse sequences for synchronously tuned traces of Heisenberg helices for the encoding by circular grating arrays, application of the slice-select linear gradients, and the implementation of coordinate frames of reference by temporally switching linear gradients of magnetic flux densities within the excited tomographic plane for the dual spatial encoding.

Unlike the digital computer domain, whose operations are controlled by a central processing unit (CPU), the layered organization of the temporally encoded analog computer domain is lacking a CPU or any hierarchical and syntactical structure. Although the thalamus forms the neuroanatomical and neuropathological key to the neocortex ([57]), there exists no specific organizationally dominant structure in the cortex cerebri.

- In the clinical MRI scanner as a temporally encoded analog quantum neurocomputer, two counterpropagating principal data streams flow across the interface between the two computer domains—timing parameters and amplitude information for controlling linear gradients—and RF excitation pulses are directed from the digital to the analog computer; temporally encoded synchronized MRI data return from the receiver back to the digital computer for algorithmic data processing.

These kinds of contrasts reflect differences in tissue biochemistry. In particular, multiple spin echo sequences provide excellent tumor discrimination via the associated increase in T_2-weighted spin–relaxation responses. For the evaluation of brain tumors, MRI is therefore the imaging method of choice typically displaying a heterogeneous mass with hemorrhage and necrosis. Glioblastoma multiforme (GBM), for instance, is seen on a neuroimaging scan as a region of the brain of high excitation–response signal intensity with central necrosis and marked edema extending along peripheral white matter tracts. As acquired by transaxial MRI scans, GBM is typically located in the cerebral hemispheres with multiple lobe involvement, ventricular rupture, and spread by way of the corpus callosum to the contralateral hemispherium cerebralis and lobus insularis, resulting in a butterfly appearance, termed *butterfly* GBM.

Although MRI does not allow for more specific diagnosis of brain gliomas than X-ray CT, major advantages include superior depiction of tumor extent, cystic and necrotic change, and anatomic relationships. The use of exogenous paramagnetic contrast enhancing agents can further improve the capability of the method to delineate tumors of gliomatosis cerebri, along ependyma and meninges, for instance, for an application of MRI-assisted neuronavigation in minimally invasive neurosurgery. The image artifact of multiple spin echo sequences, referred to as a mirror image, can be avoided by decreasing stimulated magnetization components with phase alternating image protocols.

The advantage of superconducting magnets is their high magnetic flux density up to 10 T combined with a high homogeneity of the magnetic field of 15 ppm within a sphere of diameter of 50 cm which can be achieved by a single cryogen-active shield magnet under spherical volume shimming conditions. In state-of-the-art superconducting MRI scanners, a closed cycle cryogenic refrigeration head is attached to the hard superconductor, which is a type II superconductor with a large magnetic hysteresis that uses helium gas as a refrigerant. The cryogen reliquifying procedure both reduces the helium boil-off rate and obviates the need for a liquid nitrogen cryostat. The spaces surrounding the liquid helium and, in the older designs, the liquid nitrogen are both evacuated to minimize heat leaks into the cryogenic chambers. If even a small region of the niobium–titanium wire is heated above the critical temperature T_c, it will begin to dissipate heat, and this causes a further increase in temperature. The result can be a self-propagating process leading to a magnet quench, wherein the entire stored energy in the magnetic field is converted into heat. This raises the temperature of the liquid helium above its boiling point, and the liquid helium evaporates as the magnetic field collapses.

A typical value for the cryogen consumption of a low loss cryostat is 0.09 liters per hour of liquid helium, about 10% of the early systems operating without refrigerator. The two-stage cryogenic refrigerator prolongates the liquid helium refilling interval to more than 8 months. The resulting reduction in annual cost for clinical MRI scanner systems implies that the traditional hierarchy of diagnostic imaging modalities for evaluating patients.

$$\text{Ultrasonography} \implies \text{X-ray CT} \implies \text{MRI},$$

is not longer valid for choosing the most efficient and cost saving procedure for routine clinical radiological examinations and that pulsed Fourier MRI is the modality of choice for most cases. In neurosurgery, intraoperative ultrasonography has its merits for depicting cerebral structures during neurosurgical operations ([11]), although it will be replaced in the future by stereotactic operation microscopy. Enhanced-reality systems based on MRI-guided neuronavigation will support minimally invasive neurosurgery by image fusion. In the obstetrical patient, ultrasonographic evaluation of the uterus gravidus for leiomyomas is limited because the conceptus may obscure parts of the myometrium ([45], [160], [284]). By MRI, however, gynecologic anatomy is very well displayed. Leiomyomas, whether simple or degenerated, may be clearly depicted in both the gravid and nongravid uterus ([79], [160]).

As in a nonpregnant patient, clinical MRI appears to be more accurate than ultrasonography for precise sizing and localization of leiomyomas and for differentiating ovarian masses from uterine leiomyomas. In the evaluation of the malignant neoplasms of gynecologic oncology, namely endometrial, cervical, and vaginal carcinoma ([45], [160], [162], [163], [225], [273], [284], [334]), clinical MRI has become the primary imaging approach providing soft tissue contrast beyond that obtainable by X-ray CT or ultrasonography.

For clinical images acquired in all tomographic planes—transaxial, coronal, sagittal, and parasagittal—the head and neck are still the favorite regions of the human body for Fourier MRI diagnosis. Actually X-ray CT imagery is being rapidly replaced by clinical MRI as the study of choice for the majority of lesions in the larynx, pharynx, oral cavity, tongue, nasopharynx, paranasal sinuses, and parapharyngeal space ([143], [212], [351]). Progress in high temperature superconducting magnets will support this trend in head and neck oncology toward hazard-free MRI examinations and to change the standard of practice which persists in accomplishing imaging, for instance in current hepatic imaging ([236]), via ultrasonography and X-ray CT imagery in spite of ample evidence that MRI is superior for most types of clinical imaging.

*I turn away with fear and horror from this lamentable plague of functions which do not
have derivatives.*

—Charles Hermite (1822–1901)

*For the mathematician, there is above all the question: Why a Hilbert space? After all,
he can understand Kronecker saying that God created integers, but why should He have
so intimately concerned Himself with a Hilbert space?*

—Nolan R. Wallach (1977)

*Distribution theory was one of the two great revolutions in mathematical analysis in the
20th century. It can be thought of as the completion of differential calculus, just as the
other great revolution, measure theory (or Lebesgue integration theory), can be thought
of as the completion of integral calculus.*

—Robert S. Strichartz (1994)

2.8   KERNEL DISTRIBUTIONS

The energy required to flip a proton through the angle $\theta = \pi$ in a magnetic field
of flux density 1.0 T is 2.82×10^{-26} J $= 0.176$ μeV. By the Einstein relation
this is the energy of a 42.57-MHz photon. The basic problem of MRI is to radiate
electromagnetic energy at the frequency of 42.57 MHz into the assembly of proton
spins which are ordered by the external magnetic field in such a way that by resonance
a spatially distributed magnetic spin organization is established the synchronized
connections of which are capable for corticomorphic processing. The averaging of
these spatially distributed magnetic spin assemblies is performed by distribution
theory, which has to be accommodated to the underlying quantum electrodynamic
process.

Distribution theory, usually formulated as a local extension theory in terms of open
subsets of the Euclidean vector space $\mathbb{R}^n$ or a finite dimensional C^∞-differential manifold, can be thought of as the completion of differential calculus, just as Lebesgue
integration theory can be thought of as the completion of integral calculus. Distribution theory, when applied to unitary linear representations of Lie groups G,
provides the basis for noncommutative Fourier analysis and symbol calculus. Specifically geometrical quantization gives rise to distributional harmonic analysis on the
Heisenberg nilpotent Lie group G. In pulsed Fourier MRI, distributional harmonic
analysis on the Heisenberg group G is suitable to describe relaxation-weighted spin
isochromat densities f excited in the planar coadjoint orbits $\mathbf{P}(\mathbb{R} \times \mathcal{O}_\nu)$ $(\nu \neq 0)$ of
the stratification of the unitary dual $\hat{G}$ of G in terms of the symplectically invariant
symbol calculus. The symbol calculus allows to embed the von Neumann approach to
quantum mechanics, which is based on the category of Hilbert spaces, into the Dirac
approach, which is based on complex locally convex topological vector spaces of
tempered distributions. For the preparation of the symbol calculus, some generalities
of the calculus of Schwartz kernels are needed ([308]). The full physical meaning of
the kernel distributions for the application to Fourier MRI can be appreciated in the
context of the planar coadjoint orbit stratification of the unitary dual $\hat{G}$ of the Heisen-

berg Lie group G which provides the two-dimensional Fourier analysis with an extra symplectic structure. This symplectic structure has been traced back by André Weil to Carl Ludwig Siegel's papers on the theory of quadratic forms ([367]).

For simplicity, let G denote a unimodular Lie group. Then G forms a locally compact topological group and simultaneously a finite dimensional C^∞-differential manifold such that both structures are compatible in the sense that the group operations are C^∞ mappings. In the context of the application to Fourier MRI, G and its subgroups can be thought of as a matrix group. Note, however, that the affine linear group $\mathbf{GA}(\mathbb{R})$ is not unimodular.

Let dg denote a choice of Haar measure on G. Then dg forms an element 1_G of the complex vector space $\mathcal{D}'(G)$ of distributions on G. The topological antidual of the complex vector space $\mathcal{D}(G)$ of infinitely differentiable, compactly supported, complex-valued functions on G under its canonical anti-involution of complex conjugation

$$j\colon \psi \rightsquigarrow \bar{\psi}$$

is the vector space $\mathcal{D}'(G)$ of those antilinear forms on $\mathcal{D}(G)$ which are continuous with respect to the canonical inductive limit topology of $\mathcal{D}(G)$. As a realization of the Wigner invariance theorem, the involutory antiautomorphism of $\mathcal{D}'(G)$ which is contragredient to the canonical anti-involution of $\mathcal{D}(G)$ plays a crucial role in Fourier MRI in modeling the refocusing phenomenon of phase conjugation. Note that the complex vector spaces $\mathcal{D}(G)$ and $\mathcal{D}'(G)$ form their own antispaces. Because nuclearity is preserved under countable inductive limits and Hausdorff projective limits, the complex vector spaces $\mathcal{D}(G)$ and $\mathcal{D}'(G)$ form nuclear locally convex topological vector spaces under the canonical inductive limit topology and the weak dual topology, respectively.

Let U denote a linear representation of G acting continuously on the complex Hilbert subspace $\mathcal{H}$ of $\mathcal{D}'(G)$ by Hilbert space automorphisms of $\mathcal{H}$. Then $\mathcal{H}$ forms a closed vector space of $\mathcal{D}'(G)$ under its weak dual topology in the sense that the linear injection

$$\mathcal{H} \hookrightarrow \mathcal{D}'(G)$$

forms a continuous mapping. The norm topology of $\mathcal{H}$ is finer than the topology induced on $\mathcal{H}$ by the weak dual topology of $\mathcal{D}'(G)$, the mapping

$$G \times \mathcal{H} \ni (g, \psi) \rightsquigarrow U(g)\psi \in \mathcal{H}$$

is simultaneously continuous, and the vector subspace $\mathcal{H}^{+\infty}$ of smooth vectors for the unitary linear representation U is everywhere dense in $\mathcal{H}$ with respect to the norm topology. Thus, for every element of the complex vector space $\mathcal{H}^{+\infty}$, the trajectory through $\psi \in \mathcal{H}^{+\infty}$ which is defined by the rule

$$\tilde{\psi} : g \rightsquigarrow U(g)\psi$$

forms an infinitely differentiable mapping of G in $\mathcal{H}$ ([309]). The mapping

$$\psi \rightsquigarrow \tilde{\psi}$$

defines a continuous linear embedding of $\mathcal{H}$ into the topological vector space

$$C^0(G; \mathcal{H}) \cong C^0(G) \hat{\otimes} \mathcal{H}$$

of continuous functions of G with values in the complex Hilbert space $\mathcal{H}$ under the topology of compact convergence.

For the case of the Heisenberg group G with center C and $\mathcal{H} = L^2_{\mathbb{C}}(\mathbb{R})$, the standard complex Hilbert space over the bi-infinite stratigraphic time line $\mathbb{R}$, the continuous linear embedding

$$\mathcal{H} \hookrightarrow C^0(G/C; \mathcal{H})$$

performed at resonance frequency $\nu \neq 0$ by the linear Schrödinger representation U^ν of G in $\mathcal{H}$ with projective kernel C is at the basis of the symplectically invariant symbol calculus approach to Fourier MRI because the canonical projection

$$G \longrightarrow G/C$$

allows, by passing to the quotient mod C, implementation of the phase dispersion and its compensation by phase conjugation in the laboratory coordinate frame attached to the cross section G/C to C in G.

The continuous injection $\mathcal{H} \hookrightarrow C^0(G; \mathcal{H})$ identifies $\mathcal{H}$ with a closed vector subspace $\tilde{\mathcal{H}}^0$ of $C^0(G; \mathcal{H})$ and $\mathcal{H}^{+\infty}$ with the closed vector subspace

$$\tilde{\mathcal{H}}^{+\infty} = \{\tilde{\psi} \mid U(g')\tilde{\psi}(g) = \tilde{\psi}(g'.g), \ g', \ g \in G\}$$

of $C^\infty(G; \mathcal{H})$. Notice that G defines an infinitely differentiable action on the vector space $\tilde{\mathcal{H}}^{+\infty}$ of smooth trajectories via left translations by the reflected group elements $g'^{-1} \in G$. Of course, each smooth trajectory $\tilde{\psi} \in \mathcal{H}^{+\infty}$ defines a distribution on G with values in $\mathcal{H}$ by the standard prescription

$$\tilde{\psi}(f) = \int_G \tilde{\psi}(g)f(g)\, \mathrm{d}g,$$

where $f \in \mathcal{D}(G)$ denotes an arbitrary test function on G. It is called the *trajectory distribution* associated with $\psi \in \mathcal{H}^{+\infty}$.

Let μ denote a compactly supported scalar measure on G and $\check{\mu}$ the image of μ under the involutory homeomorphism $g \rightsquigarrow g^{-1}$ of G onto itself. Then, as observed above,

$$U(g')\tilde{\psi} = \check{\varepsilon}_{g'} \star \tilde{\psi} \qquad (g' \in G)$$

for $\tilde{\psi} \in \mathcal{H}^{+\infty}$ and the Dirac measure $\varepsilon_{g'}$ located at $g' \in G$. The weak integral taken in $\mathcal{H}$,

$$U(\mu) = \int_G U(g)\,d\mu(g),$$

extends U by averaging over G. If μ is absolutely continuous with respect to dg and admits a relaxation-weighted spin isochromat density f which is integrable over G with respect to the measure dg and vanishes in a neighborhood of the point at infinity, then $U(f) = U(f\,dg)$ is given by the prescription ([367])

$$U(f) = \int_G U(g)f(g)\,dg.$$

The extension $U(\mu)$ satisfies the distributional convolution identity

$$U(\mu)\tilde{\psi} = \check{\mu} \star \tilde{\psi}$$

for all trajectory distributions $\tilde{\psi} \in \tilde{\mathcal{H}}^{+\infty}$. The elements of the complex vector space $\tilde{\mathcal{H}}^{-\infty}$ of distributions K on G with values in $\mathcal{H}$ satisfying the convolution identity

$$U(\mu)K = \check{\mu} \star K$$

for all compactly supported scalar measures μ on G are called *kernel distributions* of $\mathcal{H}$ for the given unitary linear representation U of G in $\mathcal{H}$. If the complex vector space $\tilde{\mathcal{H}}^{-\infty}$ is endowed with the locally convex topology induced by $\mathcal{D}'(G; \mathcal{H})$, the continuous inclusions

$$\tilde{\mathcal{H}}^{+\infty} \hookrightarrow \tilde{\mathcal{H}}^{0} \hookrightarrow \tilde{\mathcal{H}}^{-\infty}$$

hold. In this sequence, the vector space of trajectory distributions $\mathcal{H}^{+\infty}$ is isomorphic to $\tilde{\mathcal{H}}^{+\infty}$ of smooth vectors for U, and the vector space $\tilde{\mathcal{H}}^{0}$ is isomorphic to the representation space $\mathcal{H}$ of the unitary linear representation U of G.

The important step is to realize that the unitary representation U of G in $\mathcal{H}$ gives rise to a continuous representation $\tilde{U}$ of G in the trajectory space

$$\tilde{\mathcal{H}}^{0} \cong \mathcal{H}$$

according to the prescription

$$\tilde{U}(g') : \psi \rightsquigarrow \left(U(g')\psi\right)^{\sim} \qquad (g' \in G).$$

The polarized symbol map $\tilde{U}$ extends to an infinitely differentiable representation $g' \rightsquigarrow \tilde{U}(g')$ of G in $\mathcal{H}^{-\infty}$ by right translations. Thus

$$\tilde{U}(g')K = K \star \check{\varepsilon}_{g'}$$

for $K \in \tilde{\mathcal{H}}^{-\infty}$. In particular, it follows that

$$\tilde{U}(\mu)\tilde{\psi} = \tilde{\psi} \star \check{\mu}$$

by convolving the trajectory $\tilde{\psi} \in \tilde{\mathcal{H}}^{-\infty}$ from the right with the reflected compactly supported scalar measure μ on G. Moreover, the filter cascade identity

$$\tilde{U}(S \star T)\tilde{\psi} = \tilde{U}(S) \circ \tilde{U}(T)\tilde{\psi}$$

holds for all compactly supported distributions $S, T \in \mathcal{D}(G)$.

The kernel distribution $K \in \tilde{\mathcal{H}}^{-\infty}$ of $\mathcal{H}$ for the representation U of G is called a generating kernel distribution ([309]) provided the image $K\big(\mathcal{D}(G)\big)$ is an everywhere dense vector subspace of $\mathcal{H}$. Let U be a regular representation of G in $\mathcal{H}$ in the usual sense that the unitary group action $U(g)\psi$ of G on $\psi \in \mathcal{H}$ is given by left translations $\varepsilon_g \star \psi$ by elements $g \in G$. Then

$$U(\mu)\psi = \mu \star \psi$$

holds for each compactly supported scalar measure μ on G and each element $\psi \in \mathcal{H}$. It follows that the Schwartz kernel H of $\mathcal{H}$ in $\mathcal{D}'(G)$ is defined by convolution from the left with a uniquely defined positive definite distribution $H^\bullet$ on G. Therefore the canonical reproducing kernel of the representation U of G is defined by $\star H^\bullet$. The existence of the linear mapping

$$H : f \rightsquigarrow f \star H^\bullet$$

is a consequence of the Schwartz kernel or nuclear theorem ([308], [309]). The mapping $K \rightsquigarrow K^\bullet$ of $\tilde{\mathcal{H}}^{-\infty}$ onto the vector space

$$\mathcal{H}^{-\infty} = \big\{T \in \mathcal{D}'(G) \,|\, f \star T \in \mathcal{H}, \quad f \in \mathcal{D}(G)\big\}$$

forms a linear bijection which uniquely extends the inverse bijection

$$\tilde{\psi} \rightsquigarrow \psi$$

of $\tilde{\mathcal{H}}^0$ onto $\mathcal{H}$ and identifies the representation $\tilde{U}$ with the representation $g \rightsquigarrow U(g)$ of left translations $\varepsilon_g \star$. In particular,

$$\big(U(S)K\big)^\bullet = U(S)K^\bullet$$

holds for all kernel distributions $K \in \tilde{\mathcal{H}}^{-\infty}$ and all compactly supported complex distributions $S \in \mathcal{D}'(G)$. Moreover,

$$U(g)T = \varepsilon_g \star T$$

and

$$U(S)T = S \star T$$

hold for all elements $g \in G$ and distributions $T \in \mathcal{H}^{-\infty}$ on G.

As a consequence of the preceding reasonings, it follows that:

- There exists a bijective correspondence between the unitary regular representations of G and the positive definite distributions on G.

The contragredient representation $\check{U}$ of U is defined by the inverse of the transposed operators according to the rule

$$\check{U} : g \rightsquigarrow {}^tU\big(g^{-1}\big).$$

Therefore G acts continuously by $\check{U}$ on the topological dual $\mathcal{H}'$ of $\mathcal{H}$ under its weak dual topology. Because the canonical anti-isomorphism j of $\mathcal{H}'$ onto $\bar{\mathcal{H}}'$ transports $\check{U}$ onto the conjugate representation $\bar{U}$ acting on the topological antidual $\bar{\mathcal{H}}'$ of $\mathcal{H}$, the coefficients of $\check{U}$ are the complex conjugates of the continuous coefficient functions of U and therefore temporospatially encode important properties of the unitary linear representation U of G. In particular, the contragredient representation $\check{U}$ plays an important role in the implementation of the matched filter bank concept.

The standard L^2 Sobolev inequality establishes that the complex vector space of smooth vectors for U^ν acting on $\mathcal{H} = L^2_{\mathbb{C}}(\mathbb{R})$ is formed by the Schwartz space

$$\mathcal{H}^{+\infty} = S_{\mathbb{C}}(\mathbb{R})$$

of complex-valued smooth functions on the bi-infinite time scale $\mathbb{R}$, rapidly decreasing at infinity such that all their derivatives are also rapidly decreasing at infinity. It is well known that $\mathcal{H}^{+\infty}$ is a complex nuclear locally convex topological vector space under its canonical Fréchet space topology and that it forms a normal vector space of complex distributions on $\mathbb{R}$ in the sense that the canonical injection

$$\mathcal{D}(\mathbb{R}) \hookrightarrow \mathcal{H}^{+\infty}$$

is continuous and admits an everywhere dense image ([308]). By extension, it provides $\mathcal{H}^{+\infty}$ with its natural anti-involution. The complex vector space $\tilde{\mathcal{H}}^{-\infty}$, which is isomorphic to $\mathcal{H}^{-\infty}$ under the locally convex vector space topology induced by $\mathcal{D}'_{(G;\mathcal{H})}$, forms the Sobolev space consisting of all tempered distributions $T \in S'_{\mathbb{C}}(\mathbb{R} \oplus \mathbb{R})$ such that their symplectic convolution products satisfy

$$f \star_\nu T \in L^2_{\mathbb{C}}(\mathbb{R} \oplus \mathbb{R})$$

for all functions $f \in S_{\mathbb{C}}(\mathbb{R} \oplus \mathbb{R})$. It contains the irreducible $S_{\mathbb{C}}(\mathbb{R} \oplus \mathbb{R})$ module $S_{\mathbb{C}}(\mathbb{R} \oplus \mathbb{R})$ as well as the irreducible $L^2_{\mathbb{C}}(\mathbb{R} \oplus \mathbb{R})$ module $L^2_{\mathbb{C}}(\mathbb{R} \oplus \mathbb{R})$ in the sense of the symplectic convolution product $\star_\nu$ of $\tilde{\mathcal{H}}^{-\infty}$. Thus the continuous inclusions

$$S_{\mathbb{C}}(\mathbb{R} \oplus \mathbb{R}) \hookrightarrow L^2_{\mathbb{C}}(\mathbb{R} \oplus \mathbf{R}) \hookrightarrow \tilde{\mathcal{H}}^{-\infty} \hookrightarrow S'_{\mathbb{C}}(\mathbb{R} \oplus \mathbb{R})$$

hold. Due to the swapping symplectic matrix $\frac{1}{2}J$ associated with the Lie bracket $[\cdot, \cdot]$ of $\mathrm{Lie}(G)$, the symplectic convolution product induced by the linear Schrödinger representation U^ν on the planar coadjoint orbit $\mathbf{P}(\mathbb{R} \times \mathcal{O}_\nu)$ of G takes the explicit form

$$f \star_\nu g(x, y; \nu) = \frac{1}{2} \int_{\mathbb{R} \oplus \mathbb{R}} f(x', y'; \nu) g(x - x', y - y'; \nu) \exp\left[\pi i \nu \det\begin{pmatrix} x & y \\ x' & y' \end{pmatrix}\right] dx' dy'.$$

The normalization factor in front of the integral comes from the formal degree of the linear Schrödinger representation U^ν of G. Taking into account the iteration of smooth actions implemented by U^ν, the symplectic convolution product $f \star_\nu g$ reveals to be jointly continuous for

$$f, g \in S_{\mathbb{C}}(\mathbb{R} \oplus \mathbb{R}) \cong S_{\mathbb{C}}(\mathbb{R}) \hat{\otimes} S_{\mathbb{C}}(\mathbb{R}) \cong S_{\mathbb{C}}(\mathbb{R}; S_{\mathbb{C}}(\mathbb{R}))$$

and $\nu \neq 0$. Hence the irreducible $S_{\mathbb{C}}(\mathbb{R} \oplus \mathbb{R})$ module $S_{\mathbb{C}}(\mathbb{R} \oplus \mathbb{R})$ is a complex Fréchet algebra under the symplectic convolution. The *symplectic* Fourier transform is defined by the involutory isomorphism

$$S_{\mathbb{C}}(\mathbb{R} \oplus \mathbb{R}) \ni f \rightsquigarrow \hat{f} \in S_{\mathbb{C}}(\mathbb{R} \oplus \mathbb{R}),$$

where

$$\hat{f} = f \star_\nu (1_\nu \oplus 1_\nu).$$

The symplectic convolution with the constant distribution $1_\nu \oplus 1_\nu$ on the projectively completed, symplectic affine plane $\mathbf{P}(\mathbb{R} \times \mathcal{O}_\nu)$ explicitly reads

$$\hat{f}(x, y; \nu) = \frac{1}{2} \int_{\mathbb{R} \oplus \mathbb{R}} f(x', y'; \nu) \exp\left[\pi i \nu \det \begin{pmatrix} x & y \\ x' & y' \end{pmatrix} \right] dx' dy' \ [(x, y) \in \mathbb{R} \oplus \mathbb{R}].$$

It follows from the Stone–von Neumann theorem of quantum mechanics ([291]) or from a smooth version of the Takesaki–Takai duality theorem ([83]) applied to the dynamical system $\mathbb{R} \triangleleft G \longrightarrow \mathbb{R} \oplus \mathbb{R}$ that phase averaging of the relaxation-weighted spin isochromat density

$$f \in L_{\mathbb{C}}^2(\mathbb{R} \oplus \mathbb{R}) \hookrightarrow S_{\mathbb{C}}'(\mathbb{R} \oplus \mathbb{R})$$

by the mod C square integrable linear Schrödinger representation U^ν of G leads to the Hilbert–Schmidt integral operator

$$U^\nu(f) \in \mathcal{L}_2(\mathcal{H}),$$

realized by an integral operator of kernel in $L_{\mathbb{C}}^2(\mathbb{R} \oplus \mathbb{R})$. The integrated form $U^\nu(f)$ of U^ν extends the focal point evaluation by an average over the cross section G/C to the center C with respect to the measure $f(x, y; \nu) \, dx \otimes dy$:

- The square integrability mod C of the linear Schrödinger representation U^ν of G for $\nu \neq 0$ allows to embed, by means of the symbol calculus, the von Neumann approach to quantum mechanics, which is based on the category of Hilbert spaces into the Dirac approach, which is based on complex, locally convex topological vector spaces of tempered distributions.

Let $< \cdot, \cdot >$ denote the bracket which defines the topological vector space antiduality $\left(S_{\mathbb{C}}(\mathbb{R}), S_{\mathbb{C}}'(\mathbb{R})\right)$. It implements the involutory antiautomorphism of the complex vector space $S_{\mathbb{C}}'(\mathbb{R})$ of tempered distributions on the bi-infinite time scale $\mathbb{R}$, which is contragredient to the natural antiinvolution of $S_{\mathbb{C}}(\mathbb{R})$. Moreover, it provides $S'_{\mathbb{C}}(\mathbb{R})$ with its weak dual topology under which $S'_{\mathbb{C}}(\mathbb{R})$ forms a complex, nuclear, locally convex topological vector space ([308]):

- The complex vector spaces $S_{\mathbb{C}}(\mathbb{R})$ and $S'_{\mathbb{C}}(\mathbb{R})$ form their own antispaces, and the sesquilinear form $< \cdot, \cdot >$ is consistent with the internal scalar product of the standard complex Hilbert space $L^2_{\mathbb{C}}(\mathbb{R}) \hookrightarrow S'_{\mathbb{C}}(\mathbb{R})$.

In terms of the trace filter sweep of quantum holography, the holographic transform attached to the projectively completed, symplectic affine plane $\mathbf{P}(\mathbb{R} \times \mathcal{O}_\nu)$ at resonance frequency $\nu \neq 0$ is defined by

$$\mathcal{H}_\nu : S_{\mathbb{C}}(\mathbb{R}) \ni \psi \rightsquigarrow \left((x,y) \rightsquigarrow < U^\nu \begin{pmatrix} 1 & x & 0 \\ 0 & 1 & y \\ 0 & 0 & 1 \end{pmatrix} \psi, 1_\nu > \cdot 1_\nu \oplus 1_\nu \right).$$

The tempered distribution $1_\nu \in S'_{\mathbb{C}}(\mathbb{R})$ rotates at the frequency $\nu \neq 0$ of the unitary central character χ_ν associated with the coadjoint orbit $\mathbf{P}(\mathbb{R} \times \mathcal{O}_\nu)$. Specifically:

- The tempered distribution $1_\nu \oplus 1_\nu$ forms the central sweep of the rotating coordinate frame attached to the planar coadjoint orbit $\mathbf{P}(\mathbb{R} \times \mathcal{O}_\nu)$ at the Larmor precession frequency $\nu \neq 0$.

An application of the Paley–Wiener–Schwartz theorem allows to smooth out, on the Fourier transform side, the Poisson bracket by an expansion in terms of transvectants of the projectively completed, symplectic affine plane $\mathbf{P}(\mathbb{R} \times \mathcal{O}_\nu)$:

- For $\nu \neq 0$, the holographic transform $\mathcal{H}_\nu$ attached to the projectively completed, symplectic affine plane $\mathbf{P}(\mathbb{R} \times \mathcal{O}_\nu)$ forms a distributional analogue of the Liouville density in phase space.

Because the continuous linear mapping $\mathcal{H}_{-\nu}$ defined by the coefficient of the contragredient representation

$$\check{U}^\nu \cong U^{-\nu}$$

of G corresponding to $1_\nu \in S'_{\mathbb{C}}(\mathbb{R})$ commutes with the left regular action of G/C on $L^2_{\mathbb{C}}(G/C)$, an application of Schur's theorem ([291]) to the von Neumann algebra formed by the weakly closed commutant of $U(G)$ in the group of automorphisms of $\mathcal{H}$ yields

$$\mathcal{H}_{-\nu} \circ j \circ \mathcal{H}_\nu = \mathrm{id}_{S'_{\mathbb{C}}(\mathbb{R} \oplus \mathbb{R})},$$

and similarly

$$\mathcal{H}_\nu \circ j^{-1} \circ \mathcal{H}_{-\nu} = \mathrm{id}_{S'_{\mathbb{C}}(\mathbb{R} \oplus \mathbb{R})}.$$

Thus the matched filter bank identity

$$\bar{\mathcal{H}}_\nu' = \mathcal{H}_{-\nu}$$

holds for the inverse kernel of $\mathcal{H}_\nu$. In consistency with the Bochner–Plancherel–Schwartz characterization of positive definite distributions, the tempered distribution

$$\mathcal{H}_\nu^\bullet = 1_\nu \oplus 1_\nu$$

on the planar coadjoint orbit $\mathbf{P}(\mathbb{R} \times \mathcal{O}_\nu)$ of unitary central character χ_ν provides the uniquely defined canonical reproducing kernel $\star_\nu \mathcal{H}_\nu^\bullet$ of the linear Schrödinger representation $U^\nu(\nu \neq 0)$, of G. Notice that $\mathcal{H}_\nu^\bullet \in \tilde{\mathcal{H}}^{-\infty}$ represents the orientation class of $S_\mathbb{C}'(\mathbb{R} \oplus \mathbb{R})$. Conversely, the preceding identity and its infinitesimally generating equivalent imply the square integrability mod C of U^ν and the flatness of the planar coadjoint orbit $\mathcal{O}_\nu \hookrightarrow \mathrm{Lie}(G)^\star$ associated with the isomorphy class of U^ν in the unitary dual $\hat{G}$ ([94]):

- The flatness of the projectively completed, symplectic affine $\mathbf{P}(\mathbb{R} \times \mathcal{O}_\nu)$ $(\nu \neq 0)$ allows to identify the trace of the holographic transform $\mathcal{H}_\nu$ attached to the coadjoint orbit $\mathbf{P}(\mathbb{R} \times \mathcal{O}_\nu)$ at resonance frequency ν as follows:

$$\mathrm{tr}\, \mathcal{H}_\nu = \mathcal{H}_\nu^\bullet.$$

In terms of the exterior differential 2-form ω_ν representing the rotational curvature of $\mathbf{P}(\mathbb{R} \times \mathcal{O}_\nu)$ $(\nu \neq 0)$, the infinitesimal generator $(1/\pi i)\omega_\nu$ of the smooth dynamical system $\mathbb{R} \lhd G \longrightarrow \mathbb{R} \oplus \mathbb{R}$ reads

$$\frac{1}{\pi i} \omega_\nu = \nu\, dx \wedge dy = \tfrac{1}{2} i\nu\, dw \wedge d\bar{w}.$$

The symplectic character formula holds in the density space $\tilde{\mathcal{H}}^{-\infty}$, where (x, y) denote the differential phase-local frequency coordinates with respect to a co-ordinate frame rotating with frequency $\nu \neq 0$ and $w = x + iy \in \mathbb{C}$. The upsampling Pfaffian of the canonical symplectic form $(1/\pi i)\omega_\nu$ of the coad-joint orbit $\mathbf{P}(\mathbb{R} \times \mathcal{O}_\nu)$ of G reads

$$\mathrm{Pf}\left(\frac{1}{\pi i} \omega_\nu\right) = \nu.$$

The identity

$$U^\nu(\mu)\mathcal{H}_\nu = \mu \star_\nu \mathcal{H}_\nu,$$

which holds for all compactly supported scalar measures μ on the symplectic affine plane $\mathcal{O}_\nu$, implies

$$\mathcal{H}_\nu(\psi) = \tilde{\psi} \star_\nu \mathcal{H}_\nu^\bullet.$$

Hence

$$< \mathcal{H}_\nu(\psi), \mathcal{H}_\nu^\bullet >= \tilde{\psi}$$

for all elements $\psi \in \mathcal{H}^{-\infty}$. It follows that $\mathcal{H}_\nu(\psi) \in S_\mathbb{C}'(\mathbb{R} \oplus \mathbb{R})$ represents a reproducing kernel of $\mathcal{H} = L_\mathbb{C}^2(\mathbb{R})$ in $\mathcal{H}^{-\infty}$. The uniquely defined canonical *reproducing* kernel $\star_\nu \mathcal{H}^\bullet$, where $\mathcal{H}_\nu^\bullet \in \tilde{\mathcal{H}}^{-\infty}$, acts as the differential phase-local frequency reference of the rotating coordinate frame of frequency $\nu \neq 0$ which is attached to the planar coadjoint orbit $\mathbf{P}(\mathbb{R} \times \mathcal{O}_\nu)$. It can be thought of as the reference of a Keppler configuration consisting of circular grating arrays of phase-locked isochromats inside the projectively completed, symplectic affine plane $\mathbf{P}(\mathbb{R} \times \mathcal{O}_\nu)$.

According to Harish–Chandra's philosophy, the correct way to think of characters of Lie groups is as distributions. In terms of the symplectic presentation of G, the symplectic character formula displayed above can be looked at as a generalization of the relation

$$\exp \circ \mathrm{tr} = \det \circ \exp$$

to Schwartz kernels. From the calculus of Schwartz kernels in the locally convex topological vector space $S_\mathbb{C}'(\mathbb{R} \oplus \mathbb{R})$ of tempered distributions follow the symplectic filter bank identities

$$\sqrt{\nu} \, \mathcal{H} = \sqrt{\star_\nu \mathcal{H}_\nu^\bullet} \, \mathcal{L}_2(\mathcal{H}) \qquad (\nu > 0)$$

and

$$\sqrt{-\nu} \, \mathcal{H} = \sqrt{\star_{-\nu} \mathcal{H}_{-\nu}^\bullet} \, \mathcal{L}_2(\mathcal{H}) \qquad (\nu < 0).$$

The kernel K_f^ν associated with the Hilbert–Schmidt integral operator $U^\nu(f) \in \mathcal{L}_2(\mathcal{H})$ for $f \in L_\mathbb{C}^2(\mathbb{R} \oplus \mathbb{R})$ extends from $f \in S_\mathbb{C}(\mathbb{R} \oplus \mathbb{R})$ to its antidual $S_\mathbb{C}'(\mathbb{R} \oplus \mathbb{R})$ by the rule

$$K_f^\nu(x, y) = 2e^{-\pi i \nu xy} \, f \star_\nu \mathcal{H}_\nu^\bullet(x, y) \qquad \left[(x, y) \in \mathbb{R} \oplus \mathbb{R}\right].$$

The preceding identity leads to the following result, which explains the important role played by the symplectic filter bank processing in Fourier MRI. Several methods of MRI, such as the spin presaturation technique by gradient spoiling for motion artifact reduction in variable-thickness slabs, are based on symplectic filter bank processing:

- The generating kernel distribution K_f^ν with respect to the rotating coordinate frame attached to the projectively completed symplectic affine plane $\mathbf{P}(\mathbb{R} \times \mathcal{O}_\nu)$ obtains by symplectic filtering of the relaxation-weighted spin is isochromat density f with the uniquely defined canonical reproducing kernel $\star_\nu \mathcal{H}_\nu^\bullet$, associated with the holographic transform $\mathcal{H}_\nu$ at resonance frequency $\nu \neq 0$.

The irreducible unitary linear representation V^ν of G satisfying the resonance condition of the unitary central character and therefore attached to the same planar coadjoint orbit $\mathcal{O}_\nu \hookrightarrow \mathrm{Lie}(G)^\star$ of G defines a holographic transform isomorphic to $\mathcal{H}_\nu$ by the unitary action σ of the metaplectic group $\mathbf{Mp}(2, \mathbb{R})$ on the Hilbert space $\mathcal{H} = L^2_{\mathbb{C}}(\mathbb{R})$ and therefore a generating kernel distribution isomorphic to K^ν_f.

In order to express the Schwartz kernel $K_f(\cdot, \cdot; 1)$ in the synchronized spatial coordinates of a two-dimensional laboratory coordinate frame cross section implemented by orthogonal local magnetic field in-plane linear gradients at the isocenter (x, y) inside the symplectic manifold $(\mathcal{O}_1, \omega_1)$, the kernel distribution K_f in the gauge of the rotating coordinate frame synchronously revolving through azimuth angle ϑ at the Larmor reference frequency $\nu = (1/2\pi)\dot{\vartheta} = 1$ of synchronized spin precession inside $(\mathcal{O}_1, \omega_1)$ has to be transformed into its symplectically invariant Weyl symbol

$$\sigma(K_f)(x, y; 1) = e^{2\pi i xy} \bar{\mathcal{F}}^2_{\mathbb{R} \oplus \mathbb{R}} K_f(x, y; 1) \qquad [(x, y) \in \mathbb{R} \oplus \mathbb{R}] .$$

- The quantum holograms of Fourier MRI form a horizontally stacked plot of phase-encoded ray traces of tuned-in Heisenberg helices with vertical offsets. The Weyl symbol $\sigma(K_f)(\cdot, \cdot; \nu)$ gives rise to the partial mapping

$$K_x: y \rightsquigarrow \sigma(K_f)(x, y; \nu) \qquad (x \in \mathbb{R})$$

in local frequency twist acquisition, and the affine Lagrangian lines

$$L_y : x \rightsquigarrow \sigma(K_f)(x, y; \nu) \qquad (y \in \mathbb{R})$$

result in differential phase acquisition of the quantum phase hologram within the tomographic slice $\mathbf{P}(\mathbb{R} \times \mathcal{O}_\nu) \hookrightarrow \mathbb{R}(\mathbb{R} \times \mathrm{Lie}(G)^\star)$.

According to the tempered Schwartz kernel theorem ([308]), the Weyl symbol $\sigma(K_f)(\cdot, \cdot; \nu) \in S'_{\mathbb{C}}(\mathbb{R} \oplus \mathbb{R})$ can be identified with the learning matrix of the mappings

$$\mathbb{R} \ni x \rightsquigarrow K_x \in S'_{\mathbb{C}}(\mathbb{R})$$

and

$$\mathbb{R} \ni y \rightsquigarrow L_y \in S'_{\mathbb{C}}(\mathbb{R})$$

inside the tomographic slice $\mathbf{P}(\mathbb{R} \times \mathcal{O}_\nu) \hookrightarrow \mathbf{P}(\mathbb{R} \times \mathrm{Lie}(G)^\star)$.

Recall that by coordinatization with respect to the laboratory frame of reference the discrete Heisenberg group $\Gamma \hookrightarrow G$ can be expressed in terms of unipotent integral matrices

$$\Gamma = \left\{ \begin{pmatrix} 1 & x & z \\ 0 & 1 & y \\ 0 & 0 & 1 \end{pmatrix} \,\middle|\, x, y, z \in \mathbf{Z} \right\}.$$

The subgroups $\Gamma_n \hookrightarrow \Gamma$ $(n \in \mathbb{Z})$ are generated by the set of integral transvections $\{\exp_G P, \exp_G nQ, \exp_G I\}$ of the three-dimensional real vector space G so that the set of matrices with integer entries

$$\left\{ \begin{pmatrix} 1 & 1 & 0 \\ 0 & 1 & 0 \\ 0 & 0 & 1 \end{pmatrix}, \begin{pmatrix} 1 & 0 & 0 \\ 0 & 1 & n \\ 0 & 0 & 1 \end{pmatrix}, \begin{pmatrix} 1 & 0 & 1 \\ 0 & 1 & 0 \\ 0 & 0 & 1 \end{pmatrix} \right\}$$

forms a system of generators of Γ_n for $n \in \mathbb{Z}$. As non-split central group extensions of $\mathbb{Z}^2$ by $\mathbb{Z}$, they give rise to the stroboscopic lattice $\mathbb{Z} \oplus \mathbb{Z}$ of the Kepplerian configuration and to the ultrafast EPI acquisition technique:

- For all $n \in \mathbb{Z}$, the subgroup Γ_n of the discrete Heisenberg group $\Gamma \hookrightarrow G$ forms the stabilizer of the integral linear form L_n and therefore gives rise to the Kepplerian synchronization procedure of circular grating arrays of synchronously tuned traces of Heisenberg helices.

From the theory of pseudodifferential operators ([157], [230]) it is known that the Weyl symbol mapping

$$\sigma : S'_{\mathbb{C}}(\mathbb{R} \oplus \mathbb{R}) \to S'_{\mathbb{C}}(\mathbb{R} \oplus \mathbb{R})$$

defines a vector space isomorphism. The symplectic distributional Fourier transform isomorphism

$$\widehat{} : S'_{\mathbb{C}}(\mathbb{R} \oplus \mathbb{R}) \to S'_{\mathbb{C}}(\mathbb{R} \oplus \mathbb{R})$$

associated with the symplectic form $[\,\cdot\,,\cdot\,]$ of the Lie algebra $\mathrm{Lie}(G)$ is the transpose of the symplectic Fourier transform

$$\widehat{} : S_{\mathbb{C}}(\mathbb{R} \oplus \mathbb{R}) \to S_{\mathbb{C}}(\mathbb{R} \oplus \mathbb{R}),$$

which is defined by replacing the canonical bilinear form of the standard two-dimensional Fourier transform isomorphism $\mathcal{F}_{\mathbb{R} \oplus \mathbb{R}}$ by the symplectic form $\frac{1}{2}[\,\cdot\,,\cdot\,]$ on $\mathrm{Lie}(G)/\mathbb{R}I$. Explicitly, $\widehat{K}$ is given by

$$\widehat{K}(x, y) = \iint_{\mathbb{R} \oplus \mathbb{R}} K(x', y') \exp\left[\pi i \det\begin{pmatrix} x & y \\ x' & y' \end{pmatrix} \right] dx'\, dy'$$

for $K \in S_{\mathbb{C}}(\mathbb{R} \oplus \mathbb{R})$ and $(x, y) \in \mathbb{R} \oplus \mathbb{R}$.

An application of $\widehat{}$ to the symplectic manifold $(\mathcal{O}_1, \omega_1)$ yields the relaxation weighted spin isochromat density $f(\cdot, \cdot; 1)$ of the selectively excited planar tomographic slice of frequency $\nu = (1/2\pi)\dot{\vartheta} = 1$ by the coherent wavelet filter bank reconstruction formula

$$f(x, y; 1) = \tfrac{1}{2} e^{\pi i x y}\, \sigma(\widehat{K_f})\left(\tfrac{1}{2}x, \tfrac{1}{2}y; 1\right) \qquad [(x, y) \in \mathbb{R} \oplus \mathbb{R}]$$

with respect to the gauge of a cross section in the linear gradient bundle sitting over $\mathbf{P}(\mathbb{R} \times \mathcal{O}_1)$. Thus the symplectic Fourier transform isomorphism $\widehat{}$ inverts the composition $\sigma \circ K_1$ of the Weyl symbol isomorphism σ with the resonance

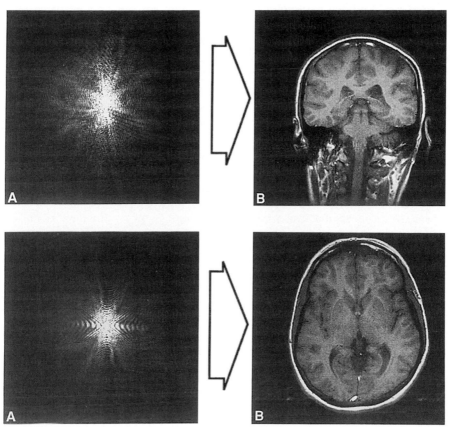

Figure 26. The transition from the raw data to the final MRI scan: Read-out A $\Longrightarrow$ B of quantum holograms via the symplectic Fourier transform algorithm. The symplectic structure of the quantum hologram can be recognized. Note that the symplectic structure of the planar coadjoint orbits of the Heisenberg Lie group G gives rise to the symplectic Fourier transform.

isomorphism K_1 and provides the adaptive filtering detection process of the Fourier MRI experiment (Figure 26).

It has been emphasized that clinical MRI is an intrinsically three-dimensional imaging modality which allows the visualization of nonplanar structures. Various clinical imaging examinations require information to be obtained from voxels than from pixels of a single plane. Particular important examples are the treatment planning and the stereotactic localization by three-dimensional MRI ([1]). Another example that is becoming progressively more important is the macrovascular imaging technique of magnetic resonance angiography (MRA). In recent etiological studies of patients with essential hypertension, for instance, MRA suggested a link between hypertension and pulsatile arterial compression of the ventrolateral medulla oblongata just below the pontomedullary junction acquired by a transaxial craniocerebral MRI scan. During the past few years, the scope of magnetic resonance angiography has progressed beyond the head and neck, such that now virtually every sizeable blood vessel of the body is accessible to macrovascular and microvascular studies. The lower biological risk associated with MRA makes it an increasingly attractive alternative to digital subtraction angiography (DSA) because DSA for the evaluation of the intracranial vasculature does carry the risks of vascular damage, systemic reactions, transient neurological deficits, and permanent neurological compromise. Moreover, DSA is relatively insensitive to the parenchymal sequelae of cerebrovascular pathology. Another alternative, the ultrasound imaging modality, cannot provide an anatomic vascular display or direct visualization of the brain parenchyma. The growth and effectiveness of clinical MRI as a vascular imaging modality can be attributed to its noninvasiveness, high flow sensitivity, multiparametric nature, and capability to evaluate the brain parenchyma directly. This evaluation can be done without repositioning the patient or significantly prolonging the examination time. Because MRA images that rival conventional angiograms are now routinely obtained, it is likely that in the near future magnetic resonance angiography will become a standard in the repertoire of noninvasive vascular radiologic examinations ([281]) and carotid bifurcation imaging.

For instance, the phase-contrast-based macrovascular magnetic resonance angiography modality relies on velocity-induced phase shifts in the presence of magnetic field gradients to distinguish blood and CSF flow from surrounding stationary tissues. The filtering measurement of the phase shift induced by flow in the transverse component of magnetization when a bipolar magnetic field gradient is applied to encode the spin velocity is performed in terms of the Liouville measure ([9]) associated with the selectively excited planar tomographic slice $\mathbf{P}\big(\mathbb{R} \times \mathcal{O}_\nu\big) \hookrightarrow \mathbf{P}(\mathbb{R} \times \mathrm{Lie}(G)^\star)$ $(\nu \neq 0)$.

Inversion of the polarity of the bipolar flow encoding gradients to receive an intravascular excitation–response signal from moving fluid by an interleaved gradient field echo sequence needs a second image acquisition. Stationary spin has zero phase shift for each polarity of the flow encoding pulse, resulting in a zero net phase shift. Thus phase contrast magnetic resonance angiography effectively subtracts out the stationary tissues leaving only the vessels and the aquaeductus cerebri, respectively, during cardiac cycle ([281]). In practice, the method actually requires three raw datasets for three-dimensional Fourier imaging acquisition of three flow encoding directions so that the total flow volume angiogram can be viewed by paging through tomographic planar slices. The method allows for direct visualization of small and complex vessels, too.

Besides phase contrast, the time-of-flight techniques of macrovascular magnetic resonance angiography which are based on motion relative to RF pulses have been applied to the intracranial vasculature (Figure 27). The time-of-flight modalities benefit from the rapid flow in the intracranial circulation to provide macrovascular contrast as opposed to subtraction in phase contrast and therefore have relatively short acquisition times T_A. The time-of-flight techniques require only a single data set, thereby avoiding the potential problems induced by eddy currents and patient motion seen with longer examinations requiring multiple image acquisitions. Time-of-flight techniques require less postprocessing and can be designed to minimize intravoxel

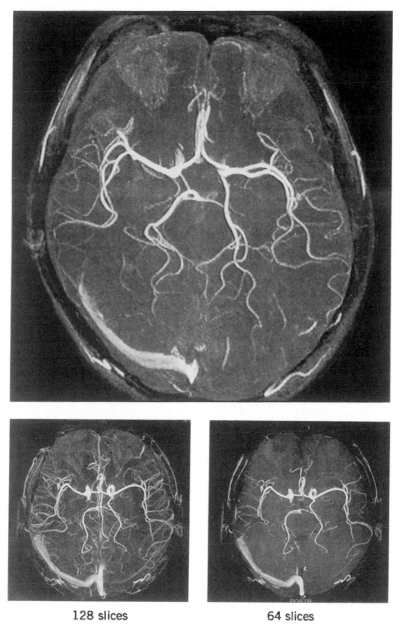

128 slices   64 slices

Figure 27. Magnetic resonance angiography of the cerebral vasculature based on the time of flight technique. The selection of 128 tomographic slices makes it possible to noninvasively depict small blood vessels. Magnetic resonance angiography is required to confirm the diagnosis in certain inoperative cerebrovascular conditions such as vertebrobasilar occlusion or dural venous sinus occlusion.

phase dispersion, which is especially problematic in the carotid siphon, bifurcation of the arteria carotis interna, horizontal arteria cerebri media, and the region of stenoses or aneurysms. Volume time-of-flight techniques allow for the use of small voxels, motion refocusing gradients for first-order flow compensation in the frequency twist and slice select directions, and short echo times T_E to reduce phase dispersion induced by motion. Small vessels with slow flow are more reliably visualized by administering an intravenous bolus injection of an exogenous paramagnetic contrast enhancing agent or by phase contrast methods.

Due to the Cavalieri principle, volume image acquisition is conceptually not far removed from planar Fourier MRI (Figure 28).

From the preceding character formula which links the Fourier transforms of the longitudinal and transversal directions, respectively, the functional self-organization by resonance of the unitary dual $\hat{G}$ of G can be recognized again. It forms the mathematical expression of the fundamental Lauterbur $\tau o \zeta \epsilon \nu \gamma \mu \alpha$ link mentioned previously.

In the planar image acquisition of conventional pulsed Fourier MRI, the RF excitation pulse and gradient pulse are turned on at the same time to coherently excite an individual tomographic planar slice of a specific thickness—the spin isochromat, where the pulse is the same as the Larmor resonance frequency $\nu = (1/2\pi)\dot{\vartheta}$ of synchronized spin precession. In the volume technique of pulsed Fourier MRI, however, RF excitation occurs for an entire volumetric data scan at the same time. The spin slice-select longitudinal linear magnetic field gradient along the axis C of the external magnetic flux density is computer controlled in such a way that a

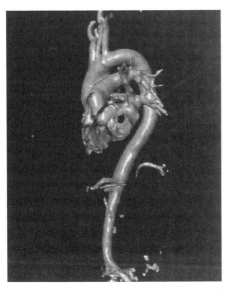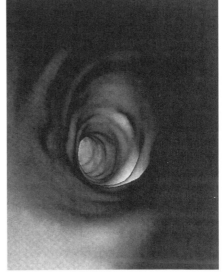

Figure 28. Three-dimensional macrovascular MRI studies: The angiograms visualize the thoraco-abdominal aorta originating from the left ventriculus cordis, and the interior of the aorta descendens. Both angiograms are based on the volumne image acquisition technique.

greater planar slab of tissue will match the on resonance condition and therefore be excited by the slab selective pulse. Spatial encoding of differential phase and local frequency occur just as they do in conventional pulsed Fourier MRI. To achieve slab-select encoding, a stepped local magnetic linear gradient must increment in the third spatial direction similar to the stepping procedure of differential phase encoding. The number of spin slice encodings performed during the clinical MRI scan determines the number of noninteractive tomographic planar slices obained from the planar slab. The amplitude of the slice encoding will determine the thickness of the slices that will ultimately be reconstructed. The reconstruction of the relaxation-weighted spin isochromat density f of the excited planar slab is performed by a three-dimensional inverse Fourier transform of the volumetric data scan

$$(x, y, z) \rightsquigarrow K_f(x, y; z)$$

with respect to the Lebesgue measure

$$\omega_\nu \wedge \frac{1}{\nu} \omega_\nu^\perp \qquad (\nu \neq 0)$$

of longitudinally dilated logarithmic part. As a consequence, the tracial character tr U^ν of the trace class operator U^ν is given by the Mellin transform of the scaled Lebesgue measure $(1/\nu)\,\mathrm{d}z\,(\nu \neq 0)$ concentrated on the center line C. Fourier inversion then provides the Plancherel measure $P_G(\nu)\,\mathrm{d}\nu$ of the Heisenberg group G.

Volumetric visualization is therefore based on voxels which are anisotropic with respect to the longitudinal direction. Volumetric visualization based on isotropic voxels needs additional acquisition time. In view of its increased image acquisition time, volume Fourier MRI is clinically viable only in conjunction with the application of fast scanning pulse sequences with short repetition period T_R. It allows for a three-dimensional visualization of the brain surface morphology, the CSF distribution, and the shape of ventricles within about 1 min. Infected lesions generating an NMR filter response intensity similar to CSF can be visualized in this way.

New excitation pulse sequences called FASTER (field echo acquisition with a short T_R and echo reduction) and FATS (fast adiabatic trajectory in a steady state) have been succesfully applied to three-dimensional imaging of the musculoskeletal system ([141]). Steady state free precession (SSFP) volume image acquisition allows for the investigation of the structures of the inner ear. Specifically, this clinical MRI modality permits visualization of aqueous components of the cochlea and ductus semicirculares of auris interna. In coronal neuroimaging of the brain, the cochlea stand out as bright objects against the dark background of invisible compact bone in the petrous region.

Although the ultrafast high speed imaging technique EPI represents a great stride forward in MRI, there are still problems when imaging a moving object in a single tomographic slice. This is particularly the case for thoracic imaging of the beating heart. During a cardiac cycle there is considerable movement in and out of the tomographic slice which cannot be followed in a single plane movie. The third axis motion is exacerbated by respiratory motion. Echo-volumar imaging (EVI) overcomes the motional problems by forming a set of nested EPI experiments where any two axes form the basis of a single planar experiment. Because the technical problems are greater and the hardware requirements are more stringent for EVI than for EPI ([142], [218]), the EVI modality is still in its infancy. Nevertheless, snapshot EVI images obtained from the thorax are already superior to clinical Doppler echocardiography ([235]).

3

APPLICATIONS AND SYNOPSIS

The contribution MRI *has made to musculoskeletal radiology is phenomenal and can be best exemplified in the knee joint.*

—Phoebe A. Kaplan (1993)

It is ironic that when MRI *was initially introduced, it was believed that it would not play a major role in the evaluation of disorders of the musculoskeletal system.*

—Peter L. Munk and A. Dale Vellet (1993)

Old habits are broken slowly and reluctantly, but we have become convinced that for nearly every indication, MRI *of the knee should replace conventional arthrography. . . . In our experience,* MRI *is as accurate as arthrography for evaluation of the menisci and more so for the extrasynovial cruciate and collateral ligaments and extensor mechanism. The fact that it is noninvasive (without the risks of arthrography or arthroscopy) and painless is important to both the arthrographer (especially in the acute situation) and to the patient (in* every *situation).*

—Jerrold H. Mink (1993)

Early MRI *in young athletes with knee pain after trauma leads to both the least expensive and most efficacious treatment path using a decision tree analysis.*

—John V. Crues, III (1995)

Please excuse the Latin, mon ami.

—Robert I. Grossman (1994)

3.1 TOMOGRAPHIC MORPHOLOGY: MRI OF THE ARTICULATIO GENUS

The articulatio genus is the largest and most complex joint in the human body. It is an extremely efficient joint allowing remarkable motion limited primarily to a single plane. The human knee accomplishes this by using an intrinsically unstable design, with a curved surface, the femoral condyles, resting on a flat surface, the tibial plateaus. Due to its complex design, the knee joint has initiated among the human joints more research from the medical, biomechanical, as well as kinematical point of view than any other large joint. The complexity of the motions performed by the normal articulatio genus, which are controlled flexions ($\geq$ 140°), minimal hyperextensions, and small rotations, prevents a full understanding of the differential geometry of the knee joint and the kinematics of its simultaneously rolling and gliding motions over the surfaces of the tibial plateaus. Therefore, the articulatio genus is a highly interesting joint from the mathematical and biophysical point of view. In view of the intellectual and clinical impact of MRI of the joints, in this text the soft tissue morphology *in vivo* and the pathology of the articulatio genus serve as an example of an application of Fourier MRI and the semantic association of its planar tomographic images acquired in transaxial, coronal, sagittal, or parasagittal slices.

In most modern medical centers, knee joint examinations have become the most common nonneurologic application of clinical MRI. Today MRI is indispensable in the work-up of patients with knee disorders. Although the articulatio genus is the joint most imaged by MRI, it should be observed that a single optimal technique for evaluating all potential knee problems has not been designed. In obtaining high quality clinical Fourier MRI scans, the experience of the imager when designing and assessing a radiodiagnostic study plays an important role in choosing a correct pulse sequence, in selectively exciting appropriate planar tomographic slices $\mathbf{P}\left(\mathbb{R} \times \mathcal{O}_\nu\right) \hookrightarrow \mathbf{P}\left(\mathbb{R} \times \mathrm{Lie}(G)^\star\right)$ ($\nu \neq 0$), and in administering an intravenous bolus injection of a suitable exogenous paramagnetic contrast enhancing agent ([95]).

As the knee joint moves from a flexed position toward extension, the femoral condyles roll on the tibial plateau and simultaneously glide anteriorly at the same rate, changing the axis of the joint through the midpoint of the condyles. Toward the end of the motion, near extension, the condylus lateralis moves slightly anteriorly and medially while the condylus medialis moves posteriorly and medially. The different movements of the medial and lateral femoral condyles generate an external rotation of the tibia relative to the femur and bring the joint into a stable locked position in extension. The muscles and tendons responsible for the major motions of the knee joint are the musculi flexor, consisting of the musculus biceps femoris, musculus semimembranosus, musculus semitendinosus, musculus sartorius, and musculus gracilis, and the extensor mechanism, consisting of the musculus quadriceps femoris, which is composed of the musculus rectus femoris, musculus vastus lateralis, musculus vastus intermedius, and musculus vastus medialis, and tendons, patella bipartita, and patellar tendon ([239]). Rather than a simple hinge joint, the human knee joint may be more properly thought of as a compound joint formed as a consequence of merging three interrelated articulations: two condylar hinge joints between the medial and lateral femoral condyles and their respective tibial plateaus and a third sellar joint gliding at the patellofemoral articulation. The structure of three articulations combined in one large joint is responsible for the pecularities of morphology and complexity of cooperative motions simultaneously performed by the articulatio genus.

The tibial plateaus over which the simultaneous rolling and gliding motions of knee kinematics are performed differ in shape. The medial tibial plateau is slightly concave, which allows for more stable weight transmission, especially in extension. The lateral tibial plateau is flat or slightly convex upward. The stabilizing components of the knee joint serve to limit excessive motion on the medial, lateral, anterior, and posterior aspects of the joint. These structures consist of the medial and lateral ligamenta collateralia, the ligamentum cruciatum genus, the ligamentum transversum genus, menisci, the patellofemoral mechanism, the joint capsule with the ligamentum popliteum arcuatum, and the adjacent muscles. Because the bones of the knee joint have little inherent stability, the stabilizing components of the articulatio genus are critical to normal function of the joint and therefore represent key structures of the knee.

As a result of the advancements in clinical MRI since its initial application in the evaluation of the normal meniscal morphology and meniscal pathology, the past few years have seen a tremendous growth in the use of MRI to diagnose, assess, and treat human knee disorders, including traumatic meniscal and ligamentous injuries, tendon abnormalities, muscle injuries, benign and malignant soft tissue neoplasms, synovial lesions, infection, hemorrhage, intra-articular and periarticular abnormalities, as well as arthritic conditions of the articulatio genus ([1], [79], [99], [141], [233], [249], [329]). Magnetic resonance imaging of the knee joint is clinically valuable because most abnormalities of the articulatio genus involve soft tissue morphology rather than the osseous components of the joint. Routine clinical MRI scans of the knee joint can be performed quickly and accurately utilizing standard spin echo sequences, the majority of radiodiagnostic images being acquired in the transaxial, coronal, or sagittal tomographic planes. They demonstrate normal cross-sectional morphology exquisitely as well as meniscal, ligamentous, and tendon abnormalities with great accuracy (Figure 29). The bone marrow of tibia and femur appears bright, and the bony cortex and medullary cavities are well visualized, as are articular cartilage, synovium genus, menisci, tendons, ligaments, and blood vessels. The condyles, trochlear notch, and undersurface of the patella are covered with hyaline cartilage. Hyaline cartilage

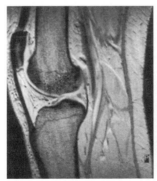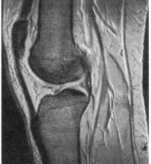

Figure 29. High resolution MRI studies of the articulatio genus visualizing the morphological details of the knee anatomy and the menisci by changing the contrast. The sagittal cross-sections have been acquired under slice selection and read-out gradients of changing polarities. Dedicated MRI scanners at low magnetic flux densities are used to improve the cost effectiveness of clinical knee examinations.

appears intermediate in response intensity on T_1-weighted scans and low in response intensity on T_2-weighted scans.

The synovium is a thin membrane that lines the joint space, excluding the articular cartilage, central portions of fibrocartilaginous menisci, and localized bare areas of the joint. These bare areas refer to the margins of the joint where the synovial membrane attaches to osseous structures covered by periosteum or perichondrium, but not cartilage. Evaluation of the synovium constitues an essential part of joint assessment on MRI examinations. Specifically, clinical MRI allows for direct visualization of synovial disorders. Improved accuracy in detecting the early stages of synovial pathology is an advantage of MRI over conventional examinations which are generally limited to demonstrating the secondary bony changes of more advanced disease.

The normal synovium is virtually imperceptible on MRI studies. The MRI depiction of the synovium as either a focal or a diffuse abnormality typically connotes a pathologic process. Synovial lesions occur with many inflammatory, infectious, neoplastic, degenerative, and idiopathic disorders. Synovial involvement may be primary, or there may be secondary synovial involvement by disease originating in adjacent tissues. The T_1- and T_2-weighted image acquisitions are useful in depicting synovial disorders. The T_1-weighted scans generally provide good morphologic display of the intra-articular morphology and have high sensitivity for detecting associated bone marrow changes such as edema. Synovial thickening due to synovitis is usually of intermediate response intensity on T_1-weighted scans, compared to lower response intensity of adjacent joint effusion. On T_2-weighted image acquisitions, an arthrographic effect occurs when the synovial thickening is of intermediate or low response intensity, outlined by hyperintense joint fluid.

The popliteal artery and vein run together through the posterior aspect of the knee and are easily identified. The arteries supplying the knee joint include the medial and lateral superior genicular arteries and the medial and lateral inferior genicular arteries. The lateral inferior genicular artery runs between the ligamentum collaterale lateralis and the lateral joint capsule. A collateral branch of this vessel is often seen on sagittal MRA scans just anterior to the anterior horn of the meniscus lateralis. The normal joint capsule is a thin structure of low response. When the capsule is thickened or irregular but still of low response, a chronic synovitis should be suspected ([79], [99], [329]).

The medial and lateral menisci of the articulatio genus are innervated dense fibrocartilaginous crescentic lamellae attached directly to the outer border of the tibia adjacent to the eminentia intercondylaria of the tibia. The menisci act to deepen the articular fossae for the femoral condyles, thus helping to stabilize the knee joint during motion.

In clinical MRI examinations, the menisci are usually imaged in sagittal and coronal tomographic slices. Strategies for meniscal protocols have not changed dramatically since the earliest reports on MRI technique in the human knee ([99]). The sagittal views are useful mainly for assessment of the integrity of the posterior and anterior horns of the menisci. On coronal views, two normal structures are often present in association with menisci of the articulatio genus: the meniscofemoral ligaments posteriorly and the transverse meniscal ligament of the knee anteriorly. The meniscofemoral ligament is a collection of fibers arising from the posterior aspect of the lateral meniscus that runs obliquely to insert on the inner surface of the medial femoral condyle. The transverse meniscal ligament is a bundle of fibers that courses horizontally and connects the anterior convex margins of the medial and lateral menisci. Normal menisci medialis and lateralis are formed of fibrocartilage which is a collagen with few mobile protons and therefore display no significant internal response on either T_1- or T_2-weighted scans but may readily be recognized by their shape on sagittal tomographic planes. Although the transaxial cross-sectional morphology of the knee joint was historically best understood, clinical coronal MRI scans should also be examined carefully for supportive evidence of meniscal tears identified on sagittal tomographic planes and to locate displaced meniscal fragments ([172], [329]).

The nervus tibialis is adjacent to the popliteal vessels and is intermediate in response intensity. The nervus peroneus communis may be identified posterolaterally, just posterior to the musculus biceps femoris. Muscle bundles are sharply outlined by surrounding planes of fat and can be distinguished from tendons by virtue of their greater response intensity on spin echo scans. Even though tendons are composed largely of water, the lack of rotational motion of the water molecules held within the triple helix of the protein that forms collagen results in tendons as well as ligaments and menisci that have extremely low response intensity on MRI on all pulse sequences. The ligamentum cruciatum genus and collateral ligaments are well resolved ([266], [329]) so that partial- and complete-thickness tears can be diagnosed. Tears of the posterior cruciate ligament occur from considerable stress on the knee and are often associated with other intra-articular injuries such as detachment of the posterior horn of the medial meniscus, medial and lateral collateral or capsular ligament tears, and avulsion of a fragment of bone from the posterior tibia at the attachment of the posterior cruciate ligament. The MRI appearance of acute posterior cruciate ligament tears is that of focal or diffuse areas of high response intensity in the ligament on T_1- and T_2-weighted scans.

The cruciate ligaments are intra-articular, intracapsular, but extrasynovial structures that perform stabilizing functions. The ligamentum cruciatum anterius and posterius prevent anterior and posterior movement of the tibia relative to the femur. Both cruciate ligaments are located adjacent to one another between the femoral condyles in the intercondylar notch. The ligamentum cruciatum anterius has its femoral attachment on the inner aspect of the condylus femoralis lateralis posteriorly and its tibial attachment into a fossa anterior and lateral to the anterior tibial spine. It is evaluated best with sagittal MRI scans. The ligamentum cruciatum posterius has its femoral attachment on the inner aspect of the condylus femoralis medialis and its tibial attachment on the far posterior aspect of the intercondylar fossa. It is generally visualized on several consecutive sagittal tomographic slices with low response on T_1- and T_2-weighted scans:

- Rupture or partial rupture of the cruciate ligaments, one of the most frequent ligament lesions among the traumatic disorders of the knee, as well as degenerative changes of the condylus femoralis and reconstruction of the ligamentum cruciatum can be visualized by a SSGE technique such as the FISP imaging modality.

The medial tibial and lateral fibular collateral ligaments stabilize the knee joint by preventing hyperextension and varus and valgus angulation of the joint. These ligaments are often partially or completely torn from trauma. There are actually three ligamentous structures that serve to stabilize the lateral knee joint: the lateral capsular ligament, the lateral collateral ligament, and the iliotibial band. The ligament that lies closest to the joint is the lateral capsular ligament. It is attached to the meniscus lateralis. There are two extracapsular ligaments that are entirely separate from the capsule and meniscus of the knee joint: the lateral collateral ligament posteriorly and the iliotibial band anteriorly. The lateral collateral ligament attaches to the posterior aspect of the condylus femoralis lateralis just above the groove for the musculus popliteus proximally, and it turns obliquely in the anteroposterior direction to insert on the head of the fibula along with the tendo biceps femoris distally. The popliteus tendon passes deep to the lateral collateral ligament. The lateral collateral ligament can usually be seen in continuity on a single coronal MRI scan as a low response intensity band extending from the lateral femur to the fibular head with a stripe of fat separating it from the underlying lateral capsular ligament and lateral meniscus. It can routinely be identified on posterior coronal MRI scans in the plane of the fibular head. The iliotibial band is seen on anterior coronal MRI scans as a vertical band of low response intensity extending from the soft tissue of the thigh to the anterolateral tibia just below the articular surface. It also has a small attachment to the proximal aspect of the condylus femoralis lateralis.

Magnetic resonance imaging is the best imaging technique for radiodiagnostic evaluation of internal derangements of the knee and can effectively supplant conventional diagnostic techniques used to evaluate pathologic processes of the knee joint, such as arthrography and arthroscopy. In summary, MRI of the knee has achieved such a high level of acceptance that in many cases orthopedists depend upon it both to determine which patients should undergo arthroscopic surgery and to guide the procedure itself. Only a decade ago, it seemed inconceivable that the MRI modality could be used for diagnosing meniscal tears in the knee. Now, the purpose of MRI of the menisci is almost always to detect tears, which are a very common cause of disability. Damage to ligaments can be diagnosed on MRI by demonstrating abnormal response intensity within or around the ligament, abnormal ligamentous morphology, or complete absence of the ligamentous structure:

- The clinical MRI modality is highly sensitive and accurate in radiodiagnosing meniscal tears. Moreover, MRI is unsurpassed in its ability to evaluate soft tissue neoplasms for size and extent and involvement of the joint or surrounding bone, muscles, tendons, ligaments, or neurovascular structures. Therefore, MRI is the noninvasive modality of choice for evaluating knee pathology.

Exclusive use of standard spin echo sequences permits a good general radiodiagnostic study of the knee joint. These sequences allow for accurate detection of pathologic process in the menisci, cruciate and collateral ligaments, bone marrow, articular cartilage, patellar tendon, and the rest of the mechanism performed by the musculus quadriceps femoris. Ischemic bone lesions, including medullary bone infarction, spontaneous femoral osteonecrosis, idiopathic or primary osteonecrosis of the tibia, medullary avascular necrosis, osteochondritis dissecans, and the osteochondroses, can be precisely evaluated as to their anatomic locations and relationship to overlying cartilage. Osteochondritis dissecans, the most common location of which is the lateral aspect of the condylus femoralis medialis, may be diagnosed and staged. Indeed, on clinical MRI scans, the focus of osteochondritis shows low response intensity on T_1- and T_2-weighted scans even prior to detection on conventional radiographs. Presence of subchondral fractures and bone contusions which are frequently associated with ligament and meniscal injuries can be diagnosed and followed. Stress fractures are visualized on T_1- and T_2-weighted scans as a linear area of low response intensity. The changes of osteoarthritis, including cartilage abnormalities, and meniscal cyst formation can be evaluated. Diffuse bone marrow disorders including hemoglobinopathies and neoplasia of the articulatio genus are well demonstrated by the use of clinical MRI techniques.

A multitude of differing malignant soft tissue neoplasms occur about the knee joint. However, the most frequent include malignant fibrous histiocytoma, liposarcoma, and synovial cell sarcoma. In addition, the most common location of primary osseous malignancies is in the distal femur and proximal tibia. These osseous neoplasms often have associated soft tissue masses. As opposed to benign soft tissue masses, MRI protocol parameters are usually nonspecific in terms of histologic diagnosis for malignant neoplasms. Typically, these lesions are isotense to muscle on T_2-weighted scans and hyperintense on scans of long repetition period T_R. Magnetic resonance imaging is also used after chemotherapy and radiation therapy to evaluate change of tumor size, extent, and image protocol parameters in response to these agents, immediately prior to surgical intervention. Decrease in tumor size and extent as well as decreased intensity on short T_R scans and increased intensity within the neoplasm on long T_R images suggests a response to therapy with edema and necrosis. After surgical resection and reconstruction clinical MRI is important to detect early recurrence, guide intervention, and evaluate for complications. Areas of edema seen as irregular and nonlocalized regions of hyperintensity on long T_R scans are usually present, resulting from surgery and radiation therapy. After intravenous administration of a paramagnetic contrast enhancing agent such as Gd–DTPA (gadolinium diethylenetriaminepentaacetic acid) dimeglumine (Magnevist), T_1-weighted scans of the articulatio genus are helpful in distinguishing vascularized tissue like neoplasm, including recurrence, inflammation, granulation tissue, or myxoid tumor component, from nonvascular components such as haemorrhage, necrosis, seroma, lymphocele, or abscess, both before and after therapy and surgery.

Clinical MRI of the knee has developed into one of the most frequently requested examinations in radiology, and MRI of the ankle and foot has become a widely used technique of radiodiagnosis and assessment ([26]). The clinical MRI scans may suffer from the magic angle spinning artifact. In this effect, an increased response intensity may be seen in normal tendons oriented obliquely with respect to the main magnetic field, an effect that is greatest when this orientation is at

$$\theta^{(2)} = \arccos \frac{1}{\sqrt{3}} = 55°$$

to that of the magnetic field ([363]). The magic angle spinning effect is greater when the MRI examination employs spin echo techniques with short echo times or gradient echo techniques. The tibialis posterior tendon, which is the largest and most anteriorly situated of the three main tendons on the medial aspect of the ankle, approximates the magic angle orientation at its site of attachment to the navicular bone, resulting in a normal appearance of increased heterogeneous response intensity in this area. Repeating the MRI examination with a foot in plantar flexion will diminish or eliminate the magic angle spinning artifact and allow the distal aspect of the tendons to be imaged optimally in cross section.

The use of clinical MRI in the evaluation of the shoulder is less widely utilized. Standard radiographic techniques demonstrate the osseous structure of the shoulder girdle but provide only limited evaluation of soft tissue morphology, including the rotator cuff, the ligamentous attachments of the glenoid labrum capsule, and the subacromial space. Conventional radiographs do not allow for direct visualization of the rotator cuff tendons, their defects and abnormalities, and their relationship to the undersurface of the acromion and the articulatio acromioclavicularis. As a result, impingement disorders are difficult to characterize on radiographic studies. Thus the complexity of morphology *in vivo*, function, and pathologic mechanism of disease in the shoulder joint pose a formidable challenge. In spite of these challenges, current evidence strongly suggests that the MRI modality possesses a unique ability to evaluate shoulder injuries, which may lead to improvements in patient care. Specifically MRI of the rotator cuff provides direct coronal oblique tomographic images parallel with the course of the supraspinatus tendon as localized on axial planar images. Axial planar images through the glenohumeral joint display capsular and labral morphology. Sagittal oblique planar images demonstrate acromial morphology and display the coracoacromial and coracohumeral ligaments ([239]). In this way, clinical MRI can reveal soft tissue morphology changes which are helpful in evaluating several important shoulder disease processes, including impingement, rotator cuff degeneration and tears, biceps tendon tears and biceps tenosynovitis, labral and capsular tears, and a spectrum of bone diseases, including fractures of the proximal humerus, avascular necrosis of the humeral head, and degenerative osteoarthritis of the glenohumeral joint ([1], [156], [325], [329], [374]). In oblique coronal tomographic slices the magic angle spinning phenomenon may occur in the distal supraspinatus tendon, suggesting a rotator cuff tear. The disappearance of the spinning artifact can be achieved by choosing different relaxation weights.

Selection is the very keel on which our mental ship is built.

—William James (1890)

Als spätester Erwerb in der Phylogenese ist die Hirnrinde praktisch allen Funktionssystemen des Gehirns als oberste Kontrollschleife überlagert und wird mit wachsender Ausschließlichkeit zur wesentlichen Bedingung dieser Funktion.

—Otto D. Creutzfeldt (1983)

Guiding principles offered for further improvements are: Analysis methods for neural data will extract more significant results, the better they mimic signal-processing strategies of the brain; neural network models adapted to the neural structures recorded from, therefore, might be powerful analysis instruments of neural multiple-channel data.

—Reinhard Eckhorn (1991)

The pattern of synchrony is never twice the same.

—Charles M. Gray (1992)

It works well: The patient moves his fingers and you see where the motor strip is. . . . The MRI camera is now much faster than the brain's hemodynamic response time. This hemodynamic latency sets the utimate limit.

—Jack W. Belliveau (1993)

The normal human brain appears to resort to anaerobic metabolism to supply the energy needed for the transient increases in neuronal activity. As a result, the amount of oxygen present in blood in the area of brain activation actually increases—a simple matter of supply exceeding demand . . . The implications for functional brain imaging with MRI are immense.

—Michael I. Posner and Marcus E. Raichle (1994)

It is important to scan the brain, particularly before the patient encounters a knife-wielding surgeon interested in making the "definitive diagnosis."

—Robert I. Grossman (1994)

3.2   *IN VIVO* DYNAMICAL MRI VISUALIZATION: THE HUMAN BRAIN FUNCTION

During the last century, neuroscience has made evident that sensory, motor, and cognitive functions can be topographically mapped to localized neuroanatomical areas of the human brain. Early neurofunctional localization was often based upon changes in function following localized brain lesions. Because cerebral lesions rarely selectively damage a specific neuroanatomical area like the lobus insularis, which in clinical transaxial MRI scans lies behind the sulcus lateralis separating the lobi temporalis and frontalis, the brain atlases used by neurosurgeons in the planning of procedures were necessarily incomplete. Therefore the imaging data of standard atlas brains have been extended by neurobiological experiments in which electrophysiological stimulation of localized neuroanatomical brain regions elicited movements, sensations, or even complex cognitive functions such as language comprehension or memory ([57]).

Until recently, the area of research of visualization of the topographic distribution of sensory responses was the domain of invasive single- and multi-unit intracerebral neurophysiological recordings with fiber microelectrodes, including digital filter processing and positron emission tomography (PET) scans. A different approach to neurofunctional topographic imaging of cognitive processing is provided by the highly sensitive multichannel superconducting quantum interference device (SQUID) imaging ([40], [103], [113]), which by contactless measurements exclusively records the event-related changes of the frequency spectrum occurring in the spectral decomposition in the magnetoencephalogram (MEG). In computer simulations, the MEG data have been cross-correlated to the corresponding electroencephalogram (EEG) data ([7]). As a result, the coupling between electrophysiological cerebral activity, metabolism, and spatially localized cerebral blood flow at the microvascular level became of particular interest.

Before the advent of modern brain imaging techniques, direct evidence had been provided that the blood flow in a specific sensory system such as the visual system changed during mental activity such as reading. Based on this observation, recent radiolabel measurements, particularly PET studies of regional cerebral blood flow and metabolism, have provided new insights into the topographic mapping of human brain functional activity. To date, magnetic resonance angiography actually has been performed more often in the cerebrovascular system than in the rest of the human body ([5], [39], [97], [272]). Although the importance of macrovascular imaging is considerable witness the current activity in magnetic resonance angiography visualization research; the mechanism by which the brain regulates and meets its needs for metabolic substrates operates at a microvascular level. Imaging techniques that can visualize, directly or indirectly, regional tissue blood flow, regional tissue microvascular volume, and local oxygen changes with high spatial resolution therefore offer important information about brain function in both normal and pathophysiological states characterized by altered metabolic needs. These include the study of brain activation during cognitive processing and the response of brain tissue to cerebrovascular or neoplastic disease. The visualization of brain function, its reaction to external cognitive stimuli, the perception and temporal encoding of sensory information, cognitive processes, the preparation for motor behavior, and the computer simulations of these neural network activities have always been of great interest both to clinical as well as cognitive neuroscience research.

Along the microvascular line of research, a very recent application of clinical MRI which is important from the temporally encoded synchronized neural network point of view has been to microvascular neurofunctional topographic imaging of cognitive processing to ascertain which neuroanatomically distinct processing areas of the human brain are engaged by place encoding in specific perceptual and motor activities of the neocortex:

- The nonlinear, nondeterministic, dynamical state vector reduction of quantum physics applied to the family of quantum holograms $\left(\mathcal{H}_1\left(h_n, h_n; \cdot, \cdot\right)\right)_{n \geq 0}$ provides the probability that the transient cluster of synchronized dynamical connections given by the associated sequence of complete bichromatic graphs $(\Gamma_{n,n})_{n\geq 0}$ of sandwhich symmetry will be observed.

From the neuroanatomical point of view, the retina forms an outpost of the cortex cerebralis so that studies of visual processing offer a direct way of forming images of the brain. In particular, vision is a good point of entry for many forms of higher mental activity, such as pattern recognition, the construction of mental images in the complete absence of outside sensory stimuli, and the semantic interpretation of symbols ([90]). The founder of the Cartesian dualism, René Descartes, who started the separation of the world into the physical and mental one, concluded in 1632 from his studies of visual imagery and the associated circuits connecting light receptors in the retina to muscles that the corpus pineale, which is situated adjacent to the thalamus as indicated by clinical transaxial MRI scans, should be the center of consciousness. The thalamus is located just above the colliculus cranialis superior, a major structure of the mesencephalon as seen in midline sagittal MRI scans, which plays a role in visual attention. In this century the neuropathologist Franz Nissl found that the key to understanding the cortex actually is in the thalamus ([57]). As a consequence, the visual cortex has been the subject of particularly intense neurophysiological, neuropharmacological, histological, and cognitive functional activity studies, although other sensory regions of the neocortex and the hippocampus ([226]) within the limbic system between the truncus encephali and the neocortex have been extensively explored. Even complex cognitive functions of the cortical lobus frontalis are being identified and localized.

In the current studies of visual imagery, the percept is assumed to be the result of photons impinging upon the retina, which sends stimuli that are further processed in the brain. During visual task performance with verbal response, various different neocortical regions of the telencephalon and subcortical structures of the thalamo-cortical system of the diencephalon take part in a complex interactive process which manifests in local metabolic and magnetic flux density changes. Visual information processing, therefore, involves not only areas in the primary visual cortex along the sulcus calcerinus along the midline of the lobus occipitalis as displayed by neurofunctional MRI data ([201]) superimposed on craniocerebral MRI scans but also extrastriate structures in the regions of the lobus parietalis, lobus temporalis, and lobus frontalis of the cerebral hemispheres (Figure 30).

The cerebral hemispheres are divided by the interhemispheric fissura longitudinalis cerebri. The lateral Sylvian fissure separates the lobus temporalis from the lobus frontalis and lobus parietalis, while the central Rolandic fissure which contains the primary motor area is bounded anteriorly by the sulcus precentralis. It is constantly identified on surface reconstruction images while the other gyri of the lobus frontalis display considerable individual variations. The superior and middle frontal gyri are best visualized on superior views of the cerebral hemispheres. The inferior gyrus frontalis, which in the dominant hemisphere contains Broca's motor speech center, is located basally and is separated from the lobus temporalis by the Sylvian fissure. The convexity of the lobus parietalis comprises the gyrus postcentralis and the superior and inferior parietal gyri. The gyrus postcentralis is located between the sulcus

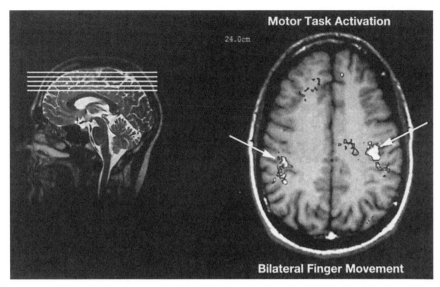

Figure 30. Neurofunctional MRI study to chart cortical areas via microvascular imaging: Motor task activation by bilateral finger movement.

centralis and postcentralis and contains the primary somatosensory region. The gyrus supramarginalis, which is located at the end of the Sylvian fissure, and the gyrus angularis are part of the inferior lobus parietalis and, in the dominant hemisphere, contain centers for selective speech function, reading, writing, calculating, and body orientation. The lateral convexity of the lobus temporalis is divided by the superior and middle sulci temporalis into the superior, middle, and inferior gyri temporalis. In the dominant hemisphere, the posterior third of the superior gyrus temporalis contains Wernicke's area, which controls comprehension of language. The lateral surface of the lobus occipitalis with the lateral gyri occipitalis contains centers for visual associative function ([24]). The scanning of visual images involves the parietal lobe, the lateral areas of the left posterior hemisphere are involved in registering the parts of an image, and the pulvinar area of the thalamus appears to be a way station used by attention to gain access to extrastriate cerebral areas.

At the interface between the human visual and language systems is the study of visual stimuli generated by passively presented word registration. The visual stimuli produce microvascular blood flow responses in multiple visual areas localized in neuroanatomical areas outside the primary visual cortex on both sides of the brain, and the mental task of giving a semantic interpretation to the visual words generates responses outside the primary visual cortex in neuroanatomical areas located along the lateral inner surface of the left hemispherium cerebralis posterior as seen in clinical transaxial MRI scans. Similar to the extrastriate area on the inner surface of the left hemisphere for visual words is Wernicke's area for auditory words ([57]). As displayed by clinical sagittal MRI scans, the Wernicke area is located anterior to the gyrus angularis where the lobi temporalis and parietalis of the left hemisphere meet.

Following the lead of Pierre Paul Broca and Carl Wernicke, language has the longest history of study within neuroscience of any cognitive system. What the neurofunctional MRI technique superimposed on craniocerebral MRI scans contributes to these studies is an exquisite picture of how a novel use of a word produces activation in the left lobus cerebralis frontalis, gyrus cinguli anterior, left lobus temporalis posterior, and right cerebellum. The verbal response involves the speech centers in the left hemispherium cerebralis, the aforementioned Wernicke sensory speech area in the left posterior temporal lobe and Broca's motor speech area of the left frontal cortex, as well as premotor, supplementary motor, and motor areas of the cerebral cortex. Note that the emergence of Broca's and Wernicke's areas was the key evolutionary step in providing the means for production and recognition of speech sounds ([78]). Subcortical structures in the nucleus caudatus and putamen of the telencephalon and in the globus pallidus and ventral thalamus of the diencephalon seen in transaxial craniocerebral MRI scans also participate, by place encoding, in the process of word perception, preparing for and executing vocalization, and semantic access ([57]).

Fast measuring techniques of MRI such as the FSE modality and the ultra-fast EPI method have demonstrated that microvascular neurofunctional topographic imaging of brain perfusion is also possible with clinical MRI. The basic mechanism behind microvascular neurofunctional MRI is that during thought processes, areas of the brain of heightened neuronal activity performing the stimulus-evoked synchronized response association increase the regional cerebral blood volume and blood flow to them. Magnetic resonance imaging allows for the measurement of cerebral blood flow by selective inversion of the proton spins ([193]). Due to the anaerobic glucose metabolism of the normal human brain, firing neurons consume no more oxygen than when they are not active. Thus the increased neuronal activity corresponds to an increase in blood volume and flow without a proportional increase in oxygen consumption. The additional regional cerebral blood volume flowing to the brain without a concomitant increase in oxygen consumption leads to a heightened concentration of oxygen in the venulae draining the firing neural assemblies. Thus the blood oxygen level has increased but the demand has not. Relative to the diamagnetic oxyhemoglobin (HbO_2), the deoxygenated hemoglobin (Hb), which becomes paramagnetic when oxygen dissociates from the hemoglobin molecule due to the ferrous iron in the Hb heme center, decreases in the concentration in tissue ([256]–[259]). Based on the discovery by Linus C. Pauling in 1935 that the amount of oxygen carried by hemoglobin intrinsically affects the magnetic properties of hemoglobin, similar to Gd–DTPA dimeglumine or dysprosium chelates but on a smaller scale, it has been found that Fourier MRI is able to topographically map the local changes from diamagnetic HbO_2 to paramagnetic Hb in the homogeneity of magnetic flux density endogenously produced with the very high spatial resolution of $0.6 \, mm^2$. This extremely elegant technique is known as blood oxygen level dependence (BOLD) neurofunctional imaging ([200], [261], [341]). Microvascular neurofunctional MRI studies are still hampered by physiological motion such as cardiac pulsation and respiration, which can lead to artifactual changes ([146]) and false activation. However, a navigator echo acquired before turning on the phase encoding and read-out gradients implementing a local laboratory coordinate frame inside a selectively excited planar tomographic slice $\mathbf{P}\left(\mathbb{R} \times \mathcal{O}_\nu\right) \hookrightarrow \mathbf{P}\left(\mathbb{R} \times \mathrm{Lie}(G)^\star\right)$ ($\nu \neq 0$) allows for the correction of the local differential phase of the subsequently acquired phase holograms. This makes BOLD a reliable dynamical imaging modality when compared against the standard of the brain pathways activated during passive visual perception:

- The bulk magnetic susceptibility difference between the microvessels and adjacent tissue caused by Hb within capillaries and venulae creates a net intravoxel dephasing of spin packets. With increased neuronal activity, a decrease in the Hb concentration reduces the intravoxel spin packet dephasing. In the BOLD modality, the shift of the local differential phase variable encoded by the clinical MRI scanner in the quantum hologram inside the selectively excited planar tomographic slice $\mathbf{P}\left(\mathbb{R} \times \mathcal{O}_\nu\right) \hookrightarrow \mathbf{P}\left(\mathbb{R} \times \mathrm{Lie}(G)^\star\right)$ ($\nu \neq 0$) detects the intravoxel spin packet dephasing.

The main advantage of the MRI modality over X-ray CT is also of importance in the field of microvascular neurofunctional MRI:

- By choosing suitable tomographic planes, transaxial, coronal, sagittal, or parasagittal, BOLD allows for also scanning the subcortical and phylogenetically older structures of the brain with equal spatial resolution and sensitivity to generate topographical maps by microvascular blood flow responses and create a mental image in the complete absence of any sensory stimulation. The mental operations involved in creating mental imagery during cognitive task performance are carried out in localized neuroanatomical areas of the brain, but different mental operations may be carried out in widely different brain areas.

Thus the procedure in dynamical neuroimaging based on inherent contrast agents reads

$$\text{Tomographic imaging} \implies \text{topographic mapping}.$$

Unfortunately the spatial resolution of microvascular neurofunctional MRI does not necessarily represent the spatial resolution for depicting the increased electrophysiological activation evoked by the sensory stimulus or cognitive processing, because the presence of large blood vessels can effectively degrade the spatial resolution in topographically mapping the microvasculature of the cerebrum ([342]). Nevertheless, even though great strides in spatial resolution have been made with MEG, microvascular neurofunctional MRI is superior over neurophysiological microelectrode extra-cellular recording devices, especially in the deeper structures of the brain.

Due to the origin of BOLD, which as stated above is why the hemodynamic and metabolic response of the brain to increased neuronal activity leads to a drop in the Hb content in the capillaries and the venous blood vessels of the activated cortical areas and hence to a detectable reduction of the intravoxel spin packet dephasing, in a way similar to the relation between the location of a neuron in the cortex and its functional properties as established by intracerebral neurophysiological multiple microelectrode recordings and digital filtering, the BOLD modality cannot keep up with the stimulus-evoked interareal synchronization process. After a sensory stimulus or cognitive operation has been turned on or off, changes in regional blood flow and oxygenation are clocked hundreds of milliseconds to several seconds later. The BOLD modality establishes, however, that sensory stimulation and changes in cognitive state produce a signal intensity change in the corresponding primary sensory cortex of the human brain. The hemodynamic properties of tissues, tissue blood flow, tissue microvascular volume, and tissue oxygenation reflect tissue metabolic changes that are initially triggered by a neuronal event. Administration of a bolus intravenous injection of the standard MRI contrast enhancing agent Gd–DTPA dimeglumine can be used as an exogenous paramagnetic tracer for regional cerebral blood volume and regional cerebral blood flow ([25], [95]) in neonates, young infants, children, and adults. Specifically, in clinical MRI scanners of high magnetic flux density, the effect of visual stimulation induces 5 to 20% of changes in signal intensity in regions of the lobus occipitalis ([31]) so that the activated regions detected in the clinical MRI scans are consistent with hemifield lateralization of the visual cortex cerebralis. In a similar way, the application of high resolution EPI sequences while carrying out a finger movement task results in a $4.3 \pm 0.3\%$ increase in signal intensity in localized regions corresponding to the motor cortex cerebralis ([14], [121], [176], [177], [340]).

As a result, for instance, of FLASH studies ([137]) of the motor cortex, left finger motion does not exclusively activate the right hemisphere in the telencephalon, but right finger task performance appears to unilaterally stimulate the left hemispherium cerebralis. More recent microvascular neurofunctional topographic imaging research of cognitive processing has invaded the auditory, speech, and language centers of the cortex cerebralis ([154], [224], [315]).

Dynamical topographic neuroimaging allows for noninvasive mappings of the neuroanatomical regions of the human brain involved in the receptive and expressive aspects of language ([154], [224]). Regions of the left frontal and temporal lobes corresponding in general to the respective locations of Broca's and Wernicke's areas only become active when two tasks are added, namely consciously assessing word meaning and choosing an appropriate response. Neuronal activity in the left inferior frontal lobe of the cortex cerebralis is greater when repeating a word than when merely listening to that word and greatest when the word is generated. In the case of semantic tasks, microvascular neurofunctional MRI studies found that attending amplified activity at several adjacent sites over frontal areas of both the left and right cortical hemispheres. An examination of the brain after training revealed that the practice of generating words completely changes the cerebral functional self-organization. Indeed, the effect of practice over many trials is that the functional activity drops away in the isocortical anterior gyrus cinguli, temporal and lateral frontal cortex, posterior cortex, and right cerebellar hemisphere:

- The temporally encoded synchronized information processing of the nervous system generates the cerebral functional self-organization principle of experience-dependent synaptic plasticity.

These and similar findings confirm earlier PET studies and support the known view that the mental operations involved in creating mental imagery are carried out in localized neuroanatomical areas but that different operations may be carried out in widely different brain areas. They also support the HERA (hemispheric encoding retrieval asymmetry) model of episodic memory to some extent. According to the HERA model, long-term memory primarily takes place in the left cortical hemisphere whereas the retrieval of the memorized information is mainly concentrated to the right cortical hemisphere ([339]). Nevertheless, it is very likely that neurofunctional MRI will soon supplant PET for microvascular neurofunctional topographic imaging due to the superior spatial and temporal resolution, repeatability, and non-invasive nature of neurofunctional MRI. Because clinical MRI avoids the use of radionuclides, the shielded gradient coils necessary for the extremely high temporal resolution afforded by the real-time EPI modality are now available at many clinical MRI centers, and even more importantly, the stimulus-evoked synchronized response association performed by MRI is closer to neurobiological plausibility than the PET scan technique—it is already a highly compelling technology:

- The microvascular neurofunctional MRI modality addresses the human brain *in vivo* on its own temporally encoded operative terms of cerebral functional self-organization. The BOLD technique opens a unique quantum physical window from which to view the cerebral areas and subareas activated by mental events. In this sense, thought and related mental operations of conscious awareness are observed in terms of their quantum physical embodiment in the living cerebrum.

Although microvascular neurofunctional topographic MRI of cognitive processing works only at a tertiary level regarding the neuronal events that are going to be visualized by regional cerebral blood volume and flow and local oxidative metabolism changes, it allows for a novel approach to a study of the human brain's synaptic plasticity ([77], [78]). Extending the effect of practice on the performance of language processing tasks, it provides evidence that temporary synchronization of distributed neural responses is crucial not only for information transmission but also for practice affected synaptic plasticity. Thus the functional role of temporary synchronized responses in experience-dependent synaptic plasticity is the same as that for neuronal assembly coding.

Moreover, microvascular neurofunctional MRI data contribute to the study of the role of the neurotransmitter dopamine (3,4–dihydroxyphenylalanine), including the catecholamines norepinephrine and epinephrine, in the brain of patients with Parkinson's disease and schizophrenia. The neurochemical messenger agent dopamine has its source inside the substantia nigra, as indicated by transaxial MRI scans of the mesencephalon. Notice that in Parkinson patients the nigral dopaminergic neurons are destroyed. Dopamine is distributed to the basal ganglia and to the lobus frontalis cerebri and is particularly important in regulating areas of the frontal lobe ([78]). Patients who were undergoing their first schizophrenic episode were found to have an abnormality in an area of the left globus pallidus, which is one of the structures of the basal ganglia, as seen in transaxial craniocerebral MRI scans, and part of a route for connecting the basal ganglia to the lobus frontalis ([57]). The basal ganglia, which appear to be among the CNS structures that are hemispherically lateralized, mediate the influence of dopamine on the anterior gyrus cinguli, which has anatomical connections to the posterior parietal lobe and to the lateral frontal lobe and controls the regulation of visual spatial attention and the semantic analysis of language. The findings in the neurochemical system of schizophrenics, which modulates mental computations, indicate an abnormal level of dopamine reaching the anterior gyrus cinguli.

The messenger agent norepinephrine is released by the locus coeruleus in the mesencephalon, which has strong connections to the lobus parietalis, the pulvinar area of the thalamus, and the colliculus cranialis superior. The data of neurofunctional MRI studies suggest that an adequate supply of norepinephrine is necessary to maintain arousal and to keep attention focused. The inability to concentrate is one major symptom of schizophrenia which can be considered as a disease of neurobiological consciousness.

Because the brains of individuals differ greatly, the scientific task of topographically mapping brain function and synaptic plasticity increasingly is dependent on individual *in vivo* studies combining MEG, SQUID imaging, and microvascular neurofunctional MRI in order to approach the difficult problem of the relation between the macroscopic quantum states of conscious awareness on the one hand and the functional activity of the cerebrum on the millisecond time scale on the other hand.

It is probably true quite generally that in the history of human thinking the most fruitful developments frequently take place at those points where two different lines of thought meet. Hence, if they actually meet, that is, if they are at least so much related to each other that a real interaction can take place, then one may hope that new and interesting developments may follow.

—Werner Heisenberg (1959)

Mögen sich andere zu ihr stellen, wie sie wollen, ich erachte es ihr gegenüber als meine Pflicht, sie, die ich in meinem Innern als wahr erkannt habe und deren Schönheit mich mit unglaublichem Entzücken erfüllt, auch nach außen hin mit allen Kräften meines Geistes zu verteidigen.

—Johann Keppler (1618)

3.3   RETROSPECT AND CONCLUSIONS

In vivo imaging and visualization in biomedical computing has rapidly emerged as a significant area of research aimed at developing approaches for radiodiagnosis and assessment of living systems and tools for testing cerebral self-organization principles. The final goal of diagnostic imaging procedures is to image the whole human body and its organ systems in a noninvasive way such that either tissue morphology or biomedical functional processes can be localized and quantified *in vivo*.

In 1895 Wilhelm Conrad Röntgen used X-ray for imaging anatomical structures in shadowgrams for the first time. The development of X-ray technology revolutionized biomedical diagnostics. Within the next decades radiologists learned to read out and interpret the overlapping density patterns of shadowgrams generated by clinical X-ray scanners on photographic films or fluorescent screens.

The history of computer-assisted diagnostic imaging started in the early 1970s, when by the concepts of projection–reconstruction and digital image processing X-ray CT was developed and made the internal cross-sectional morphology *in vivo* of the patient visible as a tomographic planar slice without over- and underlying shadows. In the CT modality, the inputs are X-ray pulses and the information being collected is spatially encoded. Unlike X-ray, diffraction filtering measurements of NMR spectroscopy carry both phase and amplitude information about the sample which is time-domain differential phase encoded.

After PET, the second major radiodiagnostic imaging technique to follow X-ray CT was MRI. The first decade of the clinical use of MRI is rapidly approaching. Whereas conventional X-ray CT is essentially a two-dimensional imaging procedure, MRI is intrinsically a three-dimensional imaging modality. The advent of MRI radiodiagnosis appears to have occurred in a startling short time, but what was actually abrupt are the perception by physicians of this technology's impact on the way radiological diagnoses are performed and the maturation of this highly sophisticated noninvasive computer-assisted radiodiagnostic imaging modality. Medical historians will no doubt equate the importance of the invention of clinical MRI at the end of the twentieth century with Röntgen's discovery of X-rays at the end of the nineteenth century, when diagnostic radiology itself was born. Because the evolution of MRI technology has been unprecedented among radiodiagnostic imaging modalities, we will look back at the first research articles and monographs on the topic of clinical MRI and be impressed by how quickly they became outdated in rapid sequence as the field of MRI burgeoned and matured.

The theoretical basis and demonstration of clinical MRI are developments of the late 1940s and, in condensed matter physics, resulted in the 1952 Nobel Prize for physics to Felix Bloch and Edward M. Purcell, a decade after their original findings ([114]). The understanding of the nucleus, which led to the conception of MRI, the discovery of superconductivity, which forms an important component of magnets used for the hardware of clinical MRI scanners, and the electronic work leading to present computer technology were developments incorporated together in the 1960s. Then MRI systems combined these three items for high resolution NMR investigations with ever-improving performance. Switching to experimental results, the fundamental *in vitro* finding by Raymond Damadian in 1971 that the T_1 spin–relaxation time measurements of malignant tumors may differ radically from those of benign soft tissue neoplasms ([61]) predicted the diagnostic value of clinical MRI. Although his suggestion was not widely adopted as a diagnostic method for differentiation of cancer tissue from noncancer tissue because it was an *in vitro* technique requiring a biopsy sample and actually did not improve on standard histopathologic methods of tissue analysis, it helped initiate efforts to distinguish normal from neoplastic states by means of clinical MRI. Nevertheless, until today imaging does not always provide histopathologic diagnosis. In 1981, the increasing clinical interest in clincial MRI grew from the almost simultaneous presentation of diagnostically informative images by the Royal Postgraduate Medical School, Hammersmith Hospital, London, and the University of California, San Francisco. What followed was a veritable explosion of interest in clinical MRI, with clinical centers almost all over the world contributing almost daily to advances in this new diagnostic area. The result is that MRI is now firmly established in the clinical workup of patients in most parts of the world by routine use of MRI whole-body scanners in the range of 0.03 to 2.0 T of magnetic flux density. For clinical MRI scanners, the hardware trend of main magnets is toward lower magnetic flux densities:

- In 1993, only 23% of MRI scanners were high field (1.0 to 2.0 T magnetic flux density) systems with 45% operating at midfield (0.2 to 0.5 T magnetic flux density) and 32% at low field (≤ 0.2 T magnetic flux density). In the future, 1.5-T units, or more ideal 2.5- or 3.0-T scanners, will carry the clinical load.

Actually the trend toward low magnetic flux density MRI units is accelerated not only for routine clinical whole-body examinations but also in the description of microvascular neurofunctional MRI techniques for noninvasive localization of functional brain areas at high spatial resolution during cognitive task performance by conventional clinical MRI scanner equipment and in MRI-assisted neuronavigation supporting minimally invasive brain surgery. Contrary to initial expectation, recent experience in morphological and neurofunctional imaging of the human brain shows that high magnetic flux density MRI/NMR spectroscopy systems at flux density of 4.0 T provide high resolution images with exquisite T_1 contrast, delineating structures especially in the basal ganglia and thalamus which until now were not observed clearly in 1.5-T clinical scans operating at 63 MHz proton frequency ([229], [342]). For microvascular neurofunctional MRI, the high magnetic flux density provides increased contribution from the venulae and the capillary bed because the susceptibility-induced alterations in the transversal spin relaxation rate from these small diameter vessels increase quadratically with the magnetic flux density. However, scans obtained with short echo times T_E at 4 T, and by implication at lower magnetic flux density with correspondingly longer T_E , are expected to be dominated by contributions from large venous vessel or in-flow effects from the large arteries. Such images are undesirable because of their poor spatial correspondence with actual sites of neuronal activity.

The speed with which the biologically safe medical high technology magnetic resonance imagers spread throughout the world was phenomenal. Innumerable innovative techniques have been created. Each development has greatly enhanced the capabilities and utilization of clinical MRI. Recently the development of spiral X-ray CT scanning techniques ([98]), which are based on the Heisenberg helix geodesic of G, has given CT a boost in the race against MRI. X-ray CT and especially spiral X-ray CT imaging are the preferred imaging modalities for pulmonary evaluation. However, unlike ultrasonic imaging or spiral CT or even double-helix X-ray CT, clinical MRI is a far more complex imaging modality demanding a detailed understanding of the soft tissue morphology contrast mechanisms and the multitude of techniques and sophisticated imaging options which are based on macroscopic quantum field phenomena. Because MRI is still at a relatively early stage of evolution, new techniques are developing rapidly in an ever more competitive clinical imaging environment. Among these new techniques, neurofunctional MRI is one of the most exciting applications to neuroscience regarding the visualization of the topographic distribution of sensory responses to local stimulation and cognitive processing. It promises to supplant PET neuroimaging in the near future due to the fact that MRI adresses *in vivo* temporally encoded synchronized neural network organizations of stimulus-evoked synchronized response association on their own temporally encoded operative terms of cerebral functional self-organization in order to create a mental image in the complete absence of any sensory stimulation. As described above, the Fourier MRI experiment consists of three processes ([86], [87]):

- the coherent preparation process of prescanning,
- the quantum holographic heterodyning process, and
- the filtering detection process.

Prescan allows for the adjustment of the transmit and receive gain and the setting of the central frequency $\nu = (1/2\pi)\dot{\vartheta}$ for a specific body part to be imaged. Transmit gain determines the RF power emitted by the transmitter and thus the excitation pulse flip angle θ. Since power absorption is patient size dependent, the transmit gain has to be adjusted individually. For optimum image quality, it is imperative that the transmit gain be set for maximum excitation–response signal intensity. Receive gain is set such that the phase-sensitive detector operates at its optimal dynamic range. The central frequency adjustment controls the position of the RF transmitter. This is complicated by the fact that protons occur in two different chemical constituents, water and triglyceride. Protons in water and triglyceride have slightly different resonance frequencies ν. The resonance frequency of water protons is higher by approximately 220 Hz at 1.5 T magnetic flux density. This chemical shift from protons in triglyceride to water may generate an image misregistration or chemical shift artifact that is of similar nature as the magnetic susceptibility artifact. As a rule, the excitation–response signal of a particular constituent is attenuated with increasing offset of the transmitter frequency from resonance. This property can be exploited for suppressing fat by centering on the water proton resonance frequency. Chemical shift selective fat suppression, however, must be distinguished from STIR. In STIR scans, fat is suppressed because of its short longitudinal spin–relaxation time T_1 rather than its chemical shift relative to water protons ([366]). In hepatic imaging, chemical shift imaging techniques seem to be superior over STIR acquisitions for detection of hepatic lipid.

The selective excitation principle for planar coadjoint orbits $\mathbf{P}(\mathbb{R} \times \mathcal{O}_\nu) \hookrightarrow \mathbf{P}(\mathbb{R} \times \mathrm{Lie}(G)^\star)(\nu \neq 0)$ of the three-dimensional Heisenberg nilpotent Lie group G localizing by resonance with the associated central characters χ_ν of frequency $\nu = (1/2\pi)\dot{\vartheta}$ the on resonance spin isochromats inside planar slabs is the basis of virtually all commercial MRI whole-body scanners currently used in the area of biomedical radiology for diagnostic planar imaging purposes. The magnetic spin echo technique of effective time reversal by the quantum teleportation phenomenon of nonlinear phase conjugation which refocuses the dissipative spin system inside the selectively excited planar coadjoint orbit $\mathbf{P}(\mathbb{R} \times \mathcal{O}_\nu) \hookrightarrow \mathbf{P}(\mathbb{R} \times \mathrm{Lie}(G)^\star)(\nu \neq 0)$ is then combined with the symplectic Fourier transform associated with the selectively excited planar coadjoint orbit $\mathbf{P}(\mathbb{R} \times \mathcal{O}_\nu)$. The square integrability mod C, or equivalently, the fact that an irreducible unitary linear representation U^ν of G of dimension greater than 1 is determined by its central character χ_ν of frequency $\nu = (1/2\pi)\dot{\vartheta}$, implies that distinct planar coadjoint orbits

$$(\mathbf{P}(\mathbb{R} \times \mathcal{O}_\nu)), \; (\mathbf{P}(\mathbb{R} \times \mathcal{O}_{\nu'})) \qquad (\nu \neq \nu')$$

in $\mathbf{P}(\mathbb{R} \times \mathrm{Lie}(G)^\star)$ are noninteractive. Therefore magnetic spin echo holograms provide diagnostically more instructive hazard-free visual information than the shadowgrams generated by clinical X-ray scanners. Moreover, the noninteractivity of different planar coadjoint orbits implies that adjacent tomographic spin slices are not affected by the selective excitation. Since a two-spin echo filtering measurement takes only 100 ms and the repetition time T_R is 1000 ms in the single-slice case, the clinical MRI scanner is idle 90% of the time. As mentioned earlier, the idle period can be used to filter measurements of excitation–response signals from other, adjacent planar coadjoint orbits once every 100 ms by using selective excitation irradiations with different frequencies. With $T_R = 1000$ ms the clinical MRI scanner generates images of 10 tomographic planar slices in the time that it would otherwise take for one. Combined with quantum holography, the multislice performance boost makes pulsed Fourier MRI viable clinically and improves the performance of the neurofunctional MRI modality.

The variability of the spin choreography of high resolution NMR studies implemented at the quantum level by the generic planar coadjoint orbit $\mathbf{P}\,(\mathbb{R} \times \mathcal{O}_1) \hookrightarrow \mathbf{P}\left(\mathbb{R} \times \mathrm{Lie}(G)^\star\right)$ of coherent signal geometry made the pulsed Fourier MRI procedure the radiodiagnostic imaging modality of first choice in noninvasive biomedical visualization and in the clinical examination of many pathologies. At the beginning of routine clinical MRI examinations, neuroradiology and intracranial pathology started to benefit from pulsed Fourier MRI. The MS lesions and posterior fossa pathology were the earliest clinical applications for which MRI became the primary radiodiagnostic tool. Magnetic resonance imaging has made tremendous contributions to MS research in the past decade, yet the precise etiology and pathophysiology of this disabling disease are still unknown. Many arguments now support the hypothesis that MS is an immune-mediated disease which tends to be a perivenular process that results in plaques of demyelination. Because histopathological verification is not usually possible, the diagnosis of MS is essentially a clinical one, requiring dissemination of the disease in time and space. Following the first description of MS seen on clinical MRI scans in 1981, many studies have shown that the hallmark of MS on clinical MRI scans is the presence of multiple asymmetric punctate periventricular white matter lesions which impair neural functions. As a result of the unique sensitivity of MRI to depict MS lesions, new insights have been gained into the natural course of the disease. Magnetic resonance imaging has proved its worth in the evaluation of therapy and is used to measure outcome in the majority of MS treatment trials ([174], [286], [343]).

The MRI modality is unequaled in detecting the plaques of demyelinating disease ([347]), the early changes associated with intracerebral infarcts, and lesions in such difficult areas as the posterior fossa ([13]) and the orbit ([333]), untroubled by bone artifacts which plague clinical X-ray CT scans at this level. The absence of compact bone in clinical MRI scans offered the first opportunity to study all of the bone marrow. Over the past few years, MRI has developed into the primary modality for the diagnosis of extra-axial fluid collections, degenerative processes of the brain ([10], [37], [134], [287], [372]), nonneoplastic space-occupying intracranial lesions such as inflammatory diseases, AIDS-related diseases, acute demyelinization, granulomas, cysts, parasites, hemorrhages, vascular anomalies, brain infarctions ([38], [173], [347]), CNS tumors and edema ([50], [166]), intraocular and intraorbital lesions ([66], [311]), ischemic disease, meningitis, MS lesions, dropped metastatis, syringomyelia, acoustic neuroma, head and neck tumor staging ([1], [10], [143], [144], [212], [286], [343], [351], [372]), cervical, thoracic, and lumbar spine diseases including intervertebral disk diseases ([1], [52], [186], [220], [266], [275], [323], [344]), and musculoskeletal neoplasms ([34], [52], [59], [329]).

Experience from recent years has shown that a wide variety of different bone and cartilage abnormalities may be demonstrated with clinical MRI, and it has come to play an important role in this regard. Actually the organ systems currently enjoying the greatest growth in MRI are the musculoskeletal system ([28], [34], [59], [141], [227], [239], [329], [353], [374]). The MRI of the musculoskeletal system allows for understanding new clinical applications of bone and joint imaging including orthopedic trauma and tumors ([68], [156], [232], [266], [267], [279], [329]).

Even occult fractures are detected on clinical Fourier MRI scans. The apparent fracture line is the result of associated edema in the underlying bone marrow. The tomographic morphologic features of the lumbosacral spine are well shown by the Fourier MRI modality. The cortical bone of the vertebrae appears dark, as do the ligaments. In fact all ligaments exhibit low signal intensity on all MRI pulse sequences because there are few mobile protons in the fibrous tissue of which they are composed. The discus intervertebralis consists of the nucleus pulposus, the annulus fibrosus, and the cartilaginous endplate. With MRI, intervertebral disks are well visualized and display a high intensity center surrounded by a lower response intensity outer ring on spin echo scans, suggesting that the annulus fibrosus is being distinguished from the nucleus pulposus. Therefore, clinical MRI is capable of supplanting myelography of herniated disks. The thecal sac and nerve roots are outlined by high intensity epidural fat which is symmetrically disposed in healthy subjects. The structure of the spinal cord itself appears relatively bright, surrounded by the lower excitation–response signal of CSF. The dura and supporting ligaments of the spine are demonstrated in either sagittal or axial tomographic images ([329], [372]). Adult studies of the hip joint show little response signal intensity from the bony cortex of acetabulum and femoral head in the articulatio coxae. The femur therefore appears as a low intensity ring surrounding a region of higher intensity arising from the excitation–response of the bone marrow in the medullary cavity. Articular cartilage, ligaments, tendons, muscles, supporting soft tissue, and the major blood vessels are spatially well resolved ([45], [239]). The excellent spatial and contrast resolution provided by clinical MRI facilitates early detection and evaluation of femoral head osteonecrosis, definition of hyaline articular cartilage in arthritis, identification of joint effusions, and characterization of osseous and soft tissue tumors about the hip ([329]).

In imaging neoplasms of the knee there is only one exception in which case X-ray CT and radiographs are more helpful than MRI, namely the evaluation of tumor components with calcification or ossification. Although X-ray CT actually did much to improve the accuracy of clinical diagnosis, its limitations are now being realized. Magnetic resonance imaging supplies a wealth of information, exceeding X-ray CT in most clinical examinations. After having conquered the brain, skull, spine, and musculoskeletal system in rapid succession, MRI has, more recently, made strong inroads in clinical neuroophthalmic imaging ([333]) and neuropediatric imaging ([15], [16], [343]), in the clinical imaging of thorax and mediastinum ([79], [281]), in the imaging of the abdomen and retroperitoneum in spite of the considerable motion ([79], [284], [313], [368]), in the male and female pelvis ([45], [79], [162], [231]) including evaluation of the gravid uterus in the obstetrical patient ([160]), and in the genitourinary tract and rectum ([45], [162], [231], [284], [326]).

In 1980 the first magnetic resonance images of the human thorax and abdomen were produced at the University of Aberdeen ([104]). Thoracic Fourier MRI revolutionized the art of chest imaging due to the ability of mapping the segmental morphology *in vivo* of the thorax in all tomographic planes, transaxial, coronal, sagittal, and parasagittal ([251], [360]). Chest imaging is routinely performed using a spin echo technique. In general, short T_E values (14 to 30 ms) and short T_R values

(250 to 500 ms) are employed. The ideal imaging slice is perpendicular to the tissue interface of interest. Sagittal and coronal scans are particularly useful in the clinical evaluation of structures such as the trachea, major airways, and great vessels and in examining such regions as the aorticopulmonary window and apices pulmonis. The lack of excitation–response signals originating from blood vessels is of great value in their distinction from hilar or mediastinal tumors without recourse to the intravenous contrast enhancing agents which are generally required for X-ray CT examinations. Spin echo pulse sequences using short T_E and T_R values provide excellent spatial resolution and morphologic details of the entire trachea, the carina tracheae, the main bronchi, and the larynx. A surface coil can be employed for studies of the cervical trachea.

The cavum mediastinale, which is one of the most important regions of the human body due to the organs, great vessels, and nerves included in the mediastinum, is ideally suited for the clinical MRI modality because of the inherent contrast between the bright signal intensity of mediastinal fat and the signal void generated by flowing blood within the heart and mediastinal vessels. Indeed, the lumens of mediastinal vessels generally show low signal intensity and are identified by their sharp contrast with high intensity mediastinal fat. The arcus aortae and its large vessels, the brachiocephalic veins, the subclavian veins, and the vena cava, are always identified. The vena azygos and arch prolongating the vena lumbalis dextra are visible in most patients. The main pulmonary artery, arteria pulmonalis dextra and sinistra, right interlobar pulmonary artery, right truncus pulmonalis anterius, and descending left pulmonary artery are all well seen, as are the large venae pulmonales. The normal hilum pulmonis consists primarily of bronchi and the pulmonary arteries and veins. The main bronchi and the bronchus intermedius are always visible on clinical MRI scans. Pulmonary nodules, when present, are often detected on MRI scans. Primary and metastatic malignancies tend to be of low signal intensity on T_1-weighted and high signal intensity on T_2-weighted scans. Other structures in the mediastinum which can consistently be identified on clinical MRI scans include normal sized mediastinal lymph nodes, the thymus gland, and the esophagus. They are intermediate in signal intensity, being less intense than fat and more intense than air-filled lung or mediastinal vessels. The ability to identify mediastinal lymph nodes in order to determine if they are enlarged and to distinguish them from vessels is an important function of any imaging modality in the cavum mediastinale. In MRI, T_1-weighted scans permit the visualization of normal sized nodes and most mediastinal nodes that are borderline in size or enlarged ([79], [210]).

As is well known from mammography, by far the most common benign tumor is the fibroadenoma followed by the lipoma, hamartoma, and papilloma. Depending on the integrity of the basal membrane, infiltrating carcinomas are distinguished from noninfiltrating ones. By far the most infiltrating carcinoma is the ductal carcinoma followed by the lobular carcinoma, medullary carcinoma, and colloid carcinoma. Conventional mammography cannot differentiate a circumscribed carcinoma from a fibroadenoma reliably. In addition, mammography cannot provide enough information about the mammary tissues which are close to the chest wall. Magnetic resonance mammography, however, is the imaging procedure of human mammary tissue morphology that gives the best diagnostic results when NDT (nondestructive testing) for breast cancer is performed by a surface mamma coil in Heisenberg solenoid or paired Helmholtz configuration with two chambers positioned at the isocenter of the superconducting magnet ([150], [151], [171], [210], [332]).

Finally, magnetic resonance angiography is expected to take the lead in the diagnosis of certain vascular disorders. The carotid bifurcation, cervical internal carotid, carotid siphon, and vertebral basal insufficiency are all well evaluated with magnetic resonance angiography (MRA). The design of ultrafast high resolution imaging techniques promises MRI to become a real-time imaging modality suited for MRA evaluation of the cardiovascular system ([71]).

The natural values of the longitudinal T_1 and transverse spin–relaxation times T_2 may be considerably modified by the presence of paramagnetic impurities in concentration as low as a few parts per million. Paramagnetic compounds have at least one unpaired electron. The magnetic moment of this electron is about 10^3 higher than the magnetic moment of a single proton. The higher magnetic moment of paramagnetic impurities improves the local energy transfer between excited protons and the excited protons and the spin-lattice and therefore changes the intensity of the echos induced by the external magnetic flux density by shortening the relaxation times T_1 and T_2. The dominant effect on T_1 or T_2 of such an exogeneous contrast agent, however, depends on baseline tissue relaxation times in the absence of the agent as well as the maximum tissue concentration achieved.

The effects of the paramagnetic ions of iron, copper, and manganese were well known to the early pioneers of NMR spectroscopy. However, these effects are greatly magnified in the transition metal ions, especially the rare earth ion gadolinium Gd^{3+}, which has spin quantum number $\frac{7}{2}$. Gadolinium occupies the central position in the lanthanide series of elements. A chelated form of the Gd ion to a ligand such as gadolinium diethylene triamine pentaacetic acid, or Gd–DTPA dimeglumine for short, in which the outer shell $4f$ electrons are rendered nonreactive, has recently been developed as a low toxicity pharmaceutical agent suitable for introduction into human subjects ([95]). Gadolinium and dysprosium chelates are nonspecific extracellular agents, analogous to iodinated vascular contrast, rather than blood-pool agents. The objective of introducing these exogenous paramagnetic compounds into MRI and MRA, which in principle are noninvasive imaging modalities, provides an opportunity of improving soft tissue image contrast by exogenous proton relaxation enhancement in situations where intrinsic image contrast is poor ([79], [163], [210], [281]). Injection of Gd–DTPA dimeglumine is indicated in adults and children to provide contrast enhancement, especially in those intracranial lesions with abnormal vascularity or abnormality in the blood-brain barrier. It facilitates visualization of intracranial lesions, including but not limited to tumors, and of lesions in the spine and associated tissues ([95]). Following the lead from brain tumor imaging, contrast-enhanced MRI provides valuable physiological information not available from unenhanced images. With the advent of improved hardware, software, clinical examination strategies, and newly developed whole-body contrast enhancing agents, the modality of contrast enhanced MRI is increasingly applied to organ systems other than the brain, spine, and CNS. When combined with Gd–DTPA dimeglumine, specifically magnetic resonance mammography can produce contrast enhancement of malignant breast tumors such as infiltrating ductal and lobular carcinomas, benign breast tumors such as fluid-filled cysts and mammary hamartomas, and normal breast parenchyma in the preoperative setting ([150], [151]). In the MRI diagnosis of prostatic carcinoma and benign prostatic hyperplasia, Gd–DTPA dimeglumine plays a similar important role ([95]). Magnetic resonance angiography in conjunction with contrast-enhanced volume MRI can provide information about orientation of flow within an intracranial aneurysm, and MRI will answer clinical and intracerebral neurophysiological questions by microvascular neurofunctional topographic imaging.

With so many directions in which to expand, clinical MRI will change dramatically over the next decade. Specifically the MRI approach to temporally encoded neural network organizations of stimulus-evoked synchronized response association by neurofunctional imaging during cognitive task performance represents a major breakthrough which is going to open up a new field of neuroscience research. Because clinical MRI embraces a multitude of research and industrial disciplines between which there is often little communication due to the jargon of each of the disciplines, it is important to provide a unifying mathematical foundation to penetrate this powerful clinical imaging modality of noninvasive computer-assisted radiological diagnosis. Symmetry principles based on Lie theory, specifically the mathematical methods of nilpotent harmonic analysis, allow for establishing that the simply connected Heisenberg nilpotent real Lie group G represents the structure group of the dissipative spin systems naturally associated with the Fourier MRI modality and the reentrant processing of synchronized temporally encoded neural networks. It is the Heisenberg Lie group G which bridges the gap to quantum physics and to temporally encoded synchronized neural network models of stimulus-response association which nonalgorithmically emulate the semantic association of planar tomographic images and dynamically perform microvascular neurofunctional topographic imaging of cognitive processing. Because the organization of dissipative systems is independent of the specific system, the range of the nilpotent harmonic analysis method goes far beyond the Fourier MRI technique and includes the study of dissipative systems without spin structure, neural gas networks, and their Feigenbaum scenarios ([298]).

Through the application to MRI, however, the power and versatility of the stratified structure of the coadjoint orbit model of two-step nilpotent harmonic analysis methods should have become clear.

The data provide strong support for the hypothesis that visual cortex can be understood as a self-organizing system. ... A consequence of this is that afferent activation patterns not matching the resonance properties of the column should produce only very little excitatory and inhibitory synaptic activity.
—Christoph von der Malsburg and Wolf Singer (1988)

Many researchers have recently focussed almost exclusively upon the existence of these synchronous oscillations. Now that the robust nature of the synchrony phenomenon has been demonstrated, a finer analysis of individual parametric features peculiar to the perceptual or cognitive codes supported by the oscillations can be carried out.
—Stephen Grossberg (1991)

After weighting the risks, I became convinced that an extensive attempt must be made to analyze consciousness in terms of its neural origins.
—Gerald M. Edelman (1989)

I believe that quantum holography is centrally important to conscious activity of the brain.
—Peter Maddock (1994)

We're pretty deep into the deeper aspects of processing.
—Robert G. Shulman (1993)

3.4 SUMMARY

In neurobiology, the brain is viewed as an organ system in which neurons respond to sensory stimuli from the environment. Other neurons in the motor cortex control muscles acting upon the environment. The link between the cerebrum and the environment is formed by a neural network in which a complex reentrant processing is going on, involving

- associative memory,
- memory storage, and
- memory retrieval.

The interaction between brain and environment is of particular importance in the development of the human brain. The role of neuronal activity is to generate a representation of the environment. This point of view implicitly presupposes the knowledge of the notion of environment together with some of its fundamental properties, such as containing visual objects, which is essential for resolving the object binding problem of early vision. In the early vision system, visual scene segmentation or figure-ground segmentation is achieved by expressing phase coherency in terms of temporary synchronization among neuronal responses of cell assemblies coding for different figures and background.

If, however, the intrinsic point of view is adopted, the environment and its fundamental properties have to be detected. The neural network obeys general self-organization principles of evolution and selection. It does so by cross-correlating information so that phase-sensitive data processing and storage remain redundant.

The environment is not assumed as a preexisting concept but rather as a reality to be detected and discovered.

Thus, in neurobiology the conventional extrinsic point of view stresses the role of nervous signals as such, whereas in cognitive neuroscience the intrinsic point of view emphasizes phase-sensitive temporal cross-correlations between phase-coherent wavelets. The intrinsic point of view, which does not focus on reactions of the brain to inputs but rather on neuronal cooperativity, corresponds to the Sherringtonian approach to creating a mental image in the complete absence of any sensory stimulation. Biological neural networks are capable of handling cooperativity by phase-sensitive temporal cross-correlations in an efficient manner: Neurons act as phase-sensitive correlation detectors because dendritic depolarizations occurring at different input synapses of the same neuron are more efficient in eliciting an output spike if they are synchronized. The neurophysiological finding that phase-sensitive temporal cross-correlations between different stimulus-evoked neural activities imply that the sensory stimuli belong together goes far beyond the classical stimulus–response relationship based on the activity of single neurons. It suggests that the recognition of stimuli is due to a particular internal spatiotemporal excitation pattern in the brain.

The paradigm shift in neurobiology which is caused by the neurophysiological finding on the nanosecond scale that temporary synchronization reflects global properties of the sensory stimulus has supplanted the place encoding principle by the temporal encoding principle. Because the stimulus-evoked interareal synchronized cooperative interaction of neural cell assemblies cannot be explained in terms of far field volume conduction, a quantum physical approach is suggested. This approach is based upon the phase-sensitive cross-correlation function which is implemented by nilpotent harmonic analysis. The phase-sensitive cross-correlation function allows for detection of the quantum teleportation phenomenon of spin packet dephasing. Nilpotent harmonic analysis adapts quantum physics by means of the stratified structure of the coadjoint orbit model $\mathbf{P}\left(\mathbb{R} \times \mathcal{O}_\nu\right) \hookrightarrow \mathbf{P}\left(\mathbb{R} \times \mathrm{Lie}(G)^\star\right)$ $(\nu \neq 0)$ of the unitary dual $\hat{G}$ of the Heisenberg nilpotent real Lie group G to massively parallel nonalgorithmic neurocomputing and visualization. The quantum theoretical approach to temporally encoded synchronized neural network organizations suggests that we consider the clinical MRI scanners of noninvasive radiological diagnostics and microvascular neurofunctional topographic imaging as temporally encoded analog quantum neurocomputers for massively parallel nonalgorithmic computation. The computing of clinical MRI scanners includes semantic association of tomographic images, macrovascular magnetic resonance angiography, and dynamical MRI visualization of microvascular neurofunctional topographic imaging of cognitive processing in order to address the human brain *in vivo* on its own temporally encoded operative terms of cerebral functional self-organization as exemplified by the retinotopic organization of the human striate cortex. The hemodynamic response time represents the limit of the temporal resolution of the microvascular neurofunctional MRI modality in the visualization studies of human cognition. The high spatial resolution of neurofunctional MRI allows the neurologist to begin understanding the neurophysiology of the psychophysics of the cerebrum as well as to analyze human brain activities by topographically imaging patterns of function reflective of behavioral propensities.

The goal of neuroimaging is to use microvascular neurofunctional MRI modalities together with cognitive neuroscience to increase the knowledge of the brain systems that support conscious awareness. Finally, maturation of neurofunctional MRI will support MRI-assisted neuronavigation as a tool of minimally invasive neurosurgery and provide a better understanding of the neurobiology of devastating mental disorders such as major depression and the assessment of attention deficit disorders such as schizophrenia. Because these disorders affect the mental life of patients in profound ways, suggestions for curing or even preventing these diseases would be of paramount importance.

In any case, the future of clinical MRI continues to be bright, with the advent of routine second and subsecond imaging techniques anticipated with the next generation of MRI scanners in the mid- to late-1990s and their application to neurofunctional dynamical topographic imaging.

Ich bin vor allem von der Existenz von perzeptuellen Karten fasziniert.
—Alain Connes (1992)

It is truly remarkable that the most complex organ so far known to exist in the universe is so arranged as to make listening in on its most closely guarded whisperings so easy.
—John S. Barlow (1993)

Wie weit diese Methoden reichen werden, muß erst die Zukunft zeigen.
—Amalie Emmy Noether (1882–1935)

BIBLIOGRAPHY

[1] F. T. Aichner, S. R. Felber, R. N. Muller, and P. A. Rinck (Eds.), *Three-dimensional magnetic resonance imaging*, Blackwell Scientific Publications, Oxford, London, Edinburgh, 1994.

[2] K. Aihara, T. Takabe, and M. Toyoda, Chaotic neural networks, *Phys. Lett.* 144A (1990), 333–340.

[3] E. J. Aiton, The elliptical orbit and the area law, in *Kepler: Four hundred years*, Proceedings of conferences held in honour of Johannes Kepler, A. Beer and P. Beer, Eds., *Vistas in Astronomy*, Vol. 18, pp. 573–583, Pergamon Press, Oxford, New York, Toronto, 1975.

[4] A. N. Akansu and R. A. Haddad, *Multiresolution signal decomposition: Transforms, subbands, and wavelets*, Academic Press, Boston, San Diego, New York, 1992.

[5] C. M. Anderson, R. R. Edelman, and P. A. Turski, *Clinical magnetic resonance angiography*, Raven Press, New York, 1993.

[6] D. K. Andes, J. C. Witham, and M. D. Miles, MAVIS: A special purpose neural computational system for ATR, *Neural Networks* 8 (1995), 1349–1358.

[7] P. A. Anninos and G. Anogianakis, Computer simulation studies to deduce the structure and function of the human brain, in *Computer simulation in brain science*, pp. 303–315, R. M. J. Cotterill, Ed., Cambridge University Press, Cambridge, New York, New Rochelle, 1988.

[8] I. P. Arlart, G. M. Bongartz, and G. Marchal (Eds.), *Magnetic resonance angiography*, Springer-Verlag, Berlin, Heidelberg, New York, 1996.

[9] M. Atiyah, *The geometry and physics of knots*, Lezioni Lincee, Cambridge University Press, Cambridge, New York, Port Chester, 1990.

[10] S. W. Atlas (Ed.), *Magnetic resonance imaging of the brain and spine*, 2nd ed., Lippincott-Raven Publishers, Philadelphia, New York, 1996.

[11] L. M. Auer and V. Van Velthoven, *Intraoperative ultrasound in neurosurgery: A comparison with* CT *and* MR *imaging*, Springer-Verlag, Berlin, Heidelberg, New York, 1989.

[12] P. Bachert, L. R. Schad, M. Bock, M. V. Knopp, M. Ebert, T. Grossmann, W. Heil, D. Hofmann, R. Surkau, and E. W. Otten, Nuclear magnetic resonance imaging of the airways in humans with use of hyperpolarized ^{3}He, *Magn. Reson. Med.* 36 (1996), 192–196.

[13] D. Balériaux, C. Matos, and W. O. Bank, MRI of intracranial tumors: State of the art in comparison with other imaging modalities, in MR *'91–4. Internationales Kernspintomographie Symposium*, pp. 379–385, J. Lissner, J. L. Doppman, and A. R. Margulis, Eds., Schnetztor-Verlag, Konstanz 1992.

[14] P. A. Bandettini, E. C. Wong, R. S. Hinks, R. S. Tikofsky, and J. S. Hyde, Time course EPI of human brain function during task activation, *Magn. Reson. Med.* 25 (1992), 390–397.

[15] A. J. Barkovich and C. L. Truwit, *Practical* MRI *atlas of neonatal brain development*, Raven Press, New York, 1990.

[16] A. J. Barkovich, *Pediatric neuroimaging*, 2nd ed., Raven Press, New York, 1995.

[17] A. J. Barkovich and T. V. Maroldo, Magnetic resonance imaging of normal and abnormal brain development, *Topics Mag. Reson. Imag.* 5 (1993), 96–122.

[18] J. S. Barlow, *The electroencephalogram: Its patterns and origins*, The MIT Press, Cambridge, MA, 1993.

[19] A. Barone and G. Paternò, *Physics and applications of the Josephson effect*, John Wiley & Sons, New York, Chichester, Brisbane, 1982.

[20] K. Baudendistel, L. R. Schad, M. Friedlinger, F. Wenz, J. Schröder, and W. J. Lorenz, Postprocessing of functional MRI data of motor cortex stimulation measured with a standard 1.5 T imager, *Mag. Reson. Imag.* 13 (1995), 701–707.

[21] M. Bauer and W. Martienssen, Coupled circle maps as a tool to model synchronization in neural networks, *Network* 2 (1991), 345–351.

[22] M. Bauer, U. Krueger, and W. Martienssen, Experimental studies of mode-locking and circle maps in inductively shunted Josephson junctions, *Europhys. Lett.* 9 (1989), 191–196.

[23] M. Bauer and W. Martienssen, Quasi-periodicity route to chaos in neural networks, *Europhys. Lett.* 10 (1989), 427–431.

[24] R. Bauer, E. van de Flierdt, K. Mörike, and C. Wagner-Manslau (Eds.), MR *tomography of the central nervous system*, 2nd ed., Gustav Fischer Verlag, Stuttgart, Jena, New York, 1993.

[25] J. W. Belliveau, D. N. Kennedy, R. C. McKinstry, B. R. Buchbinder, R. M. Weisskoff, M. S. Cohen, J. M. Vevea, T. J. Brady, and B. R. Rosen, Functional mapping of the human visual cortex by magnetic resonance imaging, *Science* 254 (1991), 716–719.

[26] J. Beltran (Ed.), The ankle and foot, *Mag. Reson. Imag. Clin. N.Am.*, 2 (1994), 1–159.

[27] J. Beltran (Ed.), *Current review of* MRI, 1st ed., CM Current Medicine, Philadelphia, PA, 1995.

[28] T. H. Berquist (Ed.), MRI *of the musculoskeletal system*, 3rd ed., Lippincott-Raven Publishers, Philadelphia, New York, 1996.

[29] W. D. Bidgood, Jr., and S. C. Horii, Introduction to the ACR–NEMA DICOM Standard, *Radiographics* 12 (1992), 345–355.

[30] J. H. Bisese and A.-M. Wang, *Pediatric cranial* MRI: *An atlas of normal development*, Springer-Verlag, New York, Berlin, Heidelberg, 1994.

[31] A. M. Blamire, S. Ogawa, K. Uğurbil, D. L. Rothman, G. McCarthy, J. M. Ellermann, F. Hyder, Z. Rattner, and R. G. Shulman, Dynamic mapping of the human visual cortex by high speed magnetic resonance imaging, *Proc. Natl. Acad. Sci. USA* 89 (1992), 11069–11073.

[32] R. J. Blattner, Pairing of half-forms, in *Géométrie Symplectique et Physique Mathématique, Colloques Internationaux du Centre de la Recherche Scientifique*, No. 237, pp. 175–186, Éditions du Centre National de la Recherche Scientifique, Paris, 1975.

[33] R. P. Boas, Jr., Summation formulas and band-limited signals, *Tôhoku Math. J.* 24 (1972), 121–125.

[34] K. Bohndorf, MR—*Tomographie des Skeletts und der peripheren Weichteile*, Springer-Verlag, Berlin, Heidelberg, New York, 1991.

[35] J. E. Bonevich, K. Harada, T. Matsuda, H. Kasai, T. Yoshida, G. Pozzi, and A. Tonomura, Electron holography observation of vortex lattices in a superconductor, *Phys. Rev. Lett.* 70 (1993), 2952–2955.

[36] A. Borel, *Représentations de groupes localement compacts, Lecture notes in mathematics*, Vol. 276, Springer-Verlag, Berlin, Heidelberg, New York, 1972.

[37] W. G. Bradley and G. Bydder, MRI *atlas of the brain*, Raven Press, New York, 1990.

[38] W. G. Bradley, Jr., *Mastering* MRI: *Central nervous system*, CD-ROM, Lippincott-Raven Publishers, Philadelphia, 1996.

[39] M. Brant-Zawadzki, O. B. Boyko, M. C. Jensen, and G. D. Gillan, MR *angiography*, Raven Press, New York, 1994.

[40] B. Bromm, Evozierte magnetische Felder in der Diagnostik afferenter Systeme (Squid–Imaging), in MR '91–4. *Internationales Kernspintomographie Symposium*, pp. 55–64, J. Lissner, J. L. Doppman, and A. R. Margulis, Eds., Schnetztor–Verlag, Konstanz, 1992.

[41] J. J. Brown, F. J. Wippold II, *Practical* MRI: *A teaching file*, Lippincott-Raven Publishers, Philadelphia, New York, 1995.

[42] P. Brunner and R. R. Ernst, Sensitivity and performance time in NMR imaging, *J. Magn. Reson.* 33 (1979), 82–106.

[43] G. M. Bydder and I. R. Young, MR imaging: Clinical use of the inversion recovery sequence, *J. Comput. Assist. Tomogr.* 9 (1985), 659–675.

[44] D. R. Cahill, M. J. Orland, and G. M. Miller, *Atlas of human cross-sectional anatomy, with* CT *and* MR *images*, 3rd ed., Wiley-Liss, New York, Chichester, Brisbane, 1995.

[45] Z. Campos, Y. Narumi, and H. Hricak, *Pocket atlas of* MRI *of the pelvis*, Raven Press, New York, 1993.

[46] G. A. Carpenter, Neural network models for pattern recognition and associative memory, *Neural Networks* 2 (1989), 243–257.

[47] E. A. Carrara, F. Pagliari, and C. Nicolini, Neural networks for the peak-picking of nuclear magnetic resonance spectra, *Neural Networks* 6 (1993), 1023–1032.

[48] H. Carswell, fMRI reveals unique aspect of Japanese language, *Diagn. Imag. Eur.*, pp. 10–12, March 1996.

[49] M. Castillo and S. Mukherji, *Imaging of the pediatric head, neck, and spine*, Lippincott-Raven Publishers, Philadelphia, New York, 1996.

[50] L. Cecconi, A. Pompili, F. Caroli, and E. Squillaci, MRI *atlas of central nervous system tumors*, Springer-Verlag, Wien, New York, 1992.

[51] A. P. Chaiyasena, Radar and sonar ambiguity functions and group theory, Ph.D. Thesis in Mathematics, The Pennsylvania State University, 1993.

[52] W. P. Chan, P. Lang, and H. K. Genant (Eds.), MRI *of the musculoskeletal system*, W. B. Saunders, Philadelphia, London, Toronto, 1994.

[53] J.-P. Changeux and A. Connes, *Gedanken-Materie*, Springer-Verlag, Berlin, Heidelberg, New York, 1992.

[54] L. P. Clarke, R. P. Velthuizen, S. Phuphanich, J. D. Schellenberg, J. A. Arrington, and M. Silbiger, MRI: Stability of three supervised segmentation techniques, *Magn. Reson. Imag.* 11 (1993), 95–106.

[55] M. S. Cohen and S. Y. Bookheimer, Localization of brain function using magnetic resonance imaging, *Trends Neurosci.* 17 (1994), 268–277.

[56] J. G. Cramer, The transactional interpretation of quantum mechanics, *Rev. Mod. Phys.* 58 (1986), 647–687.

[57] O. D. Creutzfeldt, *Cortex cerebri*, Springer-Verlag, Berlin, Heidelberg, New York, 1983.

[58] F. Crick, Function of the thalamic reticular complex: The searchlight hypothesis, *Proc. Natl. Acad. Sci. USA* 81 (1984), 4586–4590.

[59] J. V. Crues, III, *Mastering* MRI: *Musculoskeletal system,* CD-ROM, Lippincott-Raven Publishers, Philadelphia, 1996

[60] L. J. Cutrona, E. N. Leith, L. J. Porcello, and W. E. Vivian, On the application of coherent optical processing techniques to synthetic-aperture radar, *Proc.* IEEE 54 (1966), 1026–1032.

[61] R. Damadian, Tumor detection by nuclear magnetic resonance, *Science* 171 (1971), 1151–1153.

[62] H. Damasio, *Human brain anatomy in computerized images*. Oxford University Press, New York, Oxford, Athens, 1995.

[63] P. L. Davis (Ed.), Breast imaging, *Magn. Reson. Imag. Clini. N. Am.* 2 (4), (1994) 505–723.

[64] G. Deleuze, and F. Guattari, *Mille plateaux*, Les Éditions de Minuit, Paris, 1980.

[65] G. Deleuze, and F. Guattari, *Q'est–ce que la philosophie?* Les Éditions de Minuit, Paris, 1991.

[66] P. De Potter, J. A. Shields, and C. L. Shields, MRI of the eye and orbit, J. B. Lippincott Company, Philadelphia, New York, London, 1995.

[67] A. M. De Schepper (Ed.), *Imaging of soft tissue tumors,* Springer-Verlag, Berlin, Heidelberg, New York, 1996.

[68] A. L. Deutsch, J. H. Mink, and R. Kerr (Eds.), MRI *of the foot and ankle*, Raven Press, New York, 1992.

[69] R. B. Dietrich (Ed.), *Pediatric* MRI, Raven Press, New York, 1991.

[70] J. A. Dieudonné, *La géométrie des groupes classiques*, 3rd ed., Springer-Verlag, Berlin, Heidelberg, New York, 1971.

[71] A. J. Duerinckx, C. B. Higgins, and R. I. Pettigrew (Eds.), MRI *of the cardiovascular system*, Raven Press, New York, 1994.

[72] D. L. Durham, *Atlas of* MR *pathology*, W. B. Saunders, Philadelphia, London, Toronto, 1997.

[73] J. C. Eccles, New light on the mind–brain problem: How mental events could influence neural events, in *Complex systems—operational approaches to neurobiology, physics, and computers*, pp. 81–106, H. Haken, Ed., Springer-Verlag, Berlin, Heidelberg, New York, 1985.

[74] R. Eckhorn, R. Bauer, W. Jordan, M. Brosch, W. Kruse, M. Munk, and H. J. Reitböck, Coherent oscillations: A mechanism for feature linking in the visual cortex? Multiple electrode and correlation analysis in the cat, *Biol. Cybernet.* 60 (1988), 121–130.

[75] R. Eckhorn, Stimulus-specific synchronizations in the visual cortex: Linking of local features into global figures? in *Neuronal cooperativity*, pp. 184–224, J. Krüger, Ed., Springer-Verlag, Berlin, Heidelberg, New York, 1991.

[76] R. Eckhorn, P. Dicke, W. Kruse, and H. J. Reitböck, Stimulus-related facilitation and synchronization among visual cortical areas: Experiments and models, in *Nonlinear dynamics and neuronal networks, Proceedings of the 63rd W.E. Heraeus Seminar Friedrichsdorf 1990*, pp. 57–75, H.G. Schuster, Ed., VCH, Weinheim, New York, Basel, 1991.

[77] G. M. Edelman, *Neural darwinism: The theory of neuronal group selection*, Basic Books Publishers, New York, 1987.

[78] G. M. Edelman, *The remembered present: A biological theory of consciousness*, Basic Books Publishers, New York, 1989.

[79] R. R. Edelman, J. R. Hesselink, and M. B. Zlatkin (Eds.), *Clinical magnetic resonance imaging*, 2nd ed., W. B. Saunders, Philadelphia, London, Toronto, 1996.

[80] W. A. Edelstein, J. M. S. Hutchinson, G. Johnson, and T. W. Redpath, Spin-warp NMR imaging and applications to human whole-body imaging, *Phys. Med. Biol.* 25 (1980), 751–756.

[81] C. Elachi, T. Bicknell, R. L. Jordan, and C. Wu, Spaceborne synthetic-aperture imaging radars: Appications, techniques, and technology. *Proc. IEEE* 70 (1982), 1174–1209.

[82] G. Y. El–Khoury, R. A. Bergman, and W. J. Montgomery, *Sectional anatomy by MRI*, 2nd ed., Churchill Livingstone, New York, Edinburgh, London, 1995.

[83] G. A. Elliott, T. Natsume, and R. Nest, Cyclic cohomology for one-parameter smooth crossed products, *Acta Math.* 160 (1988), 285–305.

[84] A. K. Engel, P. König, A. K. Kreiter, C. M. Gray, and W. Singer, Temporal coding by coherent oscillations as a potential solution to the binding problem: Physiological evidence, in *Nonlinear dynamics and neuronal networks, Proceedings of the 63rd W.E. Heraeus Seminar Friedrichsdorf 1990*, pp. 3–25, H.G. Schuster Ed., VCH, Weinheim, New York, Basel, 1991.

[85] A. K. Engel, P. König, A. K. Kreiter, T. B. Schillen, and W. Singer, Temporal coding in the visual cortex: New vistas on integration in the nervous system, *Trends Neurosci.* 15 (1992), 218–226.

[86] R. R. Ernst, A brief account of two–dimensional NMR spectroscopy, in *Physics of NMR spectroscopy in biology and medicine, Proceedings of the International School of Physics << Enrico Fermi >>*, Course C, pp. 158–185, B. Maraviglia, Ed., North–Holland, Amsterdam, Oxford, 1988.

[87] R. R. Ernst, The multidimensional importance of time domain magnetic resonance, in *Pulsed magnetic resonance—NMR, ESR, and optics: A recognition of E. L. Hahn*, pp. 95–122, D. M. S. Bagguley, Ed., Clarendon Press, Oxford, 1992.

[88] R. R. Ernst, G. Bodenhausen, and A. Wokaun, *Principles of nuclear magnetic resonance in one and two dimensions*, Clarendon Press, Oxford, 1987.

[89] U. Essmann and H. Träuble, The direct observation of individual flux lines in type II superconductors, *Phys. Lett.* 24A (1967), 526–527.

[90] M. J. Farah, The neural bases of mental imagery, in *The cognitive neurosciences*, pp. 963–975, M. S. Gazzaniga, Ed., The MIT Press, Cambridge, MA, 1995.

[91] G. L. Farre, Representing causal relations in evolutionary systems, in *Actes du Symposium ECHO*, pp. 83–87, A. C. Ehresmann, G. L. Farre, and J.–P. Vanbremeersch, Eds., Université de Picardie Jules Verne, Amiens, 1996.

[92] G. L. Farre, The energetic structure of observation, *Am. Behav. Sci.* 40 (1997), 717–728.

[93] M. J. Feigenbaum, Quantitative universality for a class of nonlinear transformations, *J. Stat. Phys.* 19 (1978), 25–52.

[94] R. Felix, When is a Kirillov orbit a linear variety? *Proc. Am. Math. Soc.* 86 (1982), 151–152.

[95] R. Felix, A. Heshiki, N. Hosten, und H. Hricak (Herausgeber), in *Magnevist–Eine Monographie*, Blackwell Wissenschafts-Verlag, Berlin, Oxford, Edinburgh, 1994.

[96] J. P. Felmlee, R. L. Morin, J. R. Salutz, and G. B. Lund, Magnetic resonance imaging phase encoding: A pictorial essay, *Radiographics* 9 (1989), 717–722.

[97] J. P. Finn (Ed.), Magnetic resonance angiography of the body, *Magnt. Reson. Imag. Clin. N. Am.*, Vol. 1(2), (1993) 203–365.

[98] E. K. Fishman and R. B. Jeffrey, Jr. (Eds.), *Spiral CT: Principles, techniques, and clinical applications*, Raven Press, New York, 1995.

[99] S. W. Fitzgerald (Ed.), The knee, *Magnet. Reson. Imag. Clin. N. Am.*, 2(3), (1994) 325–504.

[100] J. L. Fleckenstein, J. V. Crues III, and C. D. Reimers (Eds.), *Muscle imaging in health and disease*, Springer-Verlag, New York, Berlin, Heidelberg, 1996.

[101] A. C. Fleischer, M. C. Javitt, R. B. Jeffrey, Jr., and H. W. Jones, III (Eds.), *Clinical gynecologic imaging*, Lippincott-Raven Publishers, Philadelphia, New York, 1997.

[102] H. Flohr, Qualia and brain processes, in *Emergence or reduction? Essays on the prospects of nonreductive physicalism*, pp. 220–238, A. Beckermann, H. Flohr, and J. Kim, Eds., Walter de Gruyter, Berlin, New York, 1992.

[103] V. Foglietti, Multichannel instrumentation for biomagnetism, in *Superconducting devices and their applications*, pp. 487–501, H. Koch, H. Lübbig, Eds., Springer-Verlag, Berlin, Heidelberg, New York, 1992.

[104] M. A. Foster, N. J. F. Dodd, J. M. S. Hutchison, and F. W. Smith, *Magnetic resonance in medicine and biology*, Pergamon Press, Oxford, New York, Toronto, 1984.

[105] J. Frahm, W. Hänicke, H. Bruhn, M. L. Gyngell, and K. D. Merboldt, Ultraschnelle MR-Bildgebung des Herzens mit FLASH—und STEAM—Sequenzen, in *MR '91–4. Internationales Kernspintomographie Symposium*, pp. 15–20, J. Lissner, J. L. Doppman, and A. R. Margulis, Eds., Schnetztor-Verlag, Konstanz, 1992.

[106] R. Freeman, Spin choreography, in *Pulsed magnetic resonance—NMR, ESR, and optics: A recognition of E. L. Hahn*, pp. 219–241, D. M. S. Bagguley, Ed., Clarendon Press, Oxford, 1992.

[107] R. Freeman, *Spin choreography*, Spektrum Academic Publishers, Oxford, 1997.

[108] W. J. Freeman, C. A. Skarda, Spatial EEG patterns, non-linear dynamics and perception: The Neo-Sherringtonian view, *Brain Res. Rev.* 10 (1985), 147–175.

[109] I. Fried, V. I. Nenov, S. Ojemann, and R. Woods, Functional MRI and PET imaging of motor and visual cortices for neurosurgical planning in epilepsy patients, *Epilepsia* 35, (1994), S24.

[110] K. J. Friston, A. P. Holmes, K. J. Worseley, J.-P. Poline, C. D. Frith, and R. S. J. Frackowiak, Statistical parametric maps in functional imaging, A general linear approach, *Human Brain Mapping* 2, (1995), 189–210.

[111] K. J. Friston, G. Tononi, O. Sporns, and G. M. Edelman, Characterising the complexity of neuronal interactions, *Human Brain Mapping* 3, (1995), 302–314.

[112] J. M. Fröhlich, O. Grandjean, and A. Recknagel, String vacua, supersymmetry and noncommutative geometry, in *Proc. XXI Int. Coll. Group Theoret. Meth. in Phys.*, Vol. II, 552 H. D. Doebner, W. Scherer, and C. Schulte, Eds., World Scientific, Singapore, New Jersey, London, 1997.

[113] R. D. Frostig, E. E. Lieke, A. Arieli, D.Y. Ts'o, R. Hildesheim, and A. Grinvald, Optical imaging of neuronal activity in the living brain, in *Neuronal cooperativity*, pp. 30–51, J. Krüger, Ed., Springer-Verlag, Berlin, Heidelberg, New York, 1991.

[114] E. Fukushima (Ed.), NMR *in biomedicine: The physical basis*, Key Papers in Physics, No. 2, American Institute of Physics, New York, 1989.

[115] P. Gabriel, *Matrizen, Geometrie, Lineare Algebra*, Birkhäuser, Basel, Boston, Berlin, 1996.

[116] D. G. Gadian, Proton NMR studies of brain metabolism, *Phil. Trans. R. Soc. Lond. A* 333 (1990), 561–570.

[117] D. G. Gadian, NMR *and its applications to living systems*, 2nd ed., Oxford University Press, Oxford, New York, Tokyo, 1995.

[118] L. Gao, Magnetic resonance blood flow measurement using velocity encoded phase imaging, Ph.D. Thesis in Applied Mathematics, University of California, Davis, 1993.

[119] B. Gaveau, Principe de moindre action, propagation de la chaleur et estimées sous elliptiques sur certains groupes nilpotents, *Acta Math.* 139 (1977), 95–153.

[120] A. E. George (Ed.), Neurodegenerative diseases: Alzheimer's disease and related disorders, *Neuroimag. Clin. N. Am.*, 5 (1), (1995) 41–159.

[121] A. P. Georgopoulos, Motor cortex and cognitive processing, in *The cognitive neurosciences*, pp. 507–517, M. S. Gazzaniga, Ed., The MIT Press, Cambridge, MA, 1995.

[122] R. Gilles, M. Meunier, O. Lucidarme, B. Zafrani, J.–M. Guinebretière, A. A. Tardivon, M. Le Gal, D. Vanel, S. Neuenschwander, and R. Arriagada, Clustered breast microcalcifications: Evaluation by dynamic contrast-enhanced subtraction MRI. *J. Comput. Assist. Tomogr.* 20 (1996), 9–14.

[123] R.J. Gillies (Ed.), NMR *in physiology and biomedicine*, Academic Press, San Diego, New York, Boston, 1994.

[124] E. H. Gombrich, Symmetrie, Wahrnehmung und künstlerische Gestaltung, in *Symmetrie*, R. Wille, Ed., pp. 94–119, Springer-Verlag, Berlin, Heidelberg, New York, 1988.

[125] C. M. Gray, P. König, A. K. Engel, and W. Singer, Oscillatory responses in cat visual cortex exhibit inter-columnar synchronization which reflects global stimulus properties, *Nature* 338 (1989), 334–337.

[126] C. M. Gray, A. K. Engel, P. König, and W. Singer, Synchronization of oscillatory neuronal responses in cat striate cortex: Temporal properties, *Visual Neurosci.* 8 (1992), 337–347.

[127] H. Günther, NMR–*Spektroskopie*, Vol. 3, Auflage, Georg Thieme Verlag, Stuttgart, New York, 1992.

[128] H. Guo, J. E. Odegard, M. Lang, R. A. Gopinath, I. W. Selesnick, and C. S. Burrus, Speckle reduction via wavelet shrinkage with application to SAR based ATD/R, in *Mathematical Imaging: Wavelet Applications in Signal and Image Processing, Proc.* SPIE 2303 (1994), 333–344.

[129] V. Gray Hardcastle, The binding problem and neurobiological oscillations, in *Toward a science of consciousness: The first Tucson discussions and debates*, pp. 51–65, S. R. Hameroff, A. W. Kaszniak, and A. C. Scott, Eds., The MIT Press, Cambridge, MA, 1996.

[130] S. Grossberg, and E. Mingolla, Neural dynamics of motion perception: Direction fields, apertures, and resonant grouping, *Percept. Psychophys.* 53 (1993), 243–278.

[131] S. Grossberg, E. Mingolla, and J. Williamson, Synthetic aperture radar processing by a multiple scale neural system for boundary and surface representation, *Neural Networks* 8 (1995), 1005–1028.

[132] S. Grossberg, and D. Somers, Synchronized oscillations during cooperative feature linking in a cortical model of visual perception, *Neural Networks* 4 (1991), 453–466.

[133] C. B. Grossman, *Magnetic resonance imaging and computed tomography of the head and spine*, 2nd ed., Williams & Wilkins, Baltimore, Philadelphia, London, 1996.

[134] R. I. Grossman and D. M. Yousem, *Neuroradiology: The requisites*, Mosby-Year Book, St. Louis, Baltimore, Berlin, 1994.

[135] A. Grossmann, and J. Morlet, Decomposition of functions into wavelets of constant shape, and related transforms, in *Mathematics and physics, lectures on recent results*, Vol. 1, pp. 135–165, L. Streit, Ed., World Scientific Publishing, Singapore, Philadelphia, 1985.

[136] A. Haase, Snapshot FLASH MRI. Applications to T1, T2, and chemical-shift imaging. *Magn. Reson. Med.* 13 (1990), 77–89.

[137] A. Haase, J. Frahm, D. Matthaei, W. Hänicke, and K.–D. Merboldt, FLASH imaging. Rapid NMR imaging using low flip-angle pulses. *J. Magn. Reson.* 67 (1986), 258–266.

[138] A. Haase, D. Matthaei, R. Bartkowski, E. Dühmke, and D. Heinrich, *Die Möglichkeiten des Snapshot-FLASH MR imaging. Digitale Bildgebung, Interventionelle Radiologie, Integrierte digitale Radiologie*, pp. 505–510, G.H. Schneider, E. Vogler, and K. Koćever, Eds., Blackwell Ueberreuter Wissenschaftsverlag, Berlin, 1990.

[139] E. L. Hahn, NMR and MRI in retrospect, *Phil. Trans. R. Soc. Lond.* A 333 (1990), 403–411.

[140] J. V. Hajnal, I. R. Young, and G. M. Bydder, Studies strive to place fMRI on firm foundation, *Diagn. Imag. Eur.* (November/December) 1995, 38–44.

[141] S. E. Harms, Three-dimensional and dynamic MR imaging of the musculoskeletal system, in MR *'91–4. Internationales Kernspintomographie Symposium*, pp. 103–116, J. Lissner, J. L. Doppman and A. R. Margulis, Eds., Herausgeber, Schnetztor–Verlag, Konstanz, 1992.

[142] P. R. Harvey, and P. Mansfield, Echo-volumar imaging (EVI) at 0.5 T: First whole-body volunteer studies, *Magn. Reson. Med.* 35 (1996), 80–88.

[143] A. N. Hasso, MRI *atlas of the head and neck*, Deutscher Ärzte-Verlag, Köln, 1993.

[144] A. N. Hasso, M. Shakudo, and E. Chadrycki, MRI of the brain III: Neoplastic disease, Raven Press, New York, 1991.

[145] R. E. Hendrick, P. D. Russ, and J. H. Simon (Eds.), MRI: *Principles and artifacts*, Raven Press, New York, 1993.

[146] R. M. Henkelman, and M. J. Bronskill, Artifacts in magnetic resonance imaging, *Rev. Magn. Reson. Med.* 2 (1987), 1–126.

[147] D. Hestenes, The design of linear algebra and geometry, *Acta Applicandae Math.* 23 (1991), 65–93.

[148] A. Heuck, G. Luttke, and J. W. Rohen, *MR-Atlas der Extremitäten*, F. K. Schattauer Verlagsgesellschaft, Stuttgart, New York, 1994.

[149] L. Heuser and M. Oudkerk (Eds.), *Advances in* MRI, Blackwell Science, Oxford, London, Edinburgh, 1996.

[150] S. H. Heywang–Köbrunner and R. Beck, *Contrast-enhanced* MRI *of the breast*, 2nd ed., Springer-Verlag, Berlin, Heidelberg, New York, 1996.

[151] S. H. Heywang–Köbrunner, and I. Schreer, *Bildgebende Mammadiagnostik*, Georg Thieme Verlag, Stuttgart, New York, 1996.

[152] C. B. Higgins, H. Hricak, and C. A. Helms, *Magnetic resonance imaging of the body*, 3rd ed., Lippincott-Raven Publishers, Philadelphia, New York, 1997.

[153] C. B. Higgins, N. H. Silverman, B. A. Kersting–Sommerhoff, and K. G. Schmidt, *Congenital heart disease: Echocardiography and magnetic resonance imaging*, Raven Press, New York, 1990.

[154] R. M. Hinke, X. Hu, A. E. Stillman, S.-G. Kim, H. Merkle, R. Salmi, and K. Uğurbil, Functional magnetic resonance imaging of Broca's area during internal speech, *NeuroReport* 4 (1993), 675–678.

[155] W. S. Hinshaw and A. H. Lent, An introduction to NMR imaging: From the Bloch equation to the imaging equation, *Proc.* IEEE 71 (1983), 338–350.

[156] J. Hodler, and W. Wirth, *Gelenkdiagnostik mit bildgebenden Verfahren—Schulter*, Georg Thieme Verlag, Stuttgart, New York, 1992.

[157] L. Hörmander, The Weyl calculus of pseudodifferential operators, *Comm. Pure Appl. Math.* 32 (1979), 359–443.

[158] P. Horowitz and W. Hill, *The art of electronics*, 2nd ed., Cambridge University Press, Cambridge, New York, Port Chester, 1990.

[159] H. Hosoya, Matching and symmetry of graphs, *Comp. Maths. Appls.* 12B (1986), 271–290.

[160] H. Hötzinger and L. Spätling, MRI *in der Gynäkologie und Geburtshilfe*, Springer-Verlag, Berlin, Heidelberg, New York, 1994.

[161] R. Howe, Dual pairs in physics: Harmonic oscillators, photons, electrons, and singletons, in *Applications of group theory in physics and mathematical physics*, pp. 179–207, M. Flato, P. Sally, and G. Zuckerman, Eds., *Lectures in Applied Mathematics*, Vol. 21, American Mathematical Society, Providence, RI 1985.

[162] H. Hricak and B. M. Carrington, MRI *of the pelvis: A text atlas*, Deutscher Ärzte-Verlag, Köln, 1991.

[163] H. Hricak, MR imaging in gynecologic oncology: Value of Gd–DTPA, in MR '91–4. *Internationales Kernspintomographie Symposium*, pp. 256–262, J. Lissner, J. L. Doppman and A. R. Margulis, Eds., Schnetztor–Verlag, Konstanz, 1992.

[164] F. R. Huang-Hellinger, H. C. Breiter, G. McCormack, M. S. Cohen, K. K. Kwong, J. P. Sutton, R. L. Savoy, R. M. Weisskoff, T. L. Davis, J. R. Baker, J. W. Belliveau, and B. R.

Rosen, Simultaneous functional magnetic resonance imaging and electrophysiological recording, *Human Brain Mapping* 3, (1995), 13–23.

[165] H. K. Huang, PACS, VCH Publishers, New York, Weinheim, Cambridge, 1996.

[166] W. J. Huk, G. Gademann, and G. Friedmann, *Magnetic resonance imaging of central nervous system disease*, Springer-Verlag, Berlin, Heidelberg, New York, 1989.

[167] J. Igusa, *Theta functions*, Springer-Verlag, Berlin, Heidelberg, New York, 1972.

[168] G. D. Jackson and J. S. Duncan, MRI *neuroanatomy: A new angle on the brain*, Churchill Livingstone, New York, Edinburgh, London, 1996.

[169] A. B. Jenny, P. R. Biondetti, B. Layton, and R. H. Knapp, The computer and stereotactic surgery in neuroloical surgery, *Comp. Med. Imag. Graphics* 12 (1988), 75–83.

[170] W.-I. Jung, L. Sieverding, F. Schick, S. Widmaier, M. Bunse, G. Dietze, K. Küper, and O. Lutz, Imaging of the human cardiovascular system using the rapid echo flow-rephased spin–echo technique, *Magn. Reson. Imag.* 11 (1993), 301–309.

[171] W. A. Kaiser, MR *mammography* (MRM), Springer-Verlag, Berlin, Heidelberg, New York, 1993.

[172] P. A. Kaplan and R.G. Dussault, Magnetic resonance imaging of the knee: Menisci, ligaments, tendons, *Top. Magn. Reson. Imag.* 5 (1993), 228–248.

[173] E. Kazner, S. Wende, T. Grumme, O. Stochdorph, R. Felix, and C. Claussen (Eds.), *Computed tomography and magnetic resonance of intracranial tumors—a clinical perspective*, 2nd ed., Springer-Verlag, Berlin, Heidelberg, New York, 1989.

[174] R. E. Kelley (Ed.), *Functional neuroimaging*, Futura Publishing Company, Armonk, New York, 1994.

[175] J. Kesselring, I. E. C. Ormerod, D. H. Miller, E. P. G. H. du Boulay, and W. I. McDonald, *Magnetic resonance imaging in multiple sclerosis*, Georg Thieme Verlag, Stuttgart, New York, 1989.

[176] S.-G. Kim, J. Ashe, A. P. Georgopoulos, H. Merkle, J. M. Ellermann, R. S. Menon, S. Ogawa, and K. Uğurbil, Functional imaging of the human motor cortex at high magnetic field, *J. Neurophysiol.* 69 (1993), 297–302.

[177] S.-G. Kim, J. Ashe, K. Hendrich, J. M. Ellermann, H. Merkle, K. Uğurbil, and A. P. Georgopoulos, Functional magnetic resonance imaging of motor cortex: Hemispheric asymmetry and handedness, *Science* 261 (1993), 615–617.

[178] M. King, Fourier optics and radar signal processing, in *Applications of optical fourier transforms*, pp. 209–251, H. Stark, Ed., Academic Press, Orlando, San Diego, San Francisco, 1982.

[179] H. S. Kirshner, S. I. Tsai, V. M. Runge, and A. C. Price, Magnetic resonance imaging and other techniques in the diagnosis of multiple sclerosis, *Arch. Neurol.* 42 (1985), 859–863.

[180] H. Kobayashi, T. Matsumoto, T. Yagi, and T. Shimmi, Image processing regularization filters on layered architecture, *Neural Networks* 6 (1993), 327–350.

[181] P. König and T. B. Schillen, Stimulus-dependent assembly formation of oscillatory responses: I. Synchronization, *Neural Computat.* 3 (1991), 155–166.

[182] P. König, B. Janosch, and T. B. Schillen, Stimulus-dependent assembly formation of oscillatory responses: III. Learning, *Neural Computat.* 4 (1992), 666–681.

[183] B. Kostant, Symplectic spinors, in *Geometria Simplettica e Fisica Matematica, Symposia Mathematica*, Vol. 14, pp. 139–152, Istituto Nazionale di Alta Matematica Roma, Academic Press, London, New York, 1974.

[184] A. Kozma, E. N. Leith, and N. G. Massey, Tilted–plane optical processor, *Appl. Opt.* 11 (1972), 1766–1777.

[185] H.-J. Kretschmann, and W. Weinrich, *Dreidimensionale Computergraphik neurofunktioneller Systeme: Grundlagen für die neurologisch–topische Diagnostik und die kranielle Bilddiagnostik (Magnetresonanztomographie und Computertomographie)*, Georg Thieme Verlag, Stuttgart, New York, 1996.

[186] R. Kricun and M. E. Kricun, MRI *and* CT *of the spine: Diagnostic exercises*, 2nd ed., Raven Press, New York, 1993.

[187] J. Krüger, Spike train correlations on slow time scales in monkey visual cortex, in *Neuronal cooperativity*, pp. 105–132, J. Krüger, Ed., Springer-Verlag, Berlin, Heidelberg, New York, 1991.

[188] J. Kucharczyk, M. E. Moseley, and A. J. Barkovich (Eds.), *Magnetic resonance neuroimaging*, CRC Press, Boca Raton, Ann Arbor, London, 1994.

[189] J. Kucharczyk, M. E. Moseley, T. Roberts, and W. W. Orrison (Eds.), Functional neuroimaging, *Neuroimag. Clin. N. A.*, 5 (2), (1995), 161–308.

[190] A. Kumar, D. Welti, and R. R. Ernst, NMR Fourier zeugmatography, *J. Magn. Reson.*, 18 (1975), 69–83.

[191] R. I. Kuzniecki, MRI in cerebral developmental malformations and epilepsy, *Magn. Reson. Imag.*, 13 (1995), 1137–1145.

[192] R. I. Kuzniecki and G. D. Jackson, *Magnetic resonance in epilepsy*, Raven Press, New York, 1995.

[193] K. K. Kwong, J. W. Belliveau, D. A. Chesler, I. E. Goldberg, R. M. Weisskoff, B. P. Poncelet, D. N. Kennedy, B. E. Hoppel, M. S. Cohen, R. Turner, H.-M. Cheng, T. J. Brady, and B. R. Rosen, Dynamic magnetic resonance imaging of human brain activity during primary sensory stimulation, *Proc. Natl. Acad. Sci. USA* 89 (1992), 5675–5679.

[194] A. F. Laine, Wavelet-based image processing enhances mammography, *Laser Focus World*, (December 1995), 155–156.

[195] P. Lasjaunas, *Vascular diseases in neoates, infants and children*, Springer-Verlag, Berlin, Heidelberg, New York, 1996.

[196] R. E. Latchaw and C. R. Jack (Eds.), Epilepsy: Clinical evaluation, neuroimaging, surgery, *Neuroimag. Clin. N. Am.* 5 (4), (1995) 513–738.

[197] P. C. Lauterbur, Image formation by induced local interactions: Examples employing nuclear magnetic resonance, *Nature (London)* 242 (1973), 190–191.

[198] F. W. Leberl, *Radargrammetric image processing*, Artech House, Boston, London, 1990.

[199] D. Le Bihan, MRI: New trends in functional brain imaging, in MR '93–5. *Internationales Kernspintomographie Symposium*, pp. 32–36, J. Lissner, J. L. Doppman and A.R. Margulis, Eds., Schnetztor–Verlag, Konstanz, 1994.

[200] D. Le Bihan (Ed.), *Diffusion and perfusion magnetic resonance imaging: Applications to functional* MRI, Raven Press, New York, 1995.

[201] D. Le Bihan, R. Turner, T. A. Zeffiro, C. A. Cuenod, P. Jezzard, and V. Bonnerot, Activation of human primary visual cortex during visual recall: A magnetic resonance imaging study, *Proc. Natl. Acad. Sci. USA* 90 (1993), 11802–11805.

[202] A. Leblanc, *The cranial nerves: Anatomy, imaging, vascularisation*, 2nd enlarged ed., Springer-Verlag, Berlin, Heidelberg, New York, 1995.

[203] J. K. T. Lee, S. S. Sagel, and R. J. Stanley, *Computed body tomography with* MRI *correlation*, 2nd ed., Raven Press, New York, 1989.

[204] R. R. Lee, Spinal tumors, in *Spine: State of the art reviews*, Vol. 9, pp. 261–286, Hanley & Beifus, Philadelphia, 1995.

[205] E. N. Leith, Synthetic aperture radar, in *Optical data processing applications*, pp. 89–117, D. Casasent, Ed., Springer-Verlag, Berlin, Heidelberg, New York, 1978.

[206] E. N. Leith, Optical processing of synthetic aperture radar data, in *Photonic aspects of modern radar*, pp. 381–401, H. Zmuda, and E. N. Toughlian, Eds., Artech House Publishers, Boston, London, 1994.

[207] J. Leray, *Lagrangian analysis and quantum mechanics*, The MIT Press, Massachusetts Institute of Technology, Cambridge, MA, 1981.

[208] J. Le Roux, P. Lise, E. Zerbib, and M. Foquet, A formulation in concordance with the sampling theorem for band-limited images reconstruction from projections, *Multidimen. Sys. Signal Process.* 7 (1996), 27–52.

[209] A. S. Lewis, and G. Knowles, Image compression using the 2D-wavelet transform, IEEE *Trans. Imag. Process.* 1 (1992), 244–250.

[210] J. Lissner and M. Seiderer (Eds.), *Klinische Kernspintomographie*, Vol. 2. Auflage, Ferdinand Enke Verlag, Stuttgart, 1990.

[211] D. Lu and P. M. Joseph, A matched filter echo summation technique for MRI, *Magn. Reson. Imag.* 13 (1995), 241–249.

[212] R. B. Lufkin and W. N. Hanafee (Eds.), MRI *of the head and the neck*, Raven Press, New York, 1991.

[213] R. B. Lufkin, W. G. Bradley, Jr., and M. Brant–Zawadzki (Eds.), *The Raven* MRI *teaching file on* CD–ROM. CD–ROM, Raven Press, New York, 1995.

[214] K.-L. Ma, and J. S. Painter, Parallel volume visualization on workstations, *Comput. Graphics* 17 (1993), 31–37.

[215] P. Mansfield, Multi-planar image formation using NMR spin echoes, *J. Phys. Chem.: Solid State Phys.* 10 (1977), L55–L58.

[216] P. Mansfield, Principles of NMR imaging, in *Physics of* NMR *spectroscopy in biology and medicine, Proceedings of the International School of Physics* << *Enrico Fermi* >>, *Course C*, pp. 345–369, B. Maraviglia, Ed., North-Holland, Amsterdam, Oxford, 1988.

[217] P. Mansfield, Imaging by nuclear magnetic resonance, in *Pulsed magnetic resonance-NMR, ESR, and optics: A recognition of E. L. Hahn*, pp. 317–345, D. M. S. Bagguley, Ed., Clarendon Press, Oxford, 1992.

[218] P. Mansfield, A. M. Blamire, R. Coxon, P. Gibbs, D. N. Guilfoyle, P. Harvey, and M. Symms, Snapshot echo–planar imaging methods: Current trends and future perspectives, *Phil. Trans. R. Soc. Lond. A* 333 (1990), 495–506.

[219] P. Mansfield and P.K. Grannell, NMR "diffraction" in solids, *J. Phys. C* 6 (1973), L422–L426.

[220] K. Maravilla and W. Cohen, MRI *atlas of the spine*, Deutscher Ärzte-Verlag, Köln, 1991.

[221] H. J. Markowitsch, Anatomical basis of memory disorders, in *The cognitive neurosciences*, pp. 765–779, M. S. Gazzaniga, Ed., The MIT Press, Cambridge, MA, 1995.

[222] T. Matsuda, S. Hasegawa, M. Igarashi, T. Kobayashi, M. Naito, H. Kajiyama, J. Endo, N. Osakabe, A. Tonomura, and R. Aoki, Magnetic field observation of a single flux quantum by electron–holographic interferometry, *Phys. Rev. Lett.* 62 (1989), 2519–2522.

[223] J. Mattson and M. Simon, *The pioneers of* NMR *and magnetic resonance in medicine: The story of* MRI, Bar–Ilan University Press, Ramat Gan, 1996.

[224] G. McCarthy, A. M. Blamire, D. L. Rothman, R. Gruetter, and R. G. Shulman, Echo-planar magnetic resonance imaging studies of frontal cortex activation during word generation in humans, *Proc. Natl. Acad. Sci. USA* 90 (1993), 4952–4956.

[225] S. McCarthy (Ed.), Magnetic resonance of the pelvis, *Top. Magn. Reson. Imag.* 7(1) (1995) 1–68.

[226] B. McNaughton and M. Wilson, Ensemble neural codes for spatial experience, and their reactivation during sleep, *Proceedings of the Conference Toward a Scientific Basis for Consciousness*, MIT Press, Cambridge, MA (in press).

[227] R. Meals and L. Seeger, *An atlas of forearm and hand cross-sectional anatomy, with computed tomography and magnetic resonance imaging correlation*, Deutscher Ärzte–Verlag, Köln, 1991.

[228] H.-P. Meinzer, K. Meetz, D. Scheppelmann, U. Engelmann, and H. J. Baur, The Heidelberg ray tracing model, IEEE *Comput. Graphics Appl.* 11 (1991), 34–43.

[229] R. S. Menon, S. Ogawa, D. W. Tank, and K. Uğurbil, 4 Tesla gradient recalled echo characteristics of photic stimulation induced signal changes in the human primary visual cortex, *Magn. Reson. Med.* 30 (1993), 380–387.

[230] Y. Meyer, *Wavelets: Algorithms and applications*, Society for Industrial and Applied Mathematics, Philadelphia, 1993.

[231] R. Mezrich (Ed.), The female pelvis, *Magn. Reson. Imag. Clin. N. Am.* Vol. 2 (2), (1994) 161–323.

[232] W. D. Middleton and T. L. Lawson, *Anatomy and* MRI *of the joints: A multiplanar atlas*, Raven Press, New York, 1989.

[233] J. H. Mink, M. A. Reicher, J. V. Crues III, and A. L. Deutsch, *Magnetic resonance imaging of the knee*, 2nd ed., Raven Press, New York, 1993.

[234] M. Minsky, Memoir on inventing the confocal scanning microscope, *Scanning* 10 (1988), 128–138.

[235] J. Missri, *Clinical Doppler echocardiography: Spectral and color flow imaging*, McGraw-Hill Information Services Company, Health Professions Divison, New York, St. Louis, San Francisco, 1990.

[236] D. G. Mitchell Hepatic imaging: Techniques and unique applications of magnetic resonance imaging, *Magn. Reson. Q.* 9 (1993), 84–112.

[237] E. D. Mitchell and D. A. Williams, *The way of the explorer*, G.P. Putnam's Sons Publishers, New York, 1996.

[238] M. T. Modic, T. J. Masaryk, and J. S. Ross, *Magnetic resonance imaging of the spine*, 2nd ed., Mosby-Year Book, St. Louis, Baltimore, Boston, 1994.

[239] T. B. Möller and E. Reif, MRI *atlas of the musculoskeletal system*, Blackwell Scientific Publications, Boston, Oxford, London, 1993.

[240] T. B. Möller and E. Reif, *Taschenatlas der Schnittbildanatomie, Band I und Band II*, Georg Thieme Verlag, Stuttgart, New York, 1993.

[241] R. Montgomery, Heisenberg and isoholonomic inequalities, in *Symplectic geometry and mathematical physics*, pp. 303–325, P. Donato, C. Duval, J. Elhadad, and G. M. Tuynman, Eds., Birkhäuser, Boston, Basel, Berlin, 1991.

[242] C. C. Moore, Group extensions and cohomology for locally compact groups III, *Trans. Am. Math. Soc.* 221 (1976), 1–33.

[243] C. C. Moore and J. A. Wolf, Square integrable representations of nilpotent groups, *Trans. Am. Math. Soc.* 185 (1973), 445–462.

[244] G. Morandi, Quantum Hall effect: *Topological problems in condensed matter physics*, Bibliopolis, Naples, 1988.

[245] H. Moscovici, Coherent state representation of nilpotent Lie groups, *Commun. Math. Phys.* 54 (1977), 63–68.

[246] W. Moshage, S. Achenbach, A. Weikl, G. Göhl, K. Bachmann, K. Abraham–Fuchs, and S. Schneider, Biomagnetism-clinical results: Focal ectopic activity and conduction disturbances of the heart, in MR '91–4. *Internationales Kernspintomographie Symposium*, pp. 49–54, J. Lissner, J. L. Doppman and A. R. Margulis, Eds., Schnetztor–Verlag, Konstanz, 1992.

[247] S. Mukherji and M. Castillo (Eds.), Magnetic resonance imaging of the cranial nerves, Part I: Cranial nerves I, II, III, IV, VI, *Topics Magn. Reson. Imag.* 8 (2) (1996) 73–130.

[248] S. Mukherji and M. Castillo (Eds.), Magnetic resonance imaging of the cranial nerves, Part II: Cranial nerves VII, VIII, IX, X, XI, XII, *Topics Magn. Reson. Imag.* 8 (3) (1996) 131–192.

[249] P. L. Munk, and C. A. Helms, MRI *of the knee*, 2nd ed., Lippincott-Raven Publishers, Philadelphia, New York, 1996.

[250] M. Nägele, and G. Adam, *Moderne Kniegelenkdiagnostik: Bildgebende Verfahren und klinische Aspekte*, Springer-Verlag, Berlin, Heidelberg, New York, 1995.

[251] D. P. Naidich, E. A. Zerhouni, and S. S. Siegelman, *Computed tomography and magnetic resonance of the thorax*, 2nd ed., Raven Press, New York, 1991.

[252] K. Nakanishi (Ed.), *One-dimensional and two-dimensional* NMR *spectra by modern pulse techniques*, Kodansha, Tokyo, and University Science Book, Mill Valley, CA, 1990.

[253] N. Nakasato, S. Fujita, K. Seki, T. Kawamura, A. Matani, I. Tamura, S. Fujiwara, and T. Yoshimoto, Functional localization of bilateral auditory cortices using an MRI-linked whole head magnetoencephalography (MEG) system, *Electroencephalogr. Clin. Neurophysiol.* 94 (1995), 183–190.

[254] P. T. Narasimhan and R. E. Jacobs, Neuroanatomical micromagnetic resonance imaging, in *Brain mapping: The methods*, pp. 147–167, A. W. Toga, and J. C. Mazziotta, Eds., Academic Press, San Diego, New York, Boston, 1996.

[255] G. Nicolis and I. Prigogine, *Exploring complexity*, W. H. Freeman, New York, 1989.

[256] S. Ogawa, T. M. Lee, A. R. Kay, and D. W. Tank, Brain magnetic resonance imaging with contrast dependent on blood oxygenation, *Proc. Natl. Acad. Sci. USA* 87 (1990), 9868–9872.

[257] S. Ogawa, D. W. Tank, R. S. Menon, J. M. Ellermann, S.-G. Kim, H. Merkle, and K. Uğurbil, Intrinsic signal changes accompanying sensory stimulation: Functional brain mapping using magnetic resonance imaging, *Proc. Natl. Acad. Sci. USA* 89 (1992), 5951–5955.

[258] S. Ogawa, R. S. Menon, D. W. Tank, S.-G. Kim, H. Merkle, J. M. Ellermann, and K. Uğurbil, Functional brain mapping by blood oxygenation level–dependent contrast magnetic resonance imaging, *Biophys. J.* 64 (1993), 803–812.

[259] S. Ogawa, R. Menon, and K. Uğurbil, Current topics on the mechanism of fNMRI signal changes, *Quart. Magn. Reson. Biol. Med.* 2 (1995), 43–51.

[260] A. V. Oppenheim and R. W. Schafer, *Digital signal processing*, Prentice-Hall, Englewood Cliffs, NJ, 1975.

[261] W. W. Orrison, Jr., J. D. Lewine, J. A. Sanders, and M. F. Hartshorne, *Functional brain imaging*, Mosby-Year Book, St. Louis, Baltimore, Berlin, 1995.

[262] E. K. Outwater, MR imaging of the pancreas and biliary tree, *Topics Magn. Reson. Imag.*, 8 (5) (1996) 247–320.

[263] P. Pavone and R. Passariello, MR *cholangiopancreatography*, Springer-Verlag, Berlin, Heidelberg, New York, 1996.

[264] H. G. Paretzke, Risiko für somatische Spätschäden durch ionisierende Strahlung, *Phys. Bl.* 45 (1989), 16–24.

[265] V. H. Patel, and L. Friedman, MRI *of the brain: Normal anatomy and normal variants*, W. B. Saunders, Philadelphia, London, Toronto, 1997.

[266] P. E. Peters, H. H. Matthiass, and M. Reiser (Eds.), *Magnetresonanztomographie in der Orthopädie*, Ferdinand Enke Verlag, Stuttgart, 1990.

[267] P. E. Peters, T. Vestring, G. Reuther, and G. Bongartz, MRT bei traumatischen und degenerativen Gelenkerkrankungen, in MR *'91–4. Internationales Kernspintomographie Symposium*, pp. 95–102, J. Lissner, J. L. Doppman and A. R. Margulis, Eds., Schnetztor-Verlag, Konstanz, 1992.

[268] G. Pfurtscheller and W. Klimesch, Functional topography during a visuoverbal judgment task studied with event–related desynchronization mapping, *J. Clin. Neurophysiol.* 9 (1992), 120–131.

[269] G. Pfurtscheller and C. Neuper, Simultaneous EEG 10 Hz desynchronization and 40 Hz synchronization during finger movements, *NeuroReport* 3 (1992), 1057–1060.

[270] D. C. Popescu and H. Yan, MR image compression using iterated function systems, *Magn. Reson. Imag.* 11 (1993), 727–732.

[271] K. R. Popper, *Objektive Erkenntnis*. Vierte verbesserte und ergänzte Auflage, Hoffmann und Campe Verlag, Hamburg, 1984.

[272] E. J. Potchen, E. M. Haacke, J. E. Siebert, and A. Gottschalk, *Magnetic resonance angiography: Concepts and applications*, Mosby-Year Book, St. Louis, Baltimore, Boston, 1993.

[273] M. C. Powell, B. S. Worthington, and E. M. Symonds, *Magnetic resonance imaging in obstetrics and gynaecology*, Butterworth-Heinemann, Oxford, 1994.

[274] A. Psarrou and H. Buxton, Hybrid architecture for understanding motion sequences, *Neurocomputing* 5 (1993), 221–241.

[275] R. M. Quencer (Ed.), MRI *of the spine*, Raven Press, New York, 1991.

[276] R. G. Ramsey, *Neuroradiology*, 3rd ed., W.B. Saunders, Philadelphia, London, Toronto, 1994.

[277] R. Ranga Rao, The Maslov index on the simply connected covering group and the metaplectic representation, *J. Funct. Anal.* 107 (1992), 211–233.

[278] R. Ranga Rao, On some explicit formulas in the theory of Weil representation, *Pacific J. Math.* 157 (1993), 335–371.

[279] M. A. Reicher and L. E. Kellerhouse, MRI *of the wrist and hand*, Raven Press, New York, 1990.

[280] M.A. Reicher, R. B. Lufkin, S. Smith, B. Flannigan, R. Olsen, R. Wolf, D. Hertz, J. Winter, and W. N. Hanafee, Multiple-angle, variable-interval, nonorthogonal MRI, *Am. J. Roentgenol.* 147 (1986), 363–366.

[281] M. Reiser and W. Semmler (Eds.), *Magnetresonanztomographie*, Springer-Verlag, Berlin, Heidelberg, New York, 1992.

[282] T. L. Richards, J. D. Bowen, E. C. Alvord, K. R. Maravilla, S. R. Dager, L. M. Rose, and S. Posse, Magnetic resonance spectroscopy: Basic concepts with emphasis on multiple sclerosis, *Int. J. Neuroradiol.* 2 (1996), 123–133.

[283] R. A. Roberts, and C. T. Mullis, *Digital signal processing*, Addison-Wesley Publishing Company, Reading, Menlo Park, Don Mills, 1987.

[284] P. R. Ros, and W. D. Bidgood, Jr., *Abdominal magnetic resonance imaging*, Mosby-Year Book, St. Louis, Baltimore, Boston, 1993.

[285] J. S. Ross, *Magnetic resonance angiography of the head and neck: A teaching file*, Mosby-Year Book, St. Louis, Baltimore, Berlin, 1995.

[286] V. M. Runge, *Magnetic resonance imaging: Clinical principles*, J. B. Lippincott Company, Philadelphia, New York, London, 1992.

[287] V. M. Runge, *Magnetic resonance imaging of the brain*, J. B. Lippincott Company, Philadelphia, New York, London, 1994.

[288] V. M. Runge, M. H. Awh, D. F. Bittner, and J. H. Kirsch (Eds.), *Magnetic resonance imaging of the spine*, J. B. Lippincott Company, Philadelphia, New York, London, 1995.

[289] K. Sartor, MR *imaging of the skull and brain: A correlative text-atlas*, 1st ed., Springer-Verlag, Berlin, Heidelberg, New York, 1995.

[290] W. Schempp, Gruppentheoretische Aspekte der Signalübertragung und der kardinalen Interpolationssplines I, *Math. Meth. Appl. Sci.* 5 (1983), 195–215.

[291] W. Schempp, Harmonic analysis on the Heisenberg nilpotent Lie group, with applications to signal theory, *Pitman research notes in mathematics series*, Vol. 147, Longman Scientific & Technical, London, 1986.

[292] W. Schempp, The oscillator representation of the metaplectic group applied to quantum electronics and computerized tomography, in *Stochastic processes in physics and engineering*, pp. 305–344, S. Albeverio, P. Blanchard, M. Hazewinkel, and L. Streit, Eds., D. Reidel Publishing Company, Dordrecht, Boston, London, 1988.

[293] W. Schempp, Quantum holography and neurocomputer architectures, in *Holography, commemorating the 90th anniversary of the birth of Dennis Gabor*, pp. 62–144, P. Greguss and T. H. Jeong, Eds., SPIE—The International Society for Optical Engineering Press, Bellingham, WA, 1991.

[294] W. Schempp, Quantum holography and neurocomputer architectures, in *Probabilistic and stochastic methods in analysis, with applications*, pp. 383–467, J. S. Byrnes, J. L. Byrnes, K. A. Hargreaves, and K. Berry, Eds., Kluwer Academic Publishers, Dordrecht, Boston, London, 1992.

[295] W. Schempp, Bohr's indeterminacy principle in quantum holography, self-adaptive neural network architectures, cortical self-organization, molecular computers, magnetic resonance imaging and solitonic nanotechnology, *Nanobiology* 2 (1993), 109–164.

[296] W. Schempp, Analog VLSI network models, cortical linking neural network models, and quantum holographic neural technology, in *Rethinking neural networks: Quantum fields and biological data*, pp. 233–297, K. H. Pribram, Ed., Lawrence Erlbaum Associates, Publishers, Hillsdale, NJ, and Hove, London, 1993.

[297] W. Schempp, Coherent wavelets, magnetic resonance imaging, and all that, in *Image analysis and synthesis*, pp. 347–354, W. Pölzleitner and E. Wenger, Eds., R. Oldenbourg, Wien, München, 1993.

[298] W. Schempp, Sonoluminescence, and quantum computation in ultrasonic acoustic chaos physics, to appear.

[299] W. Schempp, Gruppentheoretische Aspekte der Signalübertragung und der kardinalen Interpolationssplines II, *Math. Meth. Appl. Sci.*, to appear.

[300] W. Schempp, Quantum parallelism, in *Proc. Symposium on Alternative Models of Computation and New Routes to Parallelism,* British Computer Society, Cybernetics Machine Specialist Group, London, 1994.

[301] W. Schempp, Phase coherent wavelets, Fourier transform magnetic resonance, and synchronized time-domain neural networks, in Selected questions of mathematical physics and analysis, I, V. Volovich, Yu. N. Drozhzhinov, and A. G. Sergeev, Eds., *Proc. Steklov Inst. Math.,* Vol. 203, pp. 389–428, American Mathematics Society, Providence, RI, 1995.

[302] W. Schempp, Mysterium Cerebrotopographicum, in *Image processing and computer optics* (DIP-94), N. A. Kuznetsov and V. A. Soifer, Eds., pp. 12–30, SPIE Vol. 2363, SPIE—The International Society for Optical Engineering, Bellingham, WA, 1995.

[303] W. Schempp, Geometric analysis: The double-slit interference experiment and magnetic resonance imaging, in *Cybernetics and systems '96*, Vol. 1, R. Trappl, Ed., pp. 179–183, Austrian Society for Cybernetic Studies, University of Vienna, 1996.

[304] W. Schempp, Geometric analysis and symbol calculus: Fourier transform magnetic resonance imaging and wavelets, *Acta Appl. Math.* 48 (1997), 185–234.

[305] W. Schempp, Zu Keppler's Conchoid–Konstruktion, *Results Math.* 32 (1997), 352–390.

[306] T. B. Schillen and P. König, Stimulus-dependent assembly formation of oscillatory responses: II. Desynchronization, *Neural Computat.* 3 (1991), 167–178.

[307] T.B. Schillen and P. König, Temporal coding by coherent oscillations as a potential solution to the binding problem: Neural network simulations, in *Nonlinear dynamics and neuronal networks, Proceedings of the 63rd W. E. Heraeus Seminar Friedrichsdorf 1990*, pp. 153–171, H.G. Schuster, Ed., VCH, Weinheim, New York, Basel, 1991.

[308] L. Schwartz, Sous-espaces hilbertiens d'espaces vectoriels topologiques et noyaux associés (noyaux reproduisants), *J. Anal. Math.* 13 (1964), 115–256.

[309] L. Schwartz, Sous-espaces hilbertiens et noyaux associés; applications aux représentations des groupes de Lie, in *Deuxième Colloq. l'Anal. Fonct.*, pp. 153–163, Centre Belge Recherches Mathématiques, Librairie Universitaire, Louvain, 1964.

[310] J. Segman and W. Schempp, Two ways to incorporate scale in the Heisenberg group with an intertwining operator, *J. Math. Imag. Vision* 3 (1993), 79–94.

[311] T. Seiler, T. Bende, Magnetic resonance imaging of the eye and orbit, in *Noninvasive diagnostic techniques in ophthalmology*, pp. 17–31, B. R. Masters, Ed., Springer-Verlag, New York, Berlin, Heidelberg, 1990.

[312] R. C. Semelka, S. M. Ascher, and C. Reinhold, MRI *of the abdomen and pelvis: A text-atlas*, Wiley-Liss, New York, Chichester, Weinheim, 1987.

[313] R. C. Semelka and J. P. Shoenut, MRI *of the abdomen with* CT *correlation*, Raven Press, New York, 1993.

[314] D. S. Shucker, Square integrable representations of unimodular groups, *Proc. Am. Math. Soc.* 89 (1983), 169–172.

[315] R. G. Shulman, A. M. Blamire, D. L. Rothman, and G. McCarthy, Nuclear magnetic resonance imaging and spectroscopy of human brain function, *Proc. Natl. Acad. Sci. USA* 90 (1993), 3127–3133.

[316] W. Singer, Search for coherence: A basic principle of cortical self-organization, *Concepts Neurosci.* 1 (1990), 1–26.

[317] W. Singer, The formation of cooperative cells assemblies in the visual cortex, in *Neuronal cooperativity*, pp. 165–183, J. Krüger, Ed., Springer-Verlag, Berlin, Heidelberg, New York, 1991.

[318] W. Singer, Synchronization of cortical activity and its putative role in information processing and learning, *Annu. Rev. Physiol.* 55 (1993), 349–374.

[319] W. Singer, Putative functions of temporal correlations in neocortical processing, in Large-scale neuronal theories of the brain, pp. 201–237, C. Koch and J. L. Davis, Eds., The MIT Press, Cambridge, MA, and London, England, 1994.

[320] W. Singer, Time as a coding space in neocortical processing: A hypothesis, in *The cognitive neurosciences*, pp. 91–104, M. S. Gazzaniga, Ed., The MIT Press, Cambridge, MA, and London, England, 1995.

[321] H. B. Song, Z. H. Cho, and S. K. Hilal, Direct Fourier transform NMR tomography with modified Kumar–Welti–Ernst (MKWE) method, IEEE *Trans. Nucl. Sci.* NS–29 (1982), 493–499.

[322] A. Stäbler, D. Widenka, U. Fink, and M. Seiderer, Differenzierung knöcherner Wirbelsäulenerkrankungen durch Quantifizierung von subtraktiven GE–Bildern mit verlängerter Repetitionszeit, in MR '91–4. *Internationales Kernspintomographie Symposium*, pp. 83–89, J. Lissner, J. L. Doppman, and A. R. Margulis, Eds., Schnetztor–Verlag, Konstanz, 1992.

[323] T. E. St. Amour, S. C. Hodges, R. W. Laakman, D. E. Tamas, C. A. James, and C. M. Glasier (Eds.), MRI *of the spine*, Raven Press, New York, 1994.

[324] D. D. Stark and W. G. Bradley, Jr. (Eds.), *Magnetic resonance imaging*, 2nd ed., Mosby-Year Book, St. Louis, Baltimore, Boston, 1992.

[325] L. S. Steinbach, P. Tirman, and C. Peterfy, MRI *of the shoulder*, J. B. Lippincott Company, Philadelphia, New York, London, 1995.

[326] W. Steinbrich and G. P. Krestin (Eds.), Kernspintomographie der Abdominal-und Beckenorgane. Springer-Verlag, Berlin, Heidelberg, New York, 1990.

[327] B. Stephenson, Kepler's physical astronomy, in *Studies in the history of mathematics and physical sciences*, Vol. 13, Springer-Verlag, New York, Berlin, Heidelberg, 1987.

[328] P. Stoeter, P. Gutjahr, and K. Brühl, *Tumoren bei Kindern: Moderne Bildgebung mit* MRT *und* CT, *Band 1:* ZNS, Georg Thieme Verlag, Stuttgart, New York, 1996.

[329] D. W. Stoller, *Magnetic resonance imaging in orthopaedics & sports medicine*, 2nd ed, Lippincott-Raven Publishers, Philadelphia, New York, 1997.

[330] G. Strang, Wavelet transforms versus Fourier transforms, *Bull. (New Series) Amer. Math. Soc.* 28 (1993), 288–305.

[331] H. Strunk and P. Gutjahr, *Tumoren bei Kindern: Moderne Bildgebung mit* MRT *und* CT, *Band 2: Körperstamm und Extremitäten*, Georg Thieme Verlag, Stuttgart, New York, 1996.

[332] L. Sun, J. O. Olsen, and P.-M. L. Robitaille, Design and optimization of a breast coil for magnetic resonance imaging, *Magn. Reson. Imag.* 11 (1993), 73–80.

[333] J. L. Taveras and B. G. Haik, Magnetic resonance imaging in ophthalmology, in *Noninvasive diagnostic techniques in ophthalmology*, pp. 32–46, B.R. Masters, Ed., Springer-Verlag, New York, Berlin, Heidelberg, 1990.

[334] C. M. C. Tempany, MR *and imaging of the female pelvis*, Mosby-Year Book, St. Louis, Baltimore, Berlin, 1995.

[335] M. R. Terk, J. R. Gober, H. de Verdier, H. E. Simon, and P. M. Colletti, Evaluation of suspected musculoskeletal neoplasms using 3D T_2-weighted spectral presaturation with inversion recovery, *Magn. Reson. Imag.* 11 (1993), 931–939.

[336] A. Tonomura, *Electron holography*, Springer-Verlag, Berlin, Heidelberg, New York, 1993.

[337] K. Toyama, The structure–function problem in visual cortical circuitry studied by cross-correlation techniques and multi-channel recordings, in *Neuronal cooperativity*, pp. 5–29, J. Krüger, Ed., Springer-Verlag, Berlin, Heidelberg, New York, 1991.

[338] C. L. Truwit and T. E. Lempert, *High resolution atlas of cranial neuroanatomy*. Williams & Wilkins, Baltimore, Philadelphia, London, 1994.

[339] E. Tulving, Concepts of human memory, in *Memory: Organization and locus of change*, pp. 3–32, L. R. Squire, N. M. Weinberger, G. Lynch, and J. L. McGaugh, Eds., Oxford University Press, New York, Oxford, Athens, 1991.

[340] R. Turner, P. Jezzard, H. Wen, K. K. Kwong, D. Le Bihan, T. Zeffiro, and R. Balaban, Functional mapping of the human visual cortex at 4 and 1.5 Tesla using deoxygenation contrast EPI, *Magn. Reson. Med.* 29 (1993), 277–279.

[341] R. Turner, P. Jezzard, and K. J. Friston, Magnetic resonance functional imaging of the brain at 4 Tesla, in *Proc. of the First Nottingham Symposium on Magnetic Resonance in Medicine,* MAGMA 2, 1994.

[342] K. Uğurbil, M. Garwood, J. M. Ellermann, K. Hendrich, R. M. Hinke, X. Hu, S.-G. Kim, R. S. Menon, H. Merkle, S. Ogawa, and R. Salmi, Imaging at high magnetic fields: Initial experiences at 4 T, *Magn. Reson. Quart.* 9 (1993), 259–277.

[343] D. Uhlenbrock, *Kernspintomographie des Kopfes*, Georg Thieme Verlag, Stuttgart, New York, 1990.

[344] D. Uhlenbrock, *Kernspintomographie der Wirbelsäule und des Spinalkanals*, Georg Thieme Verlag, Stuttgart, New York, 1992.

[345] D. Uhlenbrock, MRT *und* MRA *des Kopfes*, Georg Thieme Verlag, Stuttgart, New York, 1996.

[346] P. P. Vaidyanathan, *Multirate systems and filter banks*, Prentice-Hall Signal Processing Series, Prentice-Hall, Englewood Cliffs, NJ, 1993.

[347] M. S. van der Knaap and J. Valk, *Magnetic resonance of myelin, myelination, and myelin disorders*, 2nd ed., Springer-Verlag, Berlin, Heidelberg, New York, 1995.

[348] P. van der Meulen, J. P. Groen, A. M. C. Tinus, and G. Bruntink, Contrasts in fast field echo imaging, *Magn. Reson. Imag.* 5 (1987), 554–555.

[349] M. Vetterli and J. Kovačević, Wavelets and subband coding, Prentice-Hall Signal Processing Series, Prentice-Hall, Englewood Cliffs, NJ, 1995.

[350] N. Ja. Vilenkin and A. U. Klimyk, *Representation of Lie groups and special functions*, Vol. 2: *Class I representations, special functions, and integral transforms*, Kluwer Academic Publishers, Dordrecht, Boston, London, 1993.

[351] T. J. Vogl, MRI *of the head and neck*, Springer-Verlag, Berlin, Heidelberg, New York, 1992.

[352] T. J. Vogl, MR-*Angiographie und* MR-*Tomographie des Gefäßsystems*, Springer-Verlag, Berlin, Heidelberg, New York, 1994.

[353] T.J. Vogl and D. Eberhard, MR-*Tomographie Temporomandibulargelenk*, Georg Thieme Verlag, Stuttgart, New York, 1993.

[354] T. J. Vogl, P. K. Müller, R. Hammerstingl, N. Weinhold, M. G. Mack, C. Philipp, M. Deimling, F. Beuthan, W. Pegios, H. Riess, H. P. Lemmens, and R. Felix, Malignant liver tumors treated with MR imaging-guided laser-induced thermotherapy: Technique and prospective results, *Radiology* 196 (1995), 257–265.

[355] C. von der Malsburg, Nervous structures with dynamical link, *Ber. Bunsenges. Phys. Chem.* 89 (1985), 703–710.

[356] C. von der Malsburg, Pattern recognition by labeled graph matching, *Neural Networks* 1 (1988), 141–148.

[357] C. von der Malsburg and W. Singer, Principles of cortical network organization, in *Neurobiology of neocortex*, pp. 69–99, P. Rakic and W. Singer, Eds., John Wiley & Sons, Chichester, New York, Brisbane, 1988.

[358] F. A. von Hayek, *Die Anmaßung von Wissen*, Neue Freiburger Studien, J.C.B. Mohr (Paul Siebeck), Tübingen, 1996.

[359] G. K. von Schulthess, G. McKinnon, A. Eichenberger, and V. Koechli, Cardiovascular ultrafast MRI, in *MR '93–5. Internationales Kernspintomographie Symposium*, pp. 174–180, J. Lissner, J. L. Doppman, and A. R. Margulis, Eds., Schnetztor–Verlag, Konstanz, 1994.

[360] M. Wagner and T. L. Lawson, *Atlas of chest imaging: Correlated anatomy with MRI and CT*, Raven Press, New York, 1992.

[361] B. Wallner (Ed.), MR-*Angiographie*, Georg Thieme Verlag, Stuttgart, New York, 1993.

[362] J. S. Waugh, Spin echoes and thermodynamics, in *Pulsed magnetic resonance*-NMR, ESR, *and optics: A recognition of E. L. Hahn*, pp. 174–183, D. M. S. Bagguley, Ed., Clarendon Press, Oxford, 1992.

[363] P. T. Weatherhall (Ed.), Musculoskeletal soft-tissue imaging, *Magn. Reson. Imag. Clin. N. Am.* 3 (4), (1995).

[364] D. M. Weber, Echo planar imaging, in *Progressi in RM—Note di Tecnica*, pp. 47–66, M. Cammisa and T. Scarabino, Eds., Guido Gnocchi, Naples, 1995.

[365] D. R. Wehner, *High resolution radar*, Artech House, Norwood, MA, 1987.

[366] F. W. Wehrli, *Fast-scan magnetic resonance: Principles and applications*, Raven Press, New York, 1991.

[367] A. Weil, Sur certains groupes d'opérateurs unitaires, *Acta Math.* 111 (1964), 143–211.

[368] R. Weissleder and D. D. Stark, MRI *atlas of the abdomen*, Deutscher Ärzte–Verlag, Köln, 1989.

[369] H. Weyl, *Symmetry*, Princeton University Press, Princeton, NJ, 1952.

[370] C. S. White, MR *evaluation of the pericardium, Topics Magn. Reson. Imag.* 7 (1995), 258–266.

[371] C. A. Wilson, Kepler's ellipse and area rule—their derivation from fact and conjecture, in *Kepler: Four hundred years. Proceedings of conferences held in honour of Johannes Kepler*, A. Beer and P. Beer, Eds., *Vistas in Astronomy*, Vol. 18, pp. 587–591, Pergamon Press, Oxford, New York, Toronto, 1975.

[372] D. H. Yock, Jr., *Magnetic resonance imaging of* CNS *disease: A teaching file*, Mosby-Year Book, St. Louis, Baltimore, Berlin, 1995.

[373] W. T. C. Yuh, E. T. Talι, A. K. Afifi, K. Şahinōglu, F. Gao, and R. A. Bergman, MRI of head & neck anatomy, Churchill Livingstone, New York, Edinburgh, London, 1994.

[374] M. B. Zlatkin, MRI of the shoulder, Raven Press, New York, 1991.

[375] M. Zwaan, *Moment problems in Hilbert space with applications to magnetic resonance imaging*, Academisch Proefschrift, Faculteit der Wiskunde en Informatica, Vrije Universiteit te Amsterdam, Centrum voor Wiskunde en Informatica, Amsterdam, 1991.

INDEX